MEDICAL RADIOLOGY

Diagnostic Imaging and Radiation Oncology

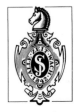

Radiation Therapy of Head and Neck Cancer

Contributors

J. D. Cox · G. H. Fletcher · D. Galinsky · D. R. Goffinet · K. L. Griem
M. L. Griem · T. W. Griffin · F. R. Hendrickson · L. Ingersoll · T. S. Kramer
G. E. Laramore · M. D. McNeese · J. Mortimer · A. A. Moss · A. K. Murthy
L. E. Olson · W. P. Shuman · J. Stitt Haas · D. Tze-Chun Chiang
W. Wisbeck

Edited by

George E. Laramore

Foreword by

Luther W. Brady and Hans-Peter Heilmann

With 123 Figures

Springer-Verlag
Berlin Heidelberg New York
London Paris Tokyo

GEORGE E. LARAMORE, Ph. D., M. D.
Professor of Radiation Oncology
Clinical Director Department of
Radiation Oncology
University of Washington
School of Medicine and University Hospital
Seattle, WA 98195
USA

MEDICAL RADIOLOGY · Diagnostic Imaging and Radiation Oncology

Continuation of
Handbuch der medizinischen Radiologie
Encyclopedia of Medical Radiology

ISBN 3-540-19360-X Springer-Verlag Berlin Heidelberg New York
ISBN 0-387-19360-X Springer-Verlag New York Berlin Heidelberg

Library of Congress Cataloging-in-Publication Data. Radiation therapy of head and neck cancer / contributors, J.D. Cox ... [et al.] ; edited by George E. Laramore ; foreword by Luther W. Brady and Hans-Peter Heilmann. p. cm. – (Medical radiology) Includes bibliographies and index.
ISBN 0-387-19360-X (U.S.)
1. Head–Cancer–Radiotherapy. 2. Neck–Cancer–Radiotherapy. I. Cox, James D. (James Daniel), 1938- . II. Laramore, George E., 1943- . III. Series.
[DNLM: 1. Head and Neck Neoplasms–radiotherapy. WE 707 R129] RC280.H4R33 1988 616.99'4910642–dc 19
DNLM/DLC

Typesetting, printing and bookbinding: Appl, Wemding
2122/3130-543210 – Printed on acid-free paper

List of Contributors

JAMES D. COX, M.D.
Professor and Chairman
Department of Radiation Oncology
Columbia Presbyterian Medical Center
622 W. 168th Street
New York, NY 100 32
USA

GILBERT H. FLETCHER, M.D.
Department of Clinical Radiotherapy
The University of Texas
M.D. Anderson Cancer Center at
Houston
Texas Medical Center
Houston, TX 77030
USA

DENNIS GALINSKY, M.D.
Section of Radiation Oncology
Department of Therapeutic Radiology
Rush Presbyterian St. Luke's Medical
Center
1753 West Congress Parkway
Chicago, IL 60612
USA

DONALD R. GOFFINET, M.D.
Professor of Radiation Oncology
Radiation Therapy Division
Department of Radiology
Stanford University Medical Center
Stanford, CA 94305
USA

KATHERINE L. GRIEM, M.D.
Department of Therapeutic Radiology
Rush Presbyterian St. Luke's Medical
Center
1753 West Congress Parkway
Chicago, IL 60612
USA

MELVIN L. GRIEM, M.D.
Professor of Radiology
Department of Therapeutic Radiology
University of Chicago, Box 442
5841 South Maryland Avenue
Chicago, IL 60637
USA

THOMAS W. GRIFFIN, M.D.
Division of Medical Oncology
Department of Medicine
University of Washington
Hospital/School of Medicine
Seattle, WA 98195
USA

FRANK R. HENDRICKSON, M.D.
Chairman, Department of Therapeutic
Radiology
Rush Presbyterian St. Luke's Medical
Center
1753 West Congress Parkway
Chicago, IL 60612
USA

LESLYE INGERSOLL, M.D.
Stanford University School
of Medicine
Stanford, CA 94305
USA

TOBY S. KRAMER, M.D.
Assistant Professor of Therapeutic
Radiology
Department of Therapeutic Radiology
Rush Presbyterian St. Luke's Medical
Center
1753 West Congress Parkway
Chicago, IL 60612
USA

GEORGE E. LARAMORE, Ph.D., M.D.
Professor of Radiation Oncology
Department of Radiation Oncology
Clinical Director
University of Washington
School of Medicine and University
Hospital
Seattle, WA 98195
USA

MARSHA D. MCNEESE, M.D.
Department of Clinical Radiotherapy
The University of Texas
M.D. Anderson Cancer Center at
Houston
Texas Medical Center
Houston, TX 77030
USA

JOANNE MORTIMER, M.D.
Division of Medical Oncology
Department of Medicine
University of Washington
Hospital/School of Medicine
Seattle, WA 98195
USA

ALBERT A. MOSS, M.D.
Department of Radiology
University Hospital
University of Washington
Seattle, WA 98195
USA

ANANTHA K. MURTHY, M.D.
Director – Section of Radiation Oncology
Department of Therapeutic Radiology
Rush Presbyterian St. Luke's Medical
Center
1753 West Congress Parkway
Chicago, IL 60612
USA

LAIRD E. OLSON, M.D.
Assistant Professor
Department of Radiation Oncology
Medical College of Wisconsin
8700 W. Wisconsin Avenue
Milwaukee, WI 53226
USA

WILLIAM P. SHUMAN, M.D.
Assistant Professor
Department of Radiology
University Hospital
University of Washington
Seattle, WA 98195
USA

JUDITH STITT HAAS, M.D.
Assistant Professor
Department of Radiation Oncology
Medical College of Wisconsin
8700 W. Wisconsin Avenue
Milwaukee, WI 53226
USA

DAVID TZE-CHUN CHIANG, M.D.
Illinois Masonic Hospital
Chicago, IL 60637
USA

WILL WISBECK, M.D.
Department of Radiation Oncology,
RC-08
University of Washington
1959 N.E. Pacific Street
Seattle, WA 98195
USA

Foreword

The contemporary management of patients with cancers of the head and neck is under careful scrutiny and major changes are being introduced in order to improve the potential not only for long-term control but also for less in the way of disfiguring and distressing complications associated with the treatment programs.

In 1988, the American Cancer Society estimates that there will be 42 400 new cases of malignant tumors of the head and neck diagnosed with 12 850 deaths.

In general, the prognosis for patients with malignant tumors of the head and neck region depends upon the site of origin, the local and regional extent of the tumor, the Karnofsky status of the patient as well as the patient's general medical condition. The potential for cure for early stage tumors is extremely high particularly for those lesions involving the vocal cord, oral cavity, and the anterior two-thirds of the tongue.

Major advances have been made in the management of head and neck cancer by the innovative utilization of surgery with radiation therapy. Small tumors can be cured by either surgery or radiation therapy with equally good results. However, far advanced tumors are more complicated and more difficult to cure requiring combined, integrated, multimodal programs of management. Therefore, the previously general poor prognosis for advanced tumors is becoming better with more aggressive treatment regimens.

The management of lymphadenopathy due to involvement with tumor can be carried out equally well by radiation therapy, radical neck dissection or a more limited neck dissection with radiation therapy. This combination of limited surgery and less aggressive radiation therapy improves the survival rate with less in the way of morbidity, physiologic dysfunction and discomfort to the patient.

Contemporary management of patients with head and neck cancer requires the combined efforts of all specialists in oncology as well as the input from highly sophisticated diagnostic techniques such as those brought to the problem by the diagnostic radiologist and the assessment of the tumor with its grave findings by the pathologist.

The purpose of the book by Professor George E. Laramore is directed toward the various aspects of the problem of head and neck cancer and designed to set forth an appropriate and proper format for more innovative management.

LUTHER W. BRADY   HANS-PETER HEILMANN
Philadelphia   Hamburg

Preface

For the last five years I have had the privilege of serving as the Chairman of the Head and Neck Cancer Committee of the Radiation Therapy Oncology Group (RTOG). During this time I had the task of coordinating the group's clinical research program in the area of head and neck cancer. This "forced" me to review both "standards of care" and ongoing research programs for various head and neck sites and put me in contact with many of the established "experts" and upcoming "innovators" in this field. My purpose in editing this book is to present what I and my colleagues feel is the best standard radiotherapy approach to the treatment of this set of diseases.

This book is designed to provide a comprehensive review suitable for both the practicing radiation oncologist and the resident in training. Approaches and treatment results from the major centers in the United States, Canada, and Europe are discussed. The intent of the book is not to toute a parochial approach characteristic of a few institutions, but rather to present a balanced picture. Both "common" and "rare" tumors are covered. The cited references are meant to be representative rather than exhaustive but should be more than adequate for the reader who wishes to review the original material that serves as background for a given chapter.

Success in treating head and neck cancer requires coordinating several different medical disciplines to evaluate the extent of tumor and to formulate a specific treatment plan. The radiation therapy aspect of treatment requires the clinician to establish appropriate field configurations and doses for the regions of diverse risk for tumor extension and generally, several changes in field geometry are required during a course of therapy. This book will aid the radiation oncologist in carrying out such a detailed plan of treatment.

Chapters 1, 2, and 3 are overviews of the head and neck cancer problem and the various diagnostic and treatment options. The epidemiological background is surveyed in Chapter 1; imaging techniques as applied to head and neck oncology and their evolving role in "clinical" staging are the subject of Chapter 2; and treatment options - particularly the interplay between surgery and radiotherapy - are discussed in Chapter 3. Chemotherapy for head and neck cancer is regarded as experimental at the present time and is discussed in a special section of Chapter 16 which is devoted to current clinical research topics.

The treatment of the regional lymphatics in the neck is the topic of Chapters 4 and 5 which discuss, respectively, the clinically negative and positive neck. The issue of elective neck dissection vs. prophylactic radiotherapy is discussed in detail. The neck staging system common to all head and neck cancer primaries is reviewed.

Chapters 6-13 focus on individual head and neck tumor sites. The particular nuances relating to a given site are discussed as well as treatment techniques of general applicability. The propensity of the various tumors to metastasize to the draining regional nodes is described as well as representative treatment fields and computer dosimetric calculations. In Chapters 6 and 7, which deal with tumors arising in the oral cavity and oropharynx, the use of radioactive implant techniques is illustrated. Chapter 8, dealing with the nasopharynx, illustrates different stage tumors with photographs taken with a wide-angle lens and discusses the large patient series from various areas of the Far East. Chapters 9 and 10 are directed towards the hypopharynx and larynx - adjacent areas anatomically but of quite different apparent radioresponsiveness. Chapter 11 deals with tumors of the nasal vestibule and paranasal sinuses which tend to be rarer than those arising in other head and neck sites. The specific treatment recommendations will hopefully be useful to the clinician who sees these lesions only occasionally. Chemodectomas are discussed in Chapter 12. These vascular tumors are of moderate radiosensitivity and can respond well – albeit slowly – to radiotherapy. The surgical approach to carotid body tumors is contrasted to the radiotherapy approach to glomus jugular tumors. Chapter 13 is devoted to tumors of the major and minor salivary glands. The combined surgery/radiotherapy approach is stressed for operable lesions. These tumors show a superb response to high LET fast neutron radiotherapy which is discussed in detail in Chapter 16. Thyroid carcinoma is the subject of Chapter 14 where the various histological subtypes and associated multiple endocrine abnormalities are described as well as the treatment of Grave's opthalmopathy. The classic problem of the squamous cell tumor presenting in the cervical neck nodes without a definite primary location is the topic of Chapter 15. Paradoxically, when properly treated, this group of patients may have a better prognosis than if the primary site is actually found. Current research topics in head and neck cancer are the subject of Chapter 16 which deals with chemotherapy, non-standard dose fractionation schemas, and high LET radiotherapy for head and neck lesions. Of these, fast neutron radiotherapy for inoperable salivary gland lesions appears to be reaching the status of "accepted" while the other treatment approaches are still experimental in the sense of definitive, phase III trials being presently in progress.

I would like to dedicate this book to my wife, Shelley, for her encouragement throughout the writing and editing process, to my sons, Gregory, Jason and Parker, and to my collaborators for their perseverence from its conception to its completion.

I would also like to thank my secretaries, Sally Seifert and Jane Timmons, for the typing and retyping of numerous chapters over the duration of the project.

GEORGE E. LARAMORE

Contents

1 Head and Neck Cancer: A General Overview

GEORGE E. LARAMORE

CONTENTS

1.1 Epidemiology

1.1.1 General

In 1987 the American Cancer Society estimates there will be 41 900 cases of head and neck cancer in the United States alone (SILVERBERG and LUBERA 1987). There will be approximately 13 200 deaths due to these malignancies. While tumors of the head and neck are uncommon compared to those arising in the lung, breast, prostate gland, or gastrointestinal tract, their diagnosis and treatment constitutes a major medical management problem. The majority of head and neck cancers are squamous cell in histology and are associated with the twin risk factors of tobacco and ethanol abuse. They generally occur in patients in the lower socioeconomic strata and such persons often wait until

GEORGE E. LARAMORE, PH. D., M. D., Department of Radiation Oncology, RC-08, University Hospital, University of Washington, Seattle, Washington 98195, USA

the tumors are quite advanced before seeking medical attention. These patients may have a marginal existence at best and often cannot cope with the cosmetic deformities of surgery and/or the rigors of radiation therapy and chemotherapy.

1.1.2 Oral Cavity and Pharynx

Some interesting patterns exist when one considers cancers arising in the oral cavity and pharynx. The most common sites of tumor origin in the oral cavity are the tongue, lip, and gum, while the tonsil and base of tongue dominate in the oropharynx (SEER Program 1973–1977). Lip cancer is distinctive in that it is associated with sun exposure as well as pipe smoking and occurs more frequently in Caucasians than in Blacks. Per 100 000 population, the incidence is 3.9 for white males and 0.3 for black males. Approximately 85% of lip cancers occur in the lower lip. Cancers of the oral cavity are strongly correlated with tobacco and alcohol use. In France, where there is greater use of these agents, the age-adjusted mortality for males is approximately 3 times higher than for the United States as a whole. In India many persons smoke an uncured form of tobacco (bidi) and also chew a paste made from the betel nut. This gives rise to an age-adjusted incidence rate for carcinomas of the oral cavity and pharynx of 33.2 for males and 12.1 for females (WATERHOUSE et al. 1976). For the United States comparable figures are 17.4 for males and 6.2 for females. The trickling of the juices down the gullet gives rise both to mucosal changes, and also increased cancer incidence in hypopharyngeal and esophageal sites. In some Asian and South American countries the reverse smoking of a cheroot gives rise to increased incidence of cancer of the hard palate (REDDY 1974). In the United States mortality among men is highest in the industrial areas of the Northeast while in women oral cancer occurs more frequently in the rural white population where use of snuff is relatively common (BLOT and FRAUMENI 1977; WINN et al. 1981). More recently, a series of studies have implicated the use of mouthwash in the development of oral cavity and pharyngeal cancers-even in a nonsmoking cohort (WEAVER et al. 1979; BLOT et al. 1983; WYNDER et al. 1983). While the evidence for a causal relationship is not conclusive, it is plausible since commercial mouthwashes contain numerous flavoring and coloring agents as well as ethanol. In the years 1950-1979, the mortality rate in white males has decreased from 6.6 to 5.2 while in non-white males it has increased from 2.0 to 2.4.

1.1.3 Larynx

Cancer of the larynx represents about 1% of all malignancies in the United States (excluding non-melanoma skin cancer) (SILVERBERG and LUBERA 1987). It is rare under age 35 and occurs mainly in persons 60 or older. In women, the average age of occurrence is somewhat younger than for men. The age adjusted incidence in the United States is about 8.6 for males compared with 1.2 for females. In the white male the mortality rate for cancer of the larynx has remained relatively constant at 2.6-2.7 from 1950-1979 while for the non-white male it has more than doubled going from 1.8 to 4.0 (McKAY et al. 1982). For both the white and non-white female it has remained relatively constant at approximately 0.4 (McKAY et al. 1982). Looking at various population subgroups, mortality rates are higher for non-whites living in the urbanized South and Northeast and but higher for whites compared to nonwhites in the rural South. The incidence of laryngeal cancer varies throughout the world in association with environmental factors and socio-economic related habits. In 1972 the highest reported incidence of laryngeal cancer in males was from Brazil (14.1) and in women was from India (2.6) (WATERHOUSE et al. 1976; ROTHMAN et al. 1980). Laryngeal cancer incidence and mortality rates correlate more with smoking patterns than ethanol use (McMICHAEL 1978). This point is discussed in more detail in the following chapter on laryngeal cancer (i.e. Chapter 10). Occupational factors associated with the development of laryngeal cancer include asbestos, diethyl sulfate, mustard gas, isopropyl alcohol, grease and oil, nickel, cadmium, chromium, and naphthalene cleaners (DECOUFLE 1982; FLANDERS et al. 1984). After controlling cohort groups for the known risk factors of tobacco and ethanol use, the relative risk factor is 4 or greater for the following occupations: sheet-metal workers, grinding wheel operators, electicians, and automobile and other mechanical trade workers.

1.1.4 Nasopharynx

Nasopharyngeal carcinoma tends to be rare within the Unites States accounting for only about 0.2% of all malignancies (excluding non-melanoma skin cancer). It ist much more common in specific areas of China and Southeast Asia. For the Canton area, in particular, the incidence is approximately 30. Even in the United States the incidence among Chinese and Filipino populations is much higher than in Caucasians and Blacks (SEER Program 1973-1977). The incidence is also quite high among the Aleute Indian population of Alaska. There is a definite correlation between nasopharyngeal cancer and increased Epstein-Barr virus blood titres, but a causal relationsship is uncertain at present. In Chinese, carcinoma of the nasopharynx is associated with an increased frequency of specific leukocyte antigen locii (HL-A2, BW46) and the latter of these is currently regarded as both a risk factor and a harbinger of a poor prognosis (SIMONS and DAY 1977). Dietary factors may also enter. HO et al. (1978) have proposed that the high levels of nitrosamines in dried salted fish (a traditional Cantonese food) is associated with the high incidence of nasopharyngeal carcinoma found there. It appears that a very complex of interplay of viral, dietary and genetic factors may be important in the development of this disease.

1.1.5 Nasal Cavity and Paranasal Sinuses

These tumors are quite rare and account for less than 0.2% of all malignancies in the United States (excluding non-melanoma skin cancer). Its frequency has been stable in the United States for the last two decades and has about equal predilection for Blacks and Causasians (REDMUND et al. 1982). Age-adjusted incidence rates are in the range of 0.3-1.0 throughout most of the world but are reported to be as high as 2.0-3.5 in parts of Africa (WATERHOUSE et al. 1976; BAUMSLAG et al. 1971). Some of this increased incidence may be due to the intranasal use of snuff that contains appreciable amounts of polycyclic hydrocarbons, nitrosamines, nickel and chromium - all known carcinogens. In the United States adenocarcinoma of the paranasal sinuses is associated with sawdust exposure in the lumber and woodworking industries (BRINTON et al. 1984).

1.1.6 Thyroid

In laboratory animals carcinoma of the thyroid develops in response to exposure to ionizing radiation or in response to excessive secretion of thyroid stimulating hormone. The latter occurs with dietary iodide insufficiency. The follicular and anaplastic types of thyroid cancer may occur at higher frequencies in regions at high risk for goiter development (CUELLO et al. 1969, WAHNER et al. 1966) but there is no clear evidence in humans that endemic iodide deficiency is casually related to the development of such tumors. Various studies have demonstrated increased incidence of papillary thyroid cancer in the atomic bomb survivors (BEEBE 1981), persons exposed to fallout from nuclear weapons testing (CONRAD 1977), radiation therapy in childhood for various benign diseases (HEMPLEMAN et al. 1975), and medical uses of radioactive iodide (DOBYNS et al. 1974). In the atomic bomb survivors the average dose to the thyroid was approximately 130 cGy while the average thyroid dose from radiation therapy for benign diseases of the head and neck was between 120–790 cGy depending on the particular entity treated. Doses in this range are thought to give rise to an increase in the absolute risk of developing thyroid cancer of between 3.4 to 3.6 per 10^6 persons per cGy (SHORE et al. 1984). The atomic bomb survivors showed a three-fold increase in the subgroup who were under age 20 at the time of detonation compared with those who were older. The minimum latency period seems to be approximately 5 years and the period of increased risk extends at least to 30 years from the time of exposure. On the other hand, very high doses of radiation in the range of 7000–10000 cGy seem to cause mainly cell death rather than a malignant transformation (BOICE and LAND 1982). Such high doses of radiation may lead, however, to the development of a sarcomatous malignancy with a latency period of 15–20 years.

1.1.7 Dietary Factors

There have been some epidemiology studies that suggest diets high in vitamins A and C convey some protection against developing epithelial tumors of the oral cavity and respiratory tract (GRAHAM et al. 1981; MARSHALL et al. 1982). After correcting cohort groups for the effects of tobacco and ethanol abuse, those with diets low in vitamins A and C had twice the risk of developing cancers in the oral cavity and larynx compared with those having a diets

high in these two vitamins. There is some physiological rationale for these findings. Ascorbic acid is an antioxidant and blocks the formation of N-nitroso compounds that are known carcinogens. Vitamin A is needed for the normal growth and maturation of epithelial tissues. A vitamin A deficiency causes a loss of the normal epithelium in the respiratory tract and causes it to be replaced by a dysplastic squamous epithelium. However, there is no evidence that dietary changes can reverse a malignant process that has already been established.

Plummer-Vinson syndrome is characterized by multiple vitamin and iron deficiencies. Its features are achlorhydria, atrophy of the tongue papillae, atrophy of the epithelial lining of the upper alimentary tract, and esophageal webs and/or strictures. Women with this syndrome have increased risk of developing cancers of the oral cavity, pharynx, and esophagus. It may be that riboflavin and iron deficiencies associated with ethanol abuse play a role in cancer development through complex changes in various enzymatic chemical processes.

1.2 Basic Pathology

1.2.1 General

Any given cell type of the body can undergo a malignant transformation. The frequency with which this occurs varies with the patient's age, sex, race, socio-economic status, occupational risk factors, and the particular region of the body under consideration – to name only a few relevant factors. The role of the pathologist is to identify the cell type involved, to establish whether the lesion is benign or malignant, and by this information give the clinician a guide to selecting the appropriate form of medical management for a given patient. In particular, the role of the pathologist is to identify various histological features of the tumor that correlate with the patient's ultimate prognosis – i.e., the relative risk of developing a local or a distant failure with a given form of treatment. Particular details relating to tumors in given head and neck sites will be discussed in the following chapters. Here we wish to give a general overview of the histopathology of squamous cell carcinomas of the head and neck region and its prognostic implications.

1.2.2 Histologic Grading

The quantitative grading of malignant neoplasms began with BRODERS (1926) who developed a scheme for determining tumor differentiation that at least was partially reproducible from observer to observer. This scheme divided squamous cell carcinomas into four categories based upon the proportion of the neoplasm that resembled normal tissue. The greater the amount of "normal-appearing" tissue, the "better differentiated" was the lesion. This approach was first applied to squamous cell carcinomas of the lip. With time, additional parameters have been incorporated into assigning a histologic "grade" to a given lesion. Such parameters are amount of keratinization and its basic pattern, number of intracellular bridges (desmosomes), nuclear pleomorphism, and frequency of mitotic figures. Today, most pathologists use a simplified version of Broder's scheme and divide squamous cell carcinomas into three grades: well differentiated, moderately differentiated, and poorly differentiated.

To get maximum information from the pathologist, adequate tissue must be submitted along with sufficient information to aid him in making a diagnosis. Age of patient, site of the biopsy, general appearance of the lesion, and suspicions of the clinician are only a few factors to be considered. While these details are generally within the purvue of the interaction between the surgeon and the pathologist, it behooves the radiation oncologist to carefully review the situation to make sure that some important detail has not been overlooked.

The light microscope and appropriate staining techniques continue to be the workhorse of the pathologist in making a diagnosis. However, the electron microscope often provides invaluable information in determining the specific type of neoplasm and is of great benefit in identifying small cell neoplasms such as "oat cell" tumors, lymphomas or esthesioneuroblastomas. Immunologic procedures – in particular, immunofluorescence and immunoperoxidase methods – characterize cellular antigenicity. Immunofluorescent techniques require fresh frozen tissues. In this technique a fluorochrome is either directly attached to the specific antibody that complexes with the cellular antigens or is attached to a second antibody that complexes with the first antibody directed against the cellular antigens. The immunoperoxidase technique utilizes bridges of antibodies that link antigens to peroxidase. The tissue is then saturated with hydrogen peroxide and a chromogen. The presence of the antigen causes the chromogen to undergo a color change at locations where the antigen is bound to the peroxidase. Antibodies against collagen demonstrate the presence or absence of the basement membrane which is a clue to the malignant nature of the cells. Particular varieties of keratin are elaborated by some malignant cells and immunologic techniques are useful in identifying them. Alterations in ABH blood group antigens occur in many squamous cell carcinomas. LIN et al. (1977) have noted a gradual loss of these antigens in laryngeal cells as they change from normal to dysplastic to frankly malignant.

Cytogenetic techniques allow one to perform karyotyping of cells and there is evidence that certain abnormal karyotypes correlate with tumor biologic behavior (WOLMAN 1984). Flow cytometry requires preparing a suspension of cells and then examining various properties as the cells flow one-by-one through a sensing area. One can measure fluorescence, electrical resistance, light scatterings, or light absorption. By appropriate monitoring of these parameters, one can measure cell size and nucleic acid levels. Fluorescent labelled antibodies can probe a variety of antigens with this technique. DNA histograms demonstrate the ploidy of tumor cells and have shown the very heterogeneous nature of most tumors. Studies are now in progress to correlate this ploidy with patient prognosis for various head and neck tumors. Finally, tritiated thymidine can be used to determine the percentage of tumor cells in the DNA synthetic phase and this often correlates with the aggressiveness of the malignancy.

1.2.3 Correlation Between Histologic Parameters and Patient Prognosis

Work correlating clinical and pathologic parameters with patient prognosis is still evolving but some results have already been demonstrated. McGAVRAN et al. 1961 divided squamous cell carcinomas into two categories: those having pushing margins and those having infiltrating margins. The infiltrative pattern of invasion correlated better with the development of lymph node metastases than tumor grad *per se*. Another study showed that all patients with regional nodal metastases came from a subgroup with demonstrated vascular space invasion in the initial biopsy specimen (POLEKSIC and KALWAIC, 1978). MARTIN et al. (1980) evaluated 108 patients with piriform sinus lesions and found that keratinization in the tumor was associated with higher rates of local/regional failure. However, the non-keratinizing group of tumors contained a greater proportion of poorly differentiated lesions and these had a higher rate of distant metastases. The pattern of invasion and the degree of inflammatory reaction at the tumor-normal tissue interface was not a predictor of local control on survival for this study group.

For carcinoma of the larynx JACOBSSON (1976) has proposed a semiquantitative grading scheme based upon observations of several parameters characterizing the tumor cell population and the tumornormal tissue interface. The parameters used include the following: structure of the neoplasm, keratinization, nuclear pleomorphism, mitotic index, pattern of invasion, vascular invasion (if any), and degree of lymphocyte and plasmocyte response. JACOBSSON (1976) noted that in early T_1 lesions the recurrences correlated best with the pattern of invasion but the degree of nuclear pleomorphism correlated better with the recurrence rate for the more advanced laryngeal tumors. Unfortunately, an attempt to apply this schema to squamous cell carcinomas of the oropharynx did not demonstrate any significant correlation between the tumor score and subsequent tumor recurrence (CRISSMAN et al. 1984). However, while the overall tumor score was not important in this study, a regression analysis on the individual parameters showed that an infiltrating pattern of invasion was associated with decreased patient survival. When only the histologic parameters were considered, then both mitotic index and pattern of invasion correlated with survival while the presence of vascular and/or lymphatic space invasion correlated with regional lymph node metastases.

The changes in the tumor with preoperative radiation have prognostic significance. For example, tumor sterilization can often be identified by the presence of keratin debris. ROLLO et al. (1981) have shown that in a group of patients with squamous cell carcinomas of the base of the tongue, a partial or complete histologic response to preoperative radiotherapy meant about a factor of 6 improvement in 5 year survival compared to patients having no obvious tumor response. Similarly, there may be a correlation between tumor histologic features and response to induction chemotherapy. YAMAMOTO et al. (1983) have noted a correlation between the pattern of invasion of squamous cell carcinomas of the oral cavity and response to bleomycin. Tumors with a "pushing" border appeared more sensitive than those with an infiltrative border. Tumor size and grade did not correlate with the observed response.

Obviously, considerably more research on these forms of correlation is needed. It is encouraging to note that the ongoing Veterans Administration Hospital Cooperative Larynx Study (CSP 268) is attempting to gather such host and tumor factors prospectively, and then to see how they correlate with local/regional control and survival.

1.3 Staging

1.3.1 General

A very concise statement of the purposes of clinical staging of tumors has been given by KEANE (1985):

a) To provide a way by which information regarding the state of a cancer can be communicated to others.
b) To assist in decisions regarding treatment.
c) To give some indication regarding prognosis.
d) To provide a mechanism for comparing the results of treatment.

In order to accomplish these ends the International Union Against Cancer (UICC) set up a special committee about 30 years ago to formulate a system. Similarly, the American Joint Committee for Cancer Staging and End Results Reporting (AJC) was established about 25 years ago. Unfortunately, the staging systems recommended by these oranizations for head and neck cancer differ in some respects and this often leads to problems in communication between various centers. To further compound the problem, there was a period of time when some of the major treatment centers, e.g., M. D. Anderson, utilized their own "in house" system and reported their results in the literature using these systems. In this book every effort will be made to constistently utilize the most recent AJC system. Unfortunately, there are some tumors and sites, e.g., chemodectomas, minor salivary glands, paranasal sinuses excluding the maxilla, etc. for which no commonly accepted staging system yet exists.

The application of any staging system consists of four basic steps (KEANE 1985):

a) Histologic confirmation of tumor
b) Clinical and radiologic examination
c) Recording of relevant information
d) Assigning a TMN stage

1.3.2 Histologic Confirmation

In general, it is not difficult to confirm the diagnosis of head and neck malignancies - particularly, of the squamous cell variety. The diagnosis of carcinoma-in-situ is an exception to this as the opinions of pathologists may differ as to what constitutes dysplasia and atypia vs. what constitutes carcinoma-in-situ. This is particularly the case for vocal cord lesions.

1.3.3 Clinical and Radiologic Examination

The main problem with clinical examination is observer reproducibility. Lesions in some regions of the head and neck are staged according to size and often it can be quite difficult to measure a moderate sized lesion – particularly in a patient with a hyperactive gag reflex. Other regions of the head and neck are staged according to sites of tumor involvement and here the question arises of interpreting areas of inflammation and/or induration.

The application of imaging techniques to the staging of head and neck cancer is an interesting subject in itself. Chapter 2 of this book is devoted entirely to this topic. It is clear that we want to gather all relevant information about the tumor status in order to best treat the patient. However, new modalities such as CT, MRI, and PET scans, while they more accurately define the tumor, are in an evolving state. For many tumor systems there is no clear correlation between an "abnormality on scan" and "histologic verification of tumor" in the context of a controlled study. It also must be recognized that more detailed studies are likely to demonstrate tumor extending beyond areas of involvement noted on simple physical examination. This staging improvement would have the net effect of improving patient survival for a given stage (by assigning higher stages to those found to have more advanced disease by the new tests) even if no improvement in treatment methods has occurred. It is important to keep this fact in mind when comparing the results of recent studies with those done before some of the newer diagnostic procedures were available.

1.3.4 Recording of Information

While this appears self-evident, unfortunately, it is not done in many cases. Hence, there is no way for someone to independently take the information and arrive at a TNM stage. This is especially frustrating when evaluating multi-institutional cooperative studies through an independent audit of the patient charts. An accurate diagram of the primary tumor and sites of nodal involvement is expecially important.

Furthermore, the AJC system asks for other information about the tumor that *at present* is not directly used in establishing a TNM stage. An example of this is a description of the tumor appearance: exophytic, superficial, moderately infiltrating, deeply infiltrating, or ulcerated. This information may be important in future staging and it is important to record it for as many tumors as possible in order to establish a large data base. Certainly, many clinicians regard exophytic tumors as more radioresponsive than deeply infiltrating tumors. Unfortunately, there are no commonly agreed upon criteria for these terms and accordingly there is considerable oberver variability.

1.3.5 Assigning TNM Stage

1.3.5.1 T Stage

This parameter refers to the primary tumor. TIS refers to carcinoma-in-situ. The frankly invasive lesions are classified as T_1, T_2, T_3, or T_4 with the lower numbers referring to the less advanced lesions. Tumors arising in the lip, parotid gland, oral cavity, and oropharynx are staged according to "size of lesion" while tumors arising in the maxillary sinus, nasopharynx, hypopharynx, and larynx are staged according to "sites of tumor involvement". The particular staging system for the various sites will be discussed in the appropriate following chapter. Here we will only point out some common threads and differences.

The T_4 category in all cases refers to a "massive" tumor with varying degrees of invasion of the adjacent tissues. Differences between the sites relate to operability criteria. For example, bony invasion makes an oropharyngeal tumor a "T_4" but does not upstage an oral cavity tumor to this degree. For tumors staged according to sites of involvement, even a small tumor may be a "T_4" and radiocurable with reasonable probability. On the other hand, a tumor that is "T_4" by virtue of massive size, may be very difficult to control with radiation alone. This is important in evaluating the results of various series that contain "selected" T_4 lesions treated in a given way.

1.3.5.2 N Stage

Squamous cell carcinomas of the head and neck frequently spread via the regional lymphatics and "N-stage" refers to this aspect of tumor involvement. Unlike the situation for the various primaries, all head and neck sites utilize the same staging for the regional nodes. This is summarized in Table 1-1. This recognizes not only the importance of size and number of involved nodes but also their location. For example, an involved node on the contralateral site of the neck generally means a higher risk of distant spread of tumor than one of the same size that is adjacent to the primary tumor. Note also that this refers to *clinical staging* and the pathologic staging after a neck dissection may differ from the clinical staging. Both stages should be recorded but it is important not to confuse the two.

Tumors from different primary sites have the propensity to spread to specific nodal groups. This can be important in searching for a small primary lesion when the patient presents first with a neck mass. While the specific nodal site does not enter directly into the determination of the N-stage, it is appropriate to utilize a standard terminology. The one used in this book is that defined by FLETCHER et al. (1978) which is illustrated in Fig. 1-1. This divides each side of the neck into nine distinct regions:

a) The *submental nodes* are located superficial to the mylohyoid muscles and anterior to the digastric muscles.
b) The *submaxillary nodes* lie along the lower border of the mandible and are contained within the submaxillary triangle. They are subdivided into three subgroups depending on their relationship to the adjacent neurovascular bundle and submaxillary salivary gland: preglandular, prevascular, and retrovascular.
c) The *subdigastric nodes* are located below the posterior belly of the digastric muscle. They are located at the level of the greater cornu of the

Table 1-1. Regional nodal staging common to all head and neck tumor sites

N_0	No clinically positive nodes
N_1	Single clinically positive homolateral node 3 cm or less in diameter
N_{2a}	Single clinically positive homolateral node between 3 and 6 cm in diameter
N_{2b}	Multiple clinically positive homolateral nodes, none of which are more than 6 cm in diameter
N_{3a}	Clinically positive homolateral node(s), one of which is more than 6 cm in diameter
N_{3b}	Bilateral clinically positive nodes. Each side of the neck should then be separately staged
N_{3c}	Only contralateral clinically positive node(s)

hyoid bone. The upper jugular nodes and the tonsillar node are contained within this group.
d) The *midjugular nodes* are located just below the hyoid bone at the bifurcation of the common carotid artery.
e) The *low jugular nodes* lie along the lower third of the internal jugular vein.
f) The *upper posterior cervical nodes* lie at the superior end of the spinal accessory chain. The uppermost node is at the tip of mastoid process beneath the sternocleidomastoid muscle.
g) The *midposterior cervical nodes* are those nodes within the spinal accessory chain that lie at the same level as the midjugular nodes.
h) The *low posterior cervical nodes* are at the lower end of the spinal accessory chain.
i) The *supraclavicular nodes* are located just above

Fig. 1-1. Nodal regions of the neck. After FLETCHER et al. (1978)

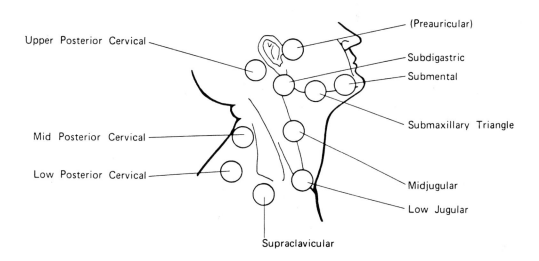

the clavicle in the transverse lymphatic chain that corrects the jugular chain with the spinal accessory chain. The anterior scalene nodes are included in this group.

In any physical examination, it is important to carefully palpate each separate region on each side of the neck. The particular nodal groups at highest risk of metastases from the various head and neck primary sites will be discussed in the subsequent chapters.

Tumors of the head and neck also can spread to the *retropharyngeal nodes* which lie along the posterior pharyngeal wall and anterior to the vertebral column. Their superior aspect lies at the base of the skull and their inferior aspect lies at the beginning of the trachea. These ar not included in any clinical staging system due to their relative inaccessability. However, these nodes often must be included in appropriately designed radiation treatment portals. The advent of ancillary radiologic scanning techniques may allow one to incorporate the status of these nodes into future staging systems.

Nodal metastases beyond the above groups are considered distant metastases.

1.3.5.3 M Stage

Tumors are staged as either M_0 or M_1 depending on whether distant metastases are absent or present. An extensive review of 5019 patients with previously untreated squamous cell carcinomas was performed by MERINO et al. (1977). These patients appeared to have localized disease at the time of presentation and were definitely treated.

A total of 546 patients subsequently developed distant metastases. The overall incidence of developing distant metastases was 10.9%. A breakdown according to primary site is given in Table 1-2. The incidence ranges from a low of 3.1% for tumors in the glottic larynx to a high of 28.1% for tumors of the nasopharynx. Of course, there is a correlation between development of distant metastases and the TN stages of the tumor. The development of distant metastases from the various primary sites will be discussed in more detail in the following chapters. Nevertheless, the information contained in Table 1-2 is important in that it gives the clinician a relative guide as to how aggressively to pursue the distant metastases workup for a given tumor.

The most common site of distant metastases was lung (52%) followed by bone (20.3%) and liver (6.0%). This relative distribution was usually the same regardless of primary tumor site, although

Table 1-2. Incidence of distant metastases from squamous cell arising from various head and neck sites. These patients all appeared to have localized disease at the time of presentation. After MERINO et al. (1977)

Primary Site	Distant Metastases (%)
Oral cavity	7.5% (116/1541)
Faucial arch	6.7% (37/550)
Oropharynx proper (tonsil, base of tongue, pharyngeal wall)	15.3% (110/717)
Nasopharynx	28.1% (63/224)
Nasal Cavity/Paranasal Sinuses	9.1% (21/230)
Supraglottic Larynx	15.0% (70/466)
Glottic Larynx	3.1% (27/858)
Hypopharynx	23.6% (102/433)
Overall	10.9% (546/5019)

there were a few exceptions to this general sequencing. For nasopharyngeal primaries that subsequently metastasized, bone lesions were more common than lung metastases (54% vs. 23.8%). Liver metastases occurred in 22% of tonsillar fossa lesions and 10.8% of tumors arising in the base of the tongue that subsequently metastasized. For glottic primaries, there was a 14.8% incidence of metastases to the mediastinal nodes in the subgroup that ultimately exhibited a distant spread.

It is mandatory that a diagnostic evaluation include a chest x-ray and blood chemistry studies that contain liver function tests, serum Ca^{+2}, and serum alkaline phosphatase. If these are normal and there is no clinical suspicion of metastases to a given site, then additional metastatic evaluation is usually not undertaken in the absence of particular protocol study requirements.

1.3.6 Stage Grouping

By convention the TNM categories are grouped according to the pattern shown in Table 1-3. The purpose of this grouping is to associate prognosis with

Table 1-3. AJC stage groupings for all squamous cell carcinomas of the head and neck sites

Stage I	$T_1\ N_0\ M_0$
Stage II	$T_2\ N_0\ M_0$
Stage III	$T_3\ N_0\ M_0$
	$T_1\ T_2\ T_3\ N_1\ M_0$
Stage IV	$T_4\ N_0\ M_0$
	Any T-stage, $N_2\ N_3\ M_0$
	Any T-stage, any N-stage, M_1

stage of disease. The assignment works well for the early stage I and II categories but the more advanced stage III and IV categories are a more heterogeneous mixture. Work is currently in progress on further refining these categories.

GRIFFIN et al. (1984) analyzed an RTOG data base consisting of 997 patients treated definitively with standard radiotherapy. They found that the primary tumor response could be modeled according to the following formula:

$$\mathrm{Ln}\,\{P/(1\text{-}P)\} = 2.100 - 0.960\,(T\text{-}2.072) \\ - 0.245\,(N\text{-}0.622) + 0.855\,(S\text{-}1.854) \\ + 0.716\,(K\text{-}1.613) \qquad (1)$$

where P is the probability of primary tumor clearance, T is the primary tumor stage ($T = 1, 2, 3, 4$), N is the stage of the neck disease ($N = 0, 1, 2, 3$). S is the location of the primary tumor site (nasopharynx $= 3$, oral cavity $= 1$, oropharynx $= 2$, larynx (glottis and supraglottis) $= 2$, and hypopharynx $= 2$), and K is the Karnofsky performance status of the patient ($K = 2$ for 90-100, $K = 1$ for 70-80, and $K = 0$ for ≤ 60). A detailed discussion of the general applicability of this formula is given in the original reference. Here it is sufficient to note that this formula was cross-checked against two other patient data bases and for most parameter sets, was found to have an accuracy of more than 90%. Moreover, those patients for whom the formula predicted a greater than 90% probability of primary tumor clearance had an 87% probability of being free of disease at two years from initiation of definitive radiotherapy. This formula clearly is not definitive since it does not incorporate tumor related parameters such as mitotic index, degree of infiltration, or amount of keratinization, but it is useful in identifying specific groups of patients that have a high probability of cure with radiotherapy alone. It is a trivial matter to enter it into any of the programmable calculators.

This formula incorporates the interaction between the indicated parameters. Note in particular, it provides a semi-quantitative description of how increasing N-stage correlates with decreasing probability of control at the primary site. Also note that better Karnofsky performance status correlates with higher probability of primary tumor control. This fact must be taken into account in comparing the results of surgical series (which often contain the patients with the better Karnofsky performance status) with the results of radiotherapy alone. Detailed tables showing the dependence of tumor control probability on Karnofsky performance status for la-

Table 1-4. RTOG proposed stage grouping system for head and neck cancer. The RTOG stages are shown in the left hand column and the corresponding TN stages are shown in the right hand column. After AL-SARRAF et al. 1984

Proposed RTOG Stage Grouping	TN Stages
I	$T_1\ N_0$
II A	$T_2\ N_0$
II B	$T_1\ N_1$; $T_2\ N_1$
III A	$T_3\ N_0$
III B	$T_1\ N_2$; $T_2\ N_2$
III C	$T_4\ N_0$
IV A	$T_1\ N_3$; $T_2\ N_3$
IV B	$T_3\ N_1$; $T_4\ N_1$
IV C	$T_3\ N_2$; $T_3\ N_3$
IV D	$T_4\ N_2$; $T_4\ N_3$

ryngeal tumors are shown in Chapter 10. The reader is encouraged to work out similar tables for the other primary sites.

MENDENHALL et al. (1984) analyzed a group of 373 patients with localized stage IV disease treated with primary radiotherapy and found there was a prognostic value into subdividing stage IV into two categories. Stage IV-A consisted of T_1, T_2, T_3, N_{2a}, N_{2b}, N_{3a} and stage IV-B consisted of T_1, T_2, T_3, N_{3b} and T_4, N_0, N_1, N_2, N_3, N_{3a}, N_{3b}. N_{3c} lesions were not considered in this study. The prognosis of stage IVA patients was substantially better than stage IV-B patients for all sites except tonsillar primaries.

AL-SARRAF et al. (1984) have recently re-examined the prognostic significance of the standard AJC stage III and IV categories for a group of 992 patients treated with definitive radiotherapy on various RTOG protocols. They found that the survival of patients with T_1, N_1 and $T_2\ N_1$ lesions was similar to those stages as $T_2\ N_0$ and that patients with $T_4\ N_0$ lesions did substantially better than those other AJC stage IV categories. They have proposed the modified stage grouping shown in Table 1-4. Stage IVD patients had a very high rate of distant metastases and, hence, may be an appropriate group of patients for aggressive chemotherapy protocols.

Only time will prove or disprove the utility of these new stage groupings, but re-examination of the problem is certainly an important step forward.

References

Al-Saraff M, Pajak TF, Laramore GE (1984) The appropriateness of the present AJC and UICC staging system for head and neck cancer for protocol design and results reporting. Proc Int Conf Head and Neck Cancer 61: 61

Baumslag N, Keen P, Petering HG (1971) Carcinoma of the maxillary antrum and its relationship to trace metal content of snuff. Arch Environ Hlth 23: 1–5

Beebe GW (1981) The Atomic bomb survivors and the problem of low-dose radiation effects. Am J Epidemiol 114: 761–783

Blot WJ, Fraumeni Jr JF (1977) Geographic patterns of oral cancer in the United States: Etiologic implications. J Chron Dis 30: 745–757

Blot WJ, Winn DM, Fraumeni Jr JF (1983) Oral cancer and mouthwash use. J Natl Cancer Inst 70: 255–260

Boice Jr JD, Land CE (1982) Ionizing radiation In: Shottenfeld D, Fraumeni Jr JF (eds) Cancer Epidemiology and Prevention, Saunders, Philadelphia, 231–253

Brinton LA, Blot WJ, Becker JA, Winn DM, Browder JA, Farmen JC, Fraumeni JF (1984) A case-control study of cancer of the nasal cavity and paranasal sinuses. Am J Epidemiol 119: 896–906

Broders AC (1926) Carcinoma: grading and practical application. Arch Path 2: 376–381

Conrad RA (1977) Summary of thyroid findings in Marshallese 22 years after exposure to radioactive fallout In: DeGroot LJ (ed) Radiation-Associated Thyroid Cancer, Grune and Stratton, New York, 241–257

Crissman JD, Liu WY, Gluckman JL, Cummings G (1984) Prognostic value of histopathologic parameters in squamous cell carcinoma of the oropharynx. Cancer 54: 2995–3001

Cuello C, Correa P, Eisenberg H (1969) Geographic pathology of thyroid carcinoma. Cancer 23: 230–239

Decoufle P (1982) Occupation In: Schottenfeld D, Fraumeni Jr JF (eds) Cancer Epidemiology and Prevention. Saunders, Philadelphia, 318–335

Dobyns BM, Sheline GF, Workman JB, Tompkins EA, McConahey WM, Becker DV (1974) Malignant and benign neoplasms of the thyroid in patients treated for hyperthyroidism: A report of the cooperative thyrotoxicosis therapy follow-up study. J Clin Endrocinol Metab 38: 976–998

Flanders WD, Cann CI, Rothman KJ, Fried MP (1984) Work-related risk factors for laryngeal cancer. Am J Epidemiol 119: 23–32

Fletcher GH, Jesse RH, Lindberg RD, Westbrook KC (1978) Neck nodes In: Fletcher GH (ed) Textbook of Radiotherapy, Lea and Febiger, Philadelphia, 249–270

Graham S, Mettlin C, Marshall J, Priore R, Rzepka T, Shedd D (1981) Dietary factors in the epidemiology of cancer of the larynx. Am J Epidemiol 113: 675–680

Griffin TW, Pajak TF, Gillespie BW, Davis LW, Brady LW, Rubin P, Marcial VA (1984) Predicting the response of head and neck cancers to radiation therapy with a multivariate modelling system: an analysis of the RTOG head and neck registry. Int J Radiat Oncol Biol Phys 10: 418–487

Hempelmann LH, Hall WJ, Phillips M, Cooper RA, Ames WR (1975) Neoplasms in persons treated with x-rays in infancy: fourth survey in 20 years. J Natl Cancer Inst 55: 519–530

Ho JHC, Huang DP, Fong YY (1978) Salted fish and nasopharyngeal carcinoma in southern Chinese. Lancet 2: 626

Jacobsson PA (1976) Histologic grading of malignancy and prognosis in glottic carcinoma of the larynx, Workshop No. 14 In: Alberti PW, Bryce DP (eds). Centennial Conference on Laryngeal Cancer. Appelton Century Crofts, New York, 847–854

Keane TJ (1985) Clinical staging of head and neck cancer In: Chretien PB, Johns ME, Shedd DP, Strong EW, Ward PH (eds) Head and Neck Cancer Volume I. Decker, Philadelphia, 89–91

Lin F, Liu PI, McGregor DH (1977) Isoantigens A, B, and H in morphologically normal mucosa and in carcinoma of the larynx. Am J Clin Path 68: 372–376

Marshall J, Graham S, Mettlin C, Shedd D, Swanson M (1982) Diet in the epidemiology of oral cancer. Nutr cancer: 3: 145–149

Martin SA, Marks JE, Lee JY, Bauer WL, Ogura JH (1980) Carcinoma of the piriform sinus: predictors of TMN relapse and survival. Cancer 46: 1974–1981

McGavran MH, Bauer WC, Ogura JH (1961) The incidence of cervical lymph node metastases from epidermoid carcinoma of the larynx and their relationship to certain characteristics of the primary tumor. Cancer 14: 55–66

McKay EW, Hanson MR, Miller RW (1982) Cancer mortality in the United States: 1950–1979, In: National Cancer Institute Mongraph No. 59 (US Government Printing Office, Washington, DC)

McMichael AJ (1978) Increases in laryngeal cancer in Britain and Australia in relation to alcohol and tobacco consumption trends. Lancet 1: 1244–1247

Mendenhall WM, Parsons JT, Million RR, Cassisi NJ, Devine JW, Greenburg BD (1984) A favorable subset of AJCC stage IV squamous cell carcinoma of the head and neck. Int J Radiat Oncol Biol Phys 10: 1841–1843

Merino OR, Lindberg RD, Fletcher GH (1977) An analysis of distant metastases from squamous cell carcinomas of the upper respiratory and digestive tracts. Cancer 40: 145–151

Poleksic S, Kalwaic HJ (1978) Prognostic value of vascular invasion in squamous cell carcinoma of the head and neck. Plast Reconstr Surg 61: 234–240

Reddy CR (1974) Carcinoma of hard palate in India in relation to reverse smoking of chuttas. J Natl Cancer Inst 53: 615–619

Redmond CK, Sass RE, Roush GC (1982) Nasal cavity and paranasal sinuses In: Schotlenfelt D, Fraumeni Jr JF (eds) Cancer Epidemiology and Prevention, Saunders, Philadelphia, 519–535

Rollo J, Rozenbom CV, Thawley S, Korba A, Ogura J, Perez CA, Powers WE, Bauer WC (1981) Squamous cell carcinoma of the base of the tongue: a clinicopathologic study of 81 cases. Cancer 43: 333–342

Rothman KJ, Cann CI, Flanders D, Fried MP (1980) Epidemiology of laryngeal cancer. Epidemiol Rev 2: 195–209

Shore RE, Woodward ED, Hemplemann LH (1984) Radiation inducted thyroid cancer In: Boice JD, Fraumeni Jr JF (eds) Radiation Carcinogenesis: Epidemiology and Biological Significance. Raven, New York, 131–138

Silverberg E, Lubera J (1987) Cancer Statistics, 1987. Ca – A Cancer Journal for Clinicians 37: 2–19

Simons MJ, Day NE (1977) Histocompatibility leukocyte antigen patterns and nasopharyngeal carcinoma. Natl Cancer Inst Monogr 47: 143–146

Wahner HW, Cuello C, Correa P, Uribe LF, Gaitan E (1966) Thyroid carcinoma in an endemic goiter area, Cali, Columbia. Am J Med 40: 58–66

Waterhouse J, Muir CS, Correa P (1976) Cancer incidence in five continents, III. Lyon, IARC Scientific Publications No 15

Weaver A, Fleming SM, Smith DP (1979) Mouthwash and oral cancer: carcinogen or coincidence? J Oral Surg 37: 250–253

Winn DM, Blot WJ, Shy CM, Pickle LW, Toledo A, Fraumeni Jr JF (1981) Snuff dipping and oral cancer among women in the southern United States. N Engl J Med 304: 745–749

Wolman SR (1984) Cytogenetics and cancer. Arch Pathol Lab Med 108: 15–19

Wynder EL, Kabat G, Rosenberg S, Levenstein M (1983) Oral cancer and mouthwash use. J Natl Cancer Inst 70: 255–260

Yamamoto E, Kohama G, Sunakawa H, Iwai M, Hiratsuka H (1983) Mode of invasion, bleomycin sensitivity and clinical course in squamous cell carcinoma of the oral cavity. Cancer 51: 2175–2180

2 Imaging Studies in Head and Neck Cancer

WILLIAM P. SHUMAN and ALBERT A. MOSS

CONTENTS

2.1 Designing the Imaging Workup of Head and Neck Tumors

Modern radiation therapy of head and neck cancer depends heavily on accurately detecting all malignant tissue present be it primary tumor, metastatic tumor, or associated adenopathy. Precise three dimensional tumor localization is critical for therapy planning so that all disease tissue is treated to tumorocidal doses while sparing as much normal adjacent tissue as possible. Fortunately, modern high technology has provided serveral ways to detect and spatially localize tumor; unfortunately high technology is expensive to apply. In this era of increasing scrutiny by governmental agencies of the cost of health care, merely ordering all conceivable imaging tests on all patients is effective but financially unacceptable. Cost effective diagnosis requires a rational sequencing of diagnostic tests based on knowledge of individual disease patterns and the latest information about the efficacy of various imaging modalities. A radiologist oriented toward oncologic practice and familiar with recent imaging developments can be of great assistance in the role of consultant for the purpose of designing an imaging workup.

WILLIAM P. SHUMAN, M.D., ALBERT A. MOSS, M.D., Department of Radiology, University Hospital, University of Washington, Seattle, WA 98 195, (206) 543-3320, USA

Much background information about an individual patient must be integrated and used to design the efficient imaging workup. Because of heavy demands on equipment, CT studies, for example, should be directed to areas of suspicion for detailed imaging, with less suspicious areas surveyed more quickly. To select and direct imaging, the history and physical exam provides the most valuable information. Type of known malignancies, previous surgical and radiation therapies, individual patient risk factors, patient signs and symptoms all provide vital directing information. The physical exam should precede any imaging studies and should be thorough, with detailed results communicated to those planning the imaging workup. In head and neck tumors, triple endoscopy with directed biopsies provides excellent assessment of tumor projecting into the lumen of any portion of the aerodigestive tract. Unfortunately, it is limited in its ability to assess submucosal spread and the extend of deep penetration of tumor, hence the need for cross-sectional imaging. Laboratory tests, such as alkaline phosphatase fractionated for bone component (indicator of bony metastases), can provide directing information. Previously performed imaging tests, such as plain radiography, ultrasound, or older CT exams should be reviewed. Once all this information is assembled, the radiation therapist and radiologist can together design a sequence of imaging exams and also design each individual exam to produce a directed, rapid, and efficient workup. Such a workup should not only provide precise extent of disease, but also tumor localization information in a form useful for therapy planning and dosimetry.

2.2 Standard Imaging Modalities

2.2.1 Plain Radiography

The utility of plain radiography has decreased with the advent of CT. It has been jokingly stated that radiographs of the skull provide no assurance of the presence of brain tissue. Likewise, radiographs of the face and neck detect only the grossest of tumors impinging on luminal air, distorting external soft tissue contours, or totally destroying bone. While plain radiography is cheap, it is no match for the markedly increased tissue contrast provided by CT in assessing malignant processes. Xeroradiography provides some improvement in soft tissue contrast, and polytomography is an improvement in spatial resolution. But neither modality can compete with the contrast and spatial resolution of CT. In the new radiology department for a 650 bed teaching hospital at the University of Washington, there is no equipment for polytomography or xeroradiography as both have been supplanted by CT. Face and neck malignancies are routinely evaluated by physical exam, endoscopy, CT, and MR.

2.2.2 Ultrasound

Early enthusiasm for specific tissue characterization by ultrasound has waned and is awaiting new technology. Ultrasound may occasionally be useful for detecting neck masses, particularly adenopathy (FRIEDMAN et al. 1983; SCHEIBLE 1981; BAKER and KRAUSE 1981). As such, it is cheap, sensitive, and easy to perform. The ability of ultrasound to differentiate cystic or necrotic from solid tissue may occasionally be helpful. Generally, however, the difficulty translating ultrasound images into three dimensional spatial localization has limited its use for radiation therapy planning.

2.2.3 Computed Tomography

Third and fourth generation CT scanners provide submillimeter spatial resolution and one or two second scan times. Motion artifact is minimized by fast scan times, and newer reconstruction algorithms decrease (although do not eliminate) streak artifacts from metal or abrupt bonysoft tissue interfaces.

2.2.3.1 Tailoring CT to Radiation Therapy Requirements

The ideal CT scanner for radiation therapy will have a large aperture and reconstruction diameter. The couch top of the scanner will be flat and match that of simulators and therapy equipment. Similar three dimensional laser light positioning devices should be available in the CT scanner room and the therapy equipment room. Fast scan and reconstruction times are important as is the capability of doing thin (1.5 mm) slices. The scanner should be able to produce high resolution scanned projection radiographs (ScoutView) as well as sagittal and coronal reconstructed images (GOITEIN 1979A; SMITH et al. 1980).

Several CT techniques can be used to produce information useful for radiation therapy. The patient should be scanned with CT in any immobilization device that will be used during therapy and in the body position to be assumed during therapy. Radio-opaque catheters can be used to outline the margins of therapy portals or select the angle of therapy beam obliquity (Fig. 2-1). Outlines of tumor margins on cross-sectional images can be marked and computer drawn on scanned projection radiograph images to aid tumor localization (Figs. 2-2 and 2-3) (SHUMAN et al. 1982). Tumor volumes can be accurately measured and compared after therapy (BRENNER et al. 1982). CT images can be transferred to therapy planning computers and contours used for dosimetry calculations. In addition CT tissue density information can be used for improving dosimetry calculations (VAN DYK 1983; HOGSTROM et al. 1979).

The use of CT in radiation therapy thus goes beyond tumor detection and staging. It can also aid selection of patient position, positioning of portals, and configuration of beams. CT can be used for dose calculations, for compensation of tissue inhomogeneity, and to follow resultant tumor regression (GOITEIN et al. 1979B). With these capabilities, numerous reports have documented the major positive impact of CT on radiation therapy planning and the results of radiation therapy (PRASAD et al. 1980; BADCOCK 1983; STEWART et al. 1978; MUNZENRIDER et al. 1977; GRIFFIN et al. 1984; VAN DYK et al. 1980; SEWCHAND et al. 1982).

2.2.3.2 CT Guided Biopsies

CT can be used to precisely localize entry point, angulation and depth for needle biopsies of deep seated head and neck tumors. Once a needle has been passed, the position of the tip in the tumor and therefore the precise tissue sampled can be confirmed by CT. Using any of a variety of 20 or 22 gauge biopsy needles, head and neck malignancies can be safely biopsied (GATENBY et al. 1983). CT can improve the safety of a biopsy by selecting an approach to tumor that avoids blood vessels and

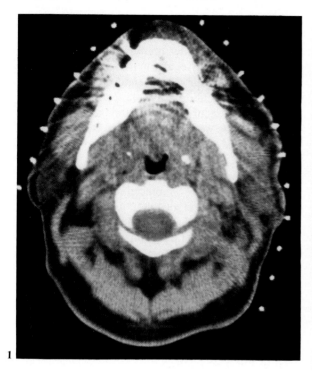

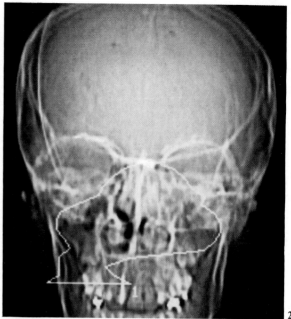

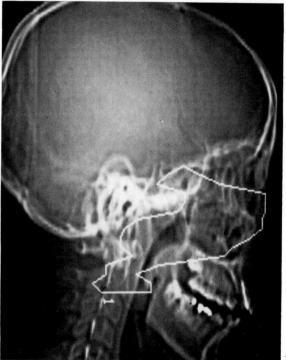

Fig. 2-1. Radiodense angiographic catheters are placed against the patient's skin at 2 cm intervals to help select obliquity of portal. As the catheter is removed the location on the skin is marked and numbered for future reference during simulation

Fig. 2-2. Using information provided to it from cross-sectional images by the operator, the computer can generate tumor outlines on the scoutview image. This is useful during simulation since the computer marked scoutview is in the same plane as the simulation radiograph

Fig. 2-3. Lateral tumor outlines on same patient as in Figure 2-2

other vital structures. Tissue obtained is usually adequate for cytological evaluation. Frequently, a core of tissue may be obtained from a cutting 22 gauge needle; this core can be stored in formalin, and later wax-mounted, sectioned and stained histologically just as with any surgical specimen.

2.2.3.3 CT Study Technique

For tumor detection in most regions of the face and neck, contiguous 5 millimeter thick sections are optimal. Thinner (1.5 mm) slices may be useful when evaluating the base of the skull or other finely detailed anatomy, particularly if sagittal or coronal reconstructions are to be performed. All images should be photographed with both soft tissue and bone centered windows. Occasionally, reconstruction of images using bone algorithms which enhance edges (rather than soft tissue algorithms which enhance subtle contrast differences) will help detect early bony erosions. Intravenous contrast should always be used and in relatively large doses. To maximally opacify vessels, prebolusing with 50–100 ml of 60% iodinated contrast followed by a rapid drip or infusion at 1 to 2 cc per second of an additional 150 ml will produce excellent visualization as well as enhancement of normal vascular anatomy and highly vascularized tumors. Scanning in more than one plane may be helpful, particularly when evaluating possible invasion of the base of the skull.

2.2.3.4 CT Evaluation of Different Regions of the Face and Neck

The Paranasal Sinuses. Squamous cell carcinoma is the most common malignancy of the sinuses, and CT is the best modality for detecting soft tissue sinus opacification from this as well as other tumors (KONDO et al. 1982; ST. PIERRE and BAKER 1983; JEANS et al. 1982). In evaluating extent of paraspinal disease, CT does well in detecting erosion through the cribiform plate into the anterior cranial fossa; invasion of the pterygopalatine fossa or infratemporal space, and direct extension into the middle cranial fossa. Direct coronal scans with bone algorithm reconstruction may be helpful in detecting subtle bony erosion, particularly in cases of ethmoidal tumor eroding into the orbits (Fig. 2-4) (LUND et al. 1983).

CT signs of malignancy in paranasal sinus tumors include irregular margins, thickened mucosa, variable contrast enhancement, and areas of necrosis (Fig. 2-5) (HASSO 1984). Bony erosion and disruption of fascial planes beyond the confines of the sinus should also be considered spreading tumor until proven otherwise (Figs. 2-6 and 2-7). CT in combination with the physical exam and endoscopy with biopsy should constitute the complete workup for extend of malignancy prior to therapy. Scanning should extend from above the base of the skull to the thoracic inlet to evaluate for adenopathy as well as primary tumor. Use of a catheter ruler during CT scanning or catheter markers of proposed portal outlines may be helpful when designing oblique fields to avoid the lens of the eye or brainstem.

After surgical and radiation therapy, CT can be helpful in following regression of disease. During the first few weeks after therapy the residual cavity or sinus may have irregular margins caused by healing and inflammation. By eight weeks, however, any focal mass, nodularity, or new bony erosions may represent recurrent tumor and biopsy of the region should be performed (BILANIUK and ZIMMERMANN 1982; HASSO 1984).

The Nasopharynx. CT evaluation of nasophyrngeal malignancies has replaced polytomography (BRANT-ZAWADZKI et al. 1982); it should be used as an adjunct to the physical and endoscopic examination. Signs of tumor include mass with submucosal infiltration (Fig. 2-8) and enlargement of the deglutinational muscle. The soft palate may be infiltrated and the eustachian tube orifice obstructed leading to serous otitis media. Involvement of the superior portion of the paraphryngeal space may affect the trigeminal nerve leading to pain, anesthesia, and masticatory muscle atrophy. Bony erosion may be seen in the base of the skull (foramen lacerum region), parasellar area, or orbital wall (Fig. 2-9) (SILVER et al. 1983A). Maxillary sinus carcinomas may extend into the nasopharynx (Fig. 2-10) and show destruction of the pterygoid plates as well (SILVER et al. 1983B). Direct coronal scanning of the nasopharynx and parapharynx and evaluation of enhancement from intravenous contrast are both helpful (HOOVER and HANAFEE 1983). After maxillectomy, CT can be used to follow for local recurrence. A baseline scan at eight weeks after surgery and repeat studies every six months for three years are useful to detect focal nodularity or bone destruction indicative of recurrence (SOM and BILLER 1983).

The Oropharynx and Parapharynx. CT should be performed after physical exam and endoscopy of the oropharynx for two reasons. First, the physical exam can be used to help design the CT exam. Second, CT may detect more tumor (particularly deep spread). In one series, CT detected some tumor volume previously undetected by physical exam in eight of twelve cases. However, CT studies of the oropharynx must be interpreted with caution. Superficial structures such as tonsillar pillars, lingual tonsils, and faucial tonsils may be quite asymmetrical; such asymmetry should not be interpreted as tumor (Fig. 2-11). Differences in tonsilar width of up to 5 mm may be normal. The cross-sectional area of the parapharyngeal space may be asymmetrical, but tumor masses there are more easily recognizeable due to disruption of fascial planes, abnor-

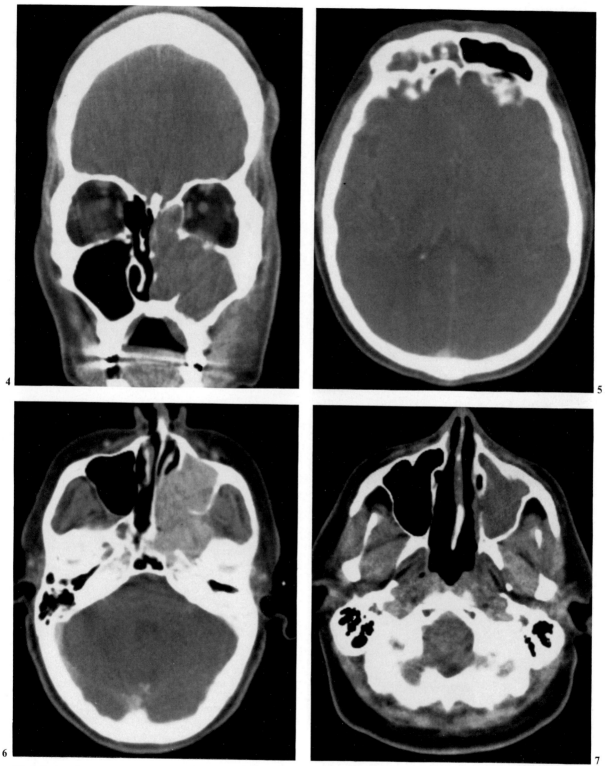

4

5

6

7

Fig. 2-4. Carcinoma of ethmoids and maxillary sinus eroding into orbit. Direct coronal scan

Fig. 2-5. Fibrous histiocytoma involving R frontal sinus

Fig. 2-6. Plasmacytoma of left maxillary antrum with bony erosion and disruption of fascial planes

Fig. 2-7. Lymphoma of left maxillary antrum destroying bone

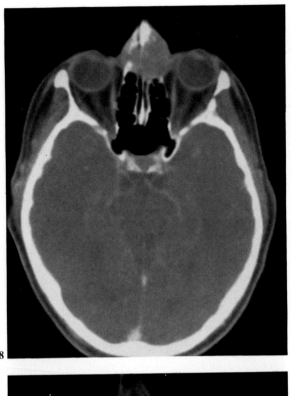

8

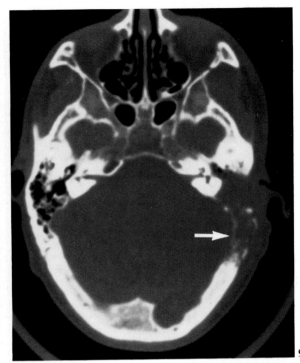

9

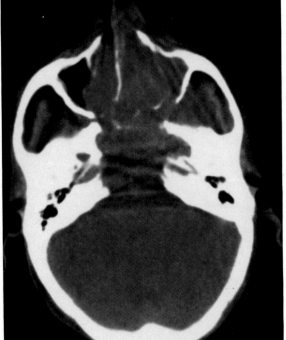

10

Fig. 2-8. Fibrous histiocytoma destroying nasal cartilage and bone

Fig. 2-9. Squamous cell carcinoma of left external auditory canal eroding mastoid bone *(arrow)*

Fig. 2-10. Squamous carcinoma of maxillary antrum extending into nasopharynx and base of skull

mal enhancement patterns, and variable density (Figs. 2-12 and 2-13) (SOM et al. 1984). The deep spaces of the floor of the month are usually symmetrical so that asymmetry of the sublingual space or tongue muscles should raise suspicion of tumor (Fig. 2-14). It should be remembered that considerable deep tumor can be present in these regions without distorting oropharynx contours or mucosal appearances, hence the value of CT to define extent of disease (Fig. 2-15).

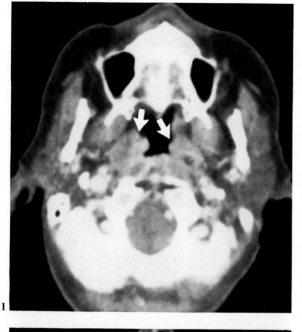

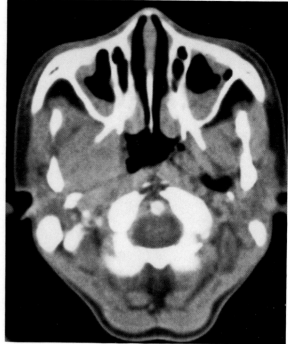

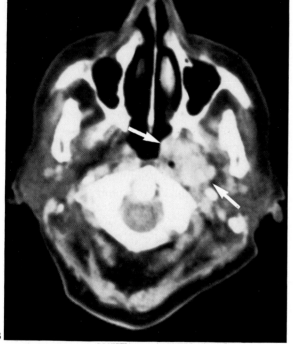

Fig. 2-11. Normal asymmetry of adenoidal tissue *(arrows)*

Fig. 2-12. Nasopharyngeal carcinoma causing asymmetry of right parapharyngeal space and disruption of fascial planes. Note maxillary mucosal disease

Fig. 2-13. Recurrent parotid tumor in left parapharyngeal space *(arrows)*. Note enhancement

The Larynx. CT does an excellent job of showing the laryngeal mucosa, cartilage, deep tissue, and associated lymphatic chain. Good CT technique involves the use of rapid scan times (2–5 seconds), thin (5 mm) sections, and high dose intravenous contrast as previously outlined (SILVERMAN et al. 1982). Scanning should extend down to the superior mediastinum and should be performed during quiet respiration since suspended respiration tends to adduct the true cords (MAFEE 1984). Scanning during phonation may help evaluate cord mobility (MANCUSO et al. 1980). In conjunction with physical exam (with mirror) and endoscopy, CT has now largely replaced laryngography (ARCHER et al. 1981; MANCUSO 1979B).

Classification of laryngeal cancer based on CT

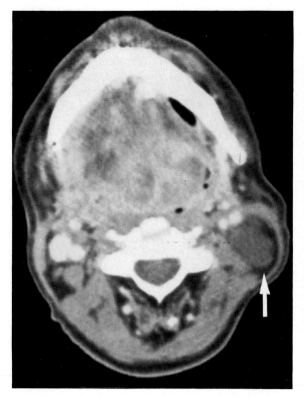

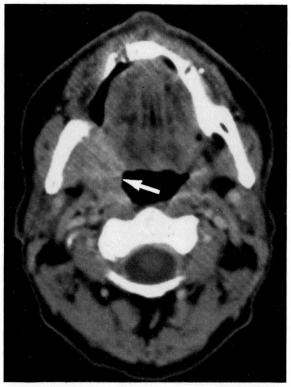

Fig. 2-14. Sarcoma of base of tongue has distorted the usual symmetry of the sublingual space. Note left neck adenopathy *(arrow)*

Fig. 2-15. Carcinoma of the right tonsillar pillar obliterates adjacent fascial planes *(arrow)*

findings seems a useful approach. CT findings closely agree with pathologic findings as to extent of disease (ARCHER et al. 1984). Use of bone reconstruction algorithms can be helpful in detecting even minimal invasion of laryngeal cartilage by the appearance of a fenestrated margin (Fig. 2-16); however, early microscopic invasion may unavoidably be missed (ARCHER et al. 1982 and 1983). While tiny mucosal lesions confined to the cords may also be missed by CT (REID 1984), phonation scans are helpful in detecting vocal cord dysfunction and pyriform sulcus tumor (GAMSU et al. 1981). CT scanning is very accurate in detecting tumor extension into the subglottic space, the preepiglottic space, and adjacent neck soft tissues (GAMSU et al. 1981; MAFEE 1983). Since pyriform sinus cancer is more often unilateral and more frequently invades the thyroid cartilage, it can often be differentiated from supraglottic laryngeal cancer by CT (LARSSON et al. 1981). Occasionally, tumor associated inflammatory changes or edema may cause CT to overestimate tumor extent (SILVERMAN et al. 1984). In general, however, CT is the modality of choice for evaluating extent of laryngeal malignancies for

therapy planning purposes (SCOTT et al. 1981; HO-ROWITZ et al. 1984; SAGEL et al. 1981).

CT has proven very helpful in evaluating for recurrence after partial laryngectomy (DI SANTIS et al. 1984A and 1984B). In one study, CT picked up recurrent tumor missed by physical exam in one-third of cases (HARNSBERGER et al. 1983). CT findings of recurrence included increased width of any remaining true cord, convexity of a surgically formed pseudocord, subglottic tumor, and extralaryngeal neck masses (DISANTIS et al. 1984A).

Parotid Tumor. CT does very well in identifying parotid pathology. Because the gland is of fatty density and most parotid tumors are of soft tissue density, most masses can be demonstrated without contrast injection in the parotid duct (Figs. 2-17 and 2-18) (RABINOV et al. 1984). Occasionally, CT after sialography may help delineate the relationship of parotid tumor to the facial nerve (MANCUSO et al. 1979A). CT sialography may also help with differentiating benign from malignant tumor growth patterns (MANCUSO et al. 1979A), but unfortunately malignant tumors may have either well circum-

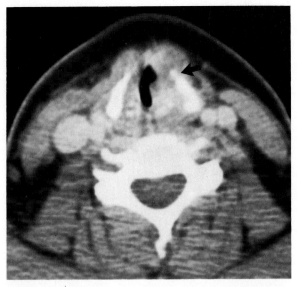

Fig. 2-16. Left supraglottic carcinoma with cartilage destruction *(arrow)*

scribed or indistinct margins. Inflammatory changes, however, are usually associated with diffuse enlargement and increase in the density of the gland (RABINOV et al. 1984). CT guided needle biopsy can be used to further characterize masses in and around the parotid gland. It should be remembered that normal submandibular glands can be quite asymmetrical in size (Fig. 2-19).

Neck Tumors and Adenopathy. In the neck CT can demonstrate and characterize extranodal spread of tumor better than the physical exam in many cases (MANCUSO et al. 1983). In about one quarter of cases CT will correctly increase the stage of disease. CT may fail to detect microscopic involvement in normal sized nodes, but this would be missed by physical exam as well. Lymph nodes larger than 1.5 centimeters have a high frequency of malignant involvement; some may show rim enhancement and areas of necrosis as well (Figs. 2-20 and 2-21) (MANCUSO et al. 1983). In the clinically normal neck in patients with squamous cell carcinoma (N_0), CT will detect adenopathy (N_1) in about 6% of cases (MANCUSO et al. 1983). CT does particularly well in evaluating the retropharyngeal lymph nodes; this area is usually beyond the limits of the physical exam. In general, the predictive value of a positive CT exam for adenopathy is about 92% (FRIEDMAN et al. 1984).

After radical neck dissection or radiation therapy, fat tissue planes in the neck may be effaced due to hemorrhage and edema for the first 8 weeks and due to fibrosis after that (SOM and BILLER 1983). Obtaining a baseline posttherapy CT can be helpful for future comparison. If a myocutaneous flap was created at surgery, it appears as a thickened layer of fatty tissue with overlying normal skin (SOM and BILLER 1983). If the fat develops infiltration with higher density or if a nodular mass develops elsewhere in the neck, abscess or recurrent tumor should be suspected and a percutaneous biopsy performed. CT guidance for biopsies is easily performed in the neck region and may be helpful in avoiding vascular structures and in confirming the location of the needle tip within the suspicious region.

2.2.4 Nuclear Medicine Studies

Bone scintigraphy has been used to evaluate for bony destruction in face and sinus malignancies (BERGSTEDT and LIND 1981). When compared to plain radiography, bone scanning detects more extensive bone involvement; no comparisons to CT have been published to date. The nonspecificity of a positive bone scintigram in the face region can be improved somewhat by gallium scanning which separates out those cases where the positive bone scan was due to osteomyelitis (SHAFER et al. 1981).

Cobalt-57 bleomycin has been used for tumor imaging in animals and humans for several years (HOU et al. 1984). Reports of series of patients with cervical and bronchogenic carcinoma are encouraging, while in testicular carcinoma results have been discouraging (NIEWEG et al. 1983; NIEWEG et al. 1984; PERTYNSKI and DURSKI 1985; MUCKERJEE 1976). Unfortunately, cobalt-57 bleomycin is also taken up in abscesses and is therefore somewhat nonspecific (WOOLFENDEN and HALL 1982). Its use in face and neck malignancies has not been reported to date.

2.2.5 Magnetic Resonance Imaging (MRI)

MR has by far the best soft tissue contrast capability of any imaging modality, considerably superior to even that of CT. In combination with the ability of MR to image directly in sagittal and coronal as well as transverse planes, this would seem to make MR a strong modality for defining extent of disease and for therapy planning (Figs. 2-22 and 2-23) (SHUMAN et al. 1985). A weakness of MR is its inability to image fine details of cortical bone anato-

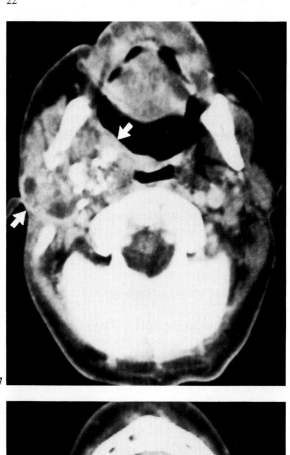

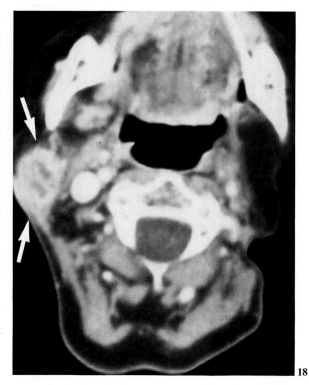

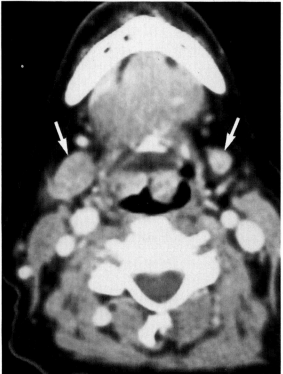

Fig. 2-17. Mixed tumor of the right parotid *(arrows)*. The right carotid artery is ocluded and there are focal dense areas of calcification in the tumor

Fig. 2-18. Adenoid cystic carcinoma of the right parotid *(arrows)*. Note previous radical neck surgery on left

Fig. 2-19. Normal asymmetry of the submandibular glands *(arrows)*

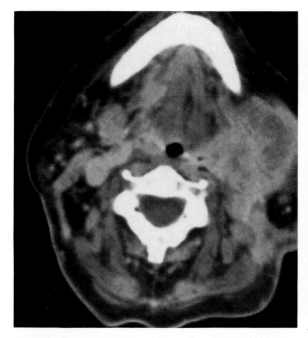

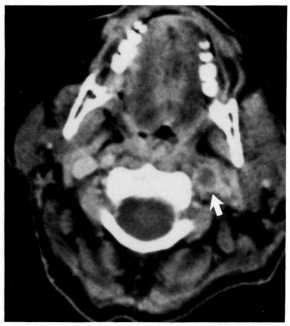

Fig. 2-20. Squamous cell carcinoma of the left neck with associated adenopathy

Fig. 2-21. Squamous cell carcinoma of the left neck. Note jugular vein thrombus *(arrow)*

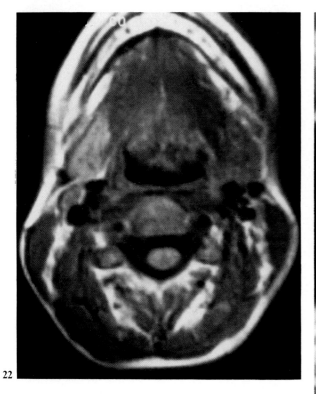

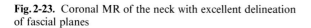

22

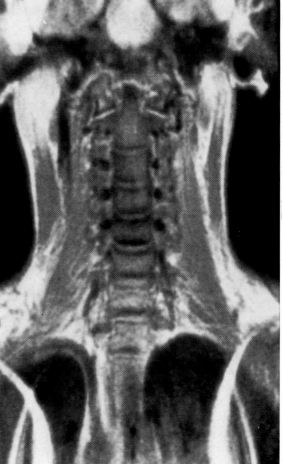

Fig. 2-22. Transverse MR of the neck. Note excellent soft tissue contrast

Fig. 2-23. Coronal MR of the neck with excellent delineation of fascial planes

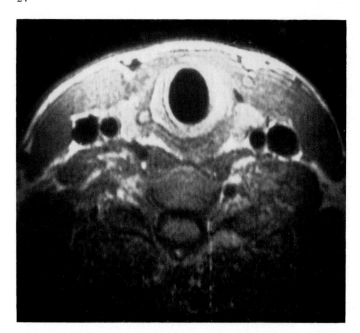

Fig. 2-24. Surface coil high resolution MR of the anterior neck showing detail of glottic region

my; however, the greater strength of MR to image abnormality adjacent to bone or bone marrow abnormality frequently makes up for this weakness.

The use of MR in imaging the nasopharynx has been reported (DILLON et al. 1984). MR was found superior to CT for displaying superficial and deep nasopharyngeal soft tissues in all normal subjects and most (10 out of 12) subjects with malignancy. In particular, MR did well in differentiating mucosa and tonsillar tissue from surrounding musculature. MR was more sensitive than CT in detecting carotid sheath, deep cervical, and retropharyngeal adenopathy. MR defined the extent of nasopharyngeal disease better than CT in the majority of patients (DILLON et al. 1984). At least one report has suggested the same may be true in the oral cavity and tongue region (UNGER 1985). In the neck region, tumors and lymph nodes have been more easily differentiated from muscle and blood vessels with MR than with CT (STARK et al. 1984). In addition, some degree of tissue characterization can be achieved, at least as far as telling cystic fluid-containing structures from solid. The early hope that MR might distinguish benign from malignant pathology has not been borne out. In the future, the advent of clinical phosphorus-31 and hydrogen spectroscopy with MR may reactivate this hope.

MR has been shown to have a major impact on the radiation therapy planning process in a substantial proportion of cases when it was employed to define extent of disease and to improve three dimensional understanding of tumor localization (SHUMAN et al. 1985). In the future, MR may become a necessary procedure prior to planning the therapy of face and neck malignancies (Fig. 2-24).

References

Archer CR, Sagel SS, Yeager VL, Martin S, Friedman WH (1981) Staging of carcinoma of the larynx. AJR 136: 571–575

Archer CR, Yeager VL (1982) Computed tomography of laryngeal cancer with histopathological correlation. Laryngoscope 92: 1173–1180

Archer CR, Yeager VL, Herbold D (1983) Improved diagnostic accuracy in the TNM staging of laryngeal cancer using a new definition of regions based on computed tomography. J Compt Assist Tomogr 7: 610–617

Archer CR, Yeager VL, Herbold DR (1984) Improved diagnostic accuracy in laryngeal cancer using a new classification based on computed tomography. Cancer 53: 44–57

Badcock PC (1983) The role of computed tomography in the planning of radiotherapy fields. Radiology 147: 241–244

Baker SR, Krause CJ (1981) Ultrasonic analysis of head and neck neoplasms - correlation with surgical findings. Ann Otol Rhinol Laryngol 90: 126–131

Bergstedt HF, Lind MG (1981) Facial bone scintigraphy. VII. Diagnosis of malignant lesions in the maxillary, ethmoidal, and palatine bones. Acta Radiol (Diagn) 22: 609–618

Bilaniuk LT, Zimmerman RA (1982) Computed tomography in evaluation of the paranasal sinuses. Radiol Clin North Amer 20: 51–66

Brant-Zawadzki MN, Minagi H, Federle MP, Rowe LD (1982) High resolution CT with image reformation in maxillofacial pathology. AJR 138: 477–483

Brenner DE, Whitley NO, Houk TL, Aisner J, Wiernik P, Whitley J (1982) Volume determinations in computed tomography. JAMA 247: 1299–1302

Dillon WP, Mills CM, Kjos B, DeGroot J, Brandt-Zawadzki MN (1984) Magnetic resonance imaging of the nasopharynx. Radiology 152: 731–738

DiSantis DJ, Balfe DM, Hayden R, Sessions D, Sagel SS (1984A) The neck after vertical hemilaryngectomy: computed tomographic study. Radiology 151: 683–687

DiSantis DJ, Balfe DM, Hayden RE, Sessions D, Lee JKT (1984B) The neck after total laryngectomy: CT study. Radiology 153: 713–717

Friedman AP, Haller JO, Goodman JD, Nagar H (1983) Sonographic evaluation of non-inflammatory neck masses in children. Radiology 147: 693–697

Friedman M, Shelton VK, Mafee M, Bellity P, Grybauskas V, Skolnik E (1984) Metastatic neck disease. Evaluation by computed tomography. Arch Otolaryngol 110: 443–447

Gamsu G, Webb WR, Shallit JB, Moss AA (1981) CT in carcinoma of the larynx and pyriform sinus: value of phonation scans. AJR 136: 577–584

Gatenby RA, Mulhern CB, Strawitz J (1983) CT guided percutaneous biopsies of head and neck masses. Radiology 146: 717–719

Goitein M (1979A) Computed tomography in planning radiation therapy. Int J Radiat Oncol Biol Phys 5: 445–447

Goitein M, Wittenbey J, Mendiondo M, Doucette J, Friedberg C, Ferrucci J, Gunderson L, Linggood R, Shipley WU, Fineberg HV (1979B) The value of CT scanning in radiation therapy planning: a prospective study. Int J Radiat Oncol Biol Phys 5: 1787–1798

Griffin BR, Shuman WP, Luk KH, Tong D (1984) LOCATE: an application of computed tomography in radiation therapy treatment planning with emphasis on tumor localization. Int J Radiat Oncol Biol Phys 10: 555–559

Harnsberger HR, Mancuso AA, Muraki AS, Perkins JL (1983) The upper aerodigestive tract and neck: CT evaluation of recurrent tumors. Radiology 149: 503–509

Hasso AN (1984) CT of tumors and tumor-like conditions of the paranasal sinuses. Radiol Clin of North Amer 22: 119–130

Hogstrom KR, Smith AR, Simon SL, Somers TW, Lone RG, Rosen II (1979) Static pion beam treatment planning of deep seated tumors using computerized tomographic scans. Int J Radiat Oncol Biol Phys 5: 875–886

Hoover LA, Hanafee WN (1983) Differential diagnosis of nasopharyngeal tumors by computed tomography scanning. Arch Otolaryngol 109: 43–47

Horowitz BL, Woodson GE, Bryan RN (1984) CT of laryngeal tumors. Radiol Clin of North Amer 22: 265–279

Hou DY, Hoch H, Johnston GS, Tsou KC, Jones AE, Miller EE, Larson SM (1984) A new tumor imaging agent - 111 In-Bleomycin complex. J Surg Oncol 27: 189–195

Jeans WD, Gilani S, Bullmore J (1982) The effect of CT scanning on staging of tumors of the paranasal sinuses. Clin Radiol 33: 173–179

Kondo M, Horiuchi M, Shiga H, Inuyama Y, Dokiya T (1982) Computed tomography of the nasal cavity and paranasal sinuses. Cancer 50: 226–231

Larsson S, Mancuso A, Hoover L, Hanafee W (1981) Differentiation of pyriform sinus cancer from supraglottic laryngeal cancer by computed tomography. Radiology 141: 427–432

Lund VJ, Howard DJ, Lloyd GAS (1983) CT evaluation of paranasal sinus tumors for cranio-facial resection. Brit J Radiol 56: 439–446

Mafee MF, Schild JA, Valvassori GE, Capek V (1983) Computed tomography of the larynx: correlation with anatomic and pathologic studies in cases of laryngeal carcinoma. Radiology 147: 123–128

Mafee MF (1984) CT of the normal larynx. Radiol Clin North Amer 22: 251–263

Mancuso AA, Rice D, Hanafee W (1979A) Computed tomography of the parotid gland during contrast sialography. Radiology 132: 211–213

Mancuso AA, Hanafee WN (1979B) A comparative evaluation of computed tomography and laryngography. Radiology 133: 131–138

Mancuso AA, Tamakawa Y, Hanafee WN (1980) CT of the fixed vocal cord. AJR 135: 529–534

Mancuso AA, Harnsberger HR, Muraki AS, Stevens MH (1983) Computed tomography of cervical and retropharyngeal lymph nodes: normal anatomy, variants of normal, and applications in staging head and neck cancer. Radiology 148: 715–723

Mukerjee MG, Mittemeyer BT (1976) Experience in staging testis tumors with bleomycin 57 cobalt. J Urol 116: 467–468

Munzenrider JE, Pilepich M, Rene-Ferrero JB, Tchakarova I, Carter BL (1977) Use of body scanner in radiotherapy treatment planning. Cancer 40: 170–179

Nieweg OE, Beekhuis H, Piers DA, Sluiter HJ, Van der wal AM, Woldring MG (1983) 57 Co-bleomycin and 67 Gacitrate in detecting and staging lung cancer. Thorax 38: 16–21

Nieweg OE, Beekhuis H, Piers DA, Sluiter HJ, Van der wal AM, Woldring MG (1984) Scintigraphy with 57 Co-bleomycin in the detection of lung cancer. Cancer 53: 1675–1681

Pertynski T, Durski K (1985) 57 Co-bleomycin scintigraphy in staging of carcinoma of the cervix. Nuklearmedizin 24: 48–51

Prasad SC, Pilepich MV, Perez CA (1980) Contribution of CT to quantitative radiation therapy planning. AJR 136: 123–128

Rabinov K, Kell T, Gordon PH (1984) CT of the salivary glands. Radiol Clin North Amer 20: 145–159

Reid MH (1984) Laryngeal carcinoma: high resolution computed tomography and thick anatomic sections. Radiology 151: 689–696

Sagel SS, AufderHeide JF, Aronberg DJ, Stanley RJ, Archer CR (1981) High resolution CT in the staging of carcinoma of the larynx. Laryngoscope 91: 292–300

Scheible W (1981) Recent advances in ultrasound: high resolution imaging of superficial structures. Head Neck Surg 4: 58–63

Scott M, Forsted DH, Rominger CJ, Brennan M (1981) Computed tomography of laryngeal neoplasms. Radiology 140: 141–144

Sewchand W, Prempree T, Patanaphan V, Whitley NO, Heidtman B, Scott RM (1982) Value of multiplanar CT images in interactive dosimetry planning of intracavitary therapy. Int J Radiat Oncol Biol Phys 8: 295–301

Shafer RB, Marlette JM, Browne GA, Elson MK (1981) The role of Tc-99m phosphate complexes and gallium-67 in the diagnosis and management of maxillofacial disease. J Nucl Med 22: 8–11

Shuman WP, Griffin BR, Haynor DR, Johnson JS, Jones

DC, Cromwell LD, Moss AA (1985) MR imaging in radiation therapy planning. Radiology 156: 143–147

Shuman WP, Griffin BR, Luk KH, Mack LA, Hanson JA (1982) CT and radiation therapy planning: the impact of LOCATE scoutview images. AJR 139: 985–989

Silver AJ, Mawad ME, Hilal SK, Sane P, Ganti SR (1983A) Computed tomography of the nasopharynx and related spaces, Part II: pathology. Radiology 147: 733–738

Silver AJ, Mawad ME, Hilal SK, Sane P, Ganti SR (1983B) Computed tomography of the nasopharynx and related spaces, Part I: anatomy. Radiology 147: 725–731

Silverman PM, Korobkin M, Thompson WM, Johnson GA, Cole TB, Fisher SR (1982) Work in progress: high-resolution thin-section computed tomography of the larynx. Radiology 145: 723–725

Silverman PM, Bossen EH, Fisher SR, Cole TB, Korobkin M, Halvorsen RA (1984) Carcinoma of the larynx and hypopharynx: computed tomographic-histopathologic correlations. Radiology 151: 697–702

Smith V, Parker DL, Stanley JH, Phillips TL, Boyd DP, Kan PT (1980) Development of a computed tomographic scanner for radiation therapy treatment planning. Radiology 136: 489–493

Som PH, Shugar JMA, Biller HF (1982) The early detection of antral malignancy in the postmaxillectomy patient. Radiology 143: 509–512

Som PM, Biller HF (1983) Computed tomography of the neck in the postoperative patient: radical neck dissection and the myocutaneous flap. Radiology 148: 157–160

Som PM, Biller HF, Lawson W, Sacher M, Lanzieri CF (1984) Parapharyngeal space masses: an updated protocol based upon 104 cases. Radiology 153: 149–156

Stark DD, Moss AA, Gamsu G, Clark OH, Gooding GAW, Webb WR (1984) Magnetic resonance imaging of the neck. Radiology 150: 455–461

Stewart JR, Hicks JA, Boone MLM, Simpson LD (1978) Int J Radiat Oncol Biol Phys 4: 313–324

St. Pierre S, Baker SR (1983) Squamous cell carcinoma of the maxillary sinus: analysis of 66 cases. Head Neck Surg 5: 508–513

Unger JM (1985) The oral cavity and tongue: magnetic resonance imaging. Radiology 155: 151–153

Van Dyk J, Battista JJ, Cunningham JR, Rider WD, Sontag MR (1980) On the impact of CT scanning on radiotherapy planning. Comput Tomogr 3: 55–65

Van Dyk J (1983) Lung dose calculations using computerized tomography: is there a need for pixel based procedures? Int J Radiat Oncol Biol Phys 9: 1035–1041

Woolfenden JM, Hall JN (1982) Cobalt-57 bleomycin uptake in experimental abscesses. Int J Radiat Oncol Biol Phys 9: 75–77

3 Overview of Treatment Options

GEORGE E. LARAMORE

CONTENTS

3.1 General Considerations

Management of the head and neck cancer patient requires the interplay of many specialists. Optimizing the technical aspects of treatment requires the interaction of the radiation oncologist, the head and neck surgeon and the medical oncologist. The choice of treatment and actually carrying it out often must take into account the socioeconomic status of the patient. Here the role of the nurse and/or social worker acting as a patient advocate is important.

Treatment decisions often reflect the personal viewpoint and previous experience of the physician having primary responsibility for the overall medical care of the patient. The initial referral from the primary care physician to the oncologic specialist is a major factor in determining the ultimate course of therapy. If the referral is to a surgeon, then it is highly likely that surgery will play a major part in the treatment plan. If the referral is to a radiation oncologist, then it is more likely that the recommendation will be definitive radiotherapy with surgery held in reserve as a salvage procedure. It is less likely that the head and neck cancer patient will be referred initially to a medical oncologist but this will become more common as more effective chemotherapeutic agents become available. It is highly desirable that all of these specialists interact in a formalized, "tumor board" setting when overall medical management plans are made. Then each specialist can present the options as he sees them and in the subsequent "discussion" appropriate references can be cited to buttress the stated opinions.

This book deals with the radiotherapeutic approach to the treatment of head and neck cancer. Every effort, however, has been made to present a balanced opinion that reflects the contributions of the surgeon and the medical oncologist to various treatment options and to cite the relevant clinical literature. The most important thing is to individualize the treatment as needed to fit the particular needs of a given patient.

3.2 Surgery

The basic principles of a surgical approach to the treatment of head and neck cancer were set forth at least 30 years ago. At that time a radical extirpation of the tumor was advocated. A fundamental concept is that clear margins must be obtained in order to cure the patient (LOOSER et al. 1978). The evidence is more direct for tumors arising within the oral cavity where positive margins are a harbinger of a local recurrence (SHAH et al. 1976) than for carcinoma of the larynx where a positive margin may not have the same significance (BAUER et al. 1975). While every effort should be made to obtain microscopically clear surgical margins, consistent with keeping to a reasonable level of attendant morbidity, all is not necessarily lost if such margins are not obtained. MANTRAVADI et al. (1983) have shown that postoperative radiotherapy given within 6 weeks of the surgical procedure is effective in preventing local tumor recurrence. When microscopic residual disease was present, the local recurrence rate was 31% and when macroscopic residual disease was present, the local recurrence rate was 50%. Presumably the recurrence rates would have been nearly 100% in the absence of adjuvant radiotherapy.

GEORGE E. LARAMORE, Ph.D., M.D., Department of Radiation Oncology, RC-08, University Hospital, University of Washington, 98195, USA

In the treatment of early stage cancer of the larynx, there has been considerable recent interest in voice conservation surgery. For tumors of the glottis, a vertical frontolateral hemilaryngectomy can be used (MOHR et al. 1983). For tumors of the supraglottis, a horizontal supraglottic procedure might be used (BOCCA et al. 1983). Although these procedures may be curative, they may leave the patient with severe dysphagia and/or aspiration problems (LOGEMAN and BYTELL 1979; DURANCEAU et al. 1976; SESSIONS et al. 1979). Technical changes in the procedures such as performing a cricopharyngeal myotomy at the time of a supraglottic laryngectomy might improve the patient's swallowing ability but the evidence on this point is not clear. Another technique of interest is the use of laser ablation surgery for early laryngeal cancer (BLAKESLEE et al. 1984). However, the 3 year disease-free survival for selected patients with T_1 lesions was only 40% using a CO_2 laser. Lasers of other wave lengths might be more effective.

Hypopharyngeal carcinomas present their own set of challenges to the surgeon. Even for small lesions, a pharyngolaryngectomy is generally required. Patients having a significant extent of tumor in the inferior direction require resection of an appreciable portion of the cervical esophagus and this may compound the difficulty of the reconstruction process. Initially a skin flap was used as pharyngeosophageal replacement tissue. Then emphasis shifted to the deltopectoral flap and more recently to the myocutaneous flap. Although the operative mortality of these procedures is low, there can be significant local complications resulting in extended hospital stays. A transposed abdominal viscus can be used to compensate for extensive resection of the esophagus (HARRISON 1979; STELL et al. 1982). The transposed viscus will often be the dose limiting structure if postoperative irradiation is needed. This is unfortunately in the range of 4500 cGy rather than the 5000–5500 cGy thought necessary to eradicate microscopic disease in a postoperative surgical field. In such cases planned preoperative radiotherapy may be a better choice.

The tongue is another organ where there is significant morbidity associated with a radical surgical excision. A limited excision of a small lesion located at the lateral aspect of the oral tongue is both effective and not associated with significant morbidity. A surgical treatment of a base of tongue lesion may, however, require sacrificing the larynx to ensure adequate surgical margins. Considerable effort has been given by the surgical community to developing reconstruction techniques to rehabilitate the

considerable cosmetic and functional deformities that result from "heroic" surgical procedures. A brief review of this work has been given by SESSIONS (1985).

Surgical resections are also possible for tumor arising in the paranasal sinuses, the external ear and middle ear. A surgical approach is routine for tumors of the maxillary sinus. The morbidity of the procedure is quite acceptable provided that enucleation of the eye is not required. Tumors of the ethmoid and sphenoid sinuses often require a "team approach" utilizing the skills of a neurosurgeon as well as the otolaryngologist. Squamous cell tumors of the external auditory canal tend to be quite aggressive and can spread to the middle ear, adjacent lymph nodes, and skull base. Postoperative radiotherapy is routinely given but its effectiveness is not certain if gross tumor has been left behind. LEWIS (1975) reported a 20% incidence of positive margins in 100 patients undergoing temporal bone resection and an additional 10% of patients were found to have grossly unresectable tumor at the time of surgery. Even with postoperative radiotherapy, the net 5-year disease free survival was only 25%. Glomus tumors of the temporal bone are also approachable if the skills of a neurosurgeon are utilized. These very vascular tumors require long operating times and the need for considerable blood infused into the patient but nevertheless have a very low mortality rate (JACKSON et al. 1982; JENKINS and FISCH 1981).

3.3 Radiotherapy

3.3.1 General Considerations

Like surgery, radiotherapy addresses the local/regional aspects of tumor control. It can be used in lieu of surgery for early-staged lesions with comparable results. For the very advanced lesions it may be the only tenable local form of treatment. For intermediate sized lesions, it is often used as an adjuvant to a surgical resection. The use of radiotherapy in these various roles for different head and neck tumors is the subject of the site-specific chapters of this book. Here we wish to give only a general overview of some of the methods of using radiotherapy and their common side effects.

The effect of a given total dose of radiation depends, of course, on how it is delivered. Unless otherwise specified, the treatment regimes discussed in this text refer to the "standard" approach utilized in the United States of treating with 180–200 cGy fractions, once-a-day, and 5 days-a-week. This schema has developed empirically to allow for the regeneration of normal tissues during the course of treatment.

The great majority of cell types respond to radiation injury through a loss of reproductive capability resulting in a clonogenic death. This is the basis of radiobiological assays of cell survival curves. There are two notable exceptions to this: lymphocytes and serous cells of salivary glands which undergo an "interphase" death that occurs shortly after irradiation. This type of death does not depend on the cell subsequently entering mitosis (KASHIMA et al. 1965). The dose-rate limiting tissue in the radiation therapeutic treatment of head and neck cancer is usually the mucosal lining of the upper aerodigestive tract. The radiation kills the stem cells in the basal layer. This has no immediate effect but several weeks later the cells in the superficial layer that are lost through normal physiological processes are not replaced and a denudation of the epithelium occurs. This denudation process causes a regenerative response in the surviving stem cells which acts to overcome the initial radiation-induced depletion. This effect varies with the individual and accounts for the variability of acute radiation reactions from patient to patient. In most patients the regenerative response can compensate for 900–1000 cGy given in 5 fractions over the course of one week and this is the origin of the "standard" fractionation schema. The skin is also rapidly a proliferating tissue and subject to the same denudation effect. However, the sparing effect of modern megavoltage radiation tends to mitigate against acute skin reactions except in the lower neck and supraclavicular fossa where "flash" results in higher superficial doses than would occur for appositional fields.

The total radiation dose is limited by the slowly proliferating tissues such as the blood vessel linings, connective tissues, bone, and central nervous system. These tissues show little change during the actual course of treatment but rather show late effects occurring several months after completion of therapy. The doses for various late complications are summarized in Table 3-1. It is important to note that the sensitivities of these "late effects" tissues are markedly dependent on the size of the radiation dose. These tissues generally have larger shoulders on their cell survival curves relative to the shoulders on the curves for the more rapidly proliferating "acute effects" tissues. Hence, larger size fractions give rise to increased late effects and in particular the "standard" European treatment schema of

Table 3-1. Total doses for specified complications in adult tissues that may be irradiated in head and neck treatment fields. Radiation doses are in cGy and should be taken only as approximate. After RUBIN et al. 1975

Organ	Injury	TD 5/5	TD 50/5
Spinal cord (10 cm)	infarction, necrosis	4500	5500
Brain (25%)	infarction, necrosis	7000	8000
Pharyngeal mucosa (50 cm²)	ulceration, mucositis	6000	7500
Skin (100 cm²)	acute and chronic dermatitis	5500	7000
Esophagus (75 cm²)	esophagitis, ulceration	6000	7500
Salivary glands	(see Figure 3-3)		
Mature cartilage or bone (10 cm²)	necrosis, fracture	6000	7500
Eye			
Retina	retinitis	5500	7000
Cornea	caratitis	5000	6000
Lens	cataracts	500	1200
Thyroid Gland	hypothyroidism	4500	15000
Pituitary Gland	hypopituitarism	4500	20000
Ear			
Middle	serous otitis	5000	7000
Vestibular	Meniere's syndrome	6000	7000
Muscle	atrophy	6000	8000
Lymphatics	sclerosis	5000	>7000
Large arteries/ veins	sclerosis	>8000	>10000

5000 cGy/4 weeks gives rise to more subcutaneous fibrosis than the more protracted United States schema. Conversely, the aim of "hyperfractionation" schemas that utilize multiple smaller fractions per day is to go to higher total doses without increasing the overall late effects.

It is not the purpose of this text to review in detail basic radiobiological concepts. However, it is thought that metastatic tumor in cervical neck nodes may contain a greater fraction of hypoxic cells than the primary lesion and this may account for the success of controlling these lesions with neutrons without there being firm evidence for improved control at the primary site (GRIFFIN et al. 1983). Similarly, hyperthermia seems to preferentially enhance the effect of radiation on low pH (i.e. hypoxic) cells and on cells in late S phase which also tend to be relatively radioresistant. High LET radiotherapy and hyperthermia are generally thought to be experimental procedures in the treatment of head and neck cancer and therefore will be discussed in chapter 16.

Radioactive implants offer both a low-dose-rate continuous form of treatment and the delivery of the irradiation to a precisely specified target volume. For properly selected cases, it is a very effective technique in boosting areas of tumor. Its place in the treatment of the various disease sites will be discussed in the following chapters.

Since cell killing by radiation is essentially an exponential function of the radiation dose, the dose required for a given level of tumor control is approximately proportional to the logarithm of the number of clonogenic cells in the tumor. Model calculations have been made by PETERS et al. (1980) and a representative result is shown in Fig. 3-1. If one knows that a given radiation dose has a certain probability of controlling a tumor of a certain size, then the dose required to yield the same tumor control for a different size tumor can be determined from the figure. This provides the rationale for the "shrinking field technique" whereby lower radiation doses are used to treat areas of subclinical disease.

The rate of tumor regression following radiotherapy depends upon factors such as the relative cellu-

lar and stromal content of the tumor, the tumor turnover rate, and the rate at which the body can remove dead cells from the tumor site. Hence, the prognostic significance of a residual mass at the end of therapy varies according to tumor histology, grade, and location. The turnover rate of most squamous cell carcinomas of the head and neck is intermediate in nature. The presence of a residual abnormality at the end of treatment is associated with a reduced tumor control probability when compared with a complete regression, but conversely, the presence of a residual clinical abnormality does not mean that the tumor will definitely recur (BARKLEY and FLETCHER 1977). They found for tumors of the oropharynx that the primary tumor recurred 30-50% of the time if there was a complete clinical response and 60-70% of the time if there was a residual abnormality at the completion of therapy. RTOG studies show that the presence of a residual abnormality 4-6 weeks after completion of therapy is a stronger correlate with ultimate tumor control than the status of the treatment site at the immediate completion of treatment (FAZEKAS et al. 1983).

In the immediate post irradiation period it is not possible to determine whether or not viable appearing tumor cells have clonogenic potential. Hence, a biopsy in this period may have little clinical information. Moreover, it may lead to significant healing problems with the development of a painful ulcer. It is best to simply closely follow a residual abnormality and not to biopsy it unless there is clinical evidence of actual tumor progression.

3.3.2 Radiation Techniques

When used as an adjuvant to surgery, radiotherapy can be used either preoperatively or postoperatively. Each sequence has its advocates. The aims of adjuvant preoperative radiotherapy are to sterilize microscopic disease outside the surgical resection field and to shrink tumor, thus making the surgery easier. It also theoretically reduces the risk of disseminating viable tumor cells at the time of surgical resection. A dose of 5000 cGy over 5-5½ weeks is usually adequate for this purpose (FLETCHER 1973, 1984).

When radiotherapy is used postoperatively, the surgical bed has a disrupted blood supply and conventional wisdom says that higher doses of radiation are needed because of the increased risk of more radioresistant hypoxic tumor cells. Generally, 5500-6000 cGy in 180-200 cGy fractions are used

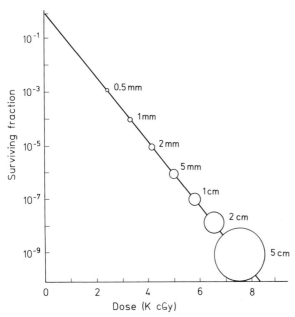

Fig. 3-1. Representative total radiation doses for fractionated radiotherapy required to achieve a certain level of cell killing for different size tumors. The "D_0" of the curve was taken to be 350 cGy and the daily dose increment taken to be 200 cGy. It was assumed that the cellular radiosensitivity and the clonogenic fraction of cells is independent of tumor size. After PETERS et al. (1980)

for microscopic disease in this setting. Postoperative radiotherapy has the advantage of being given only to those patients at significant risk for tumor recurrence as determined by a thorough review of pathological data and also allows for the planned delivery of higher radiation doses to areas of postsurgical residual disease. It has the further advantage of not delaying the surgical procedure which, for operable patients, is probably the most important treatment modality.

In an attempt to compare preoperative and postoperative radiotherapy in a controlled trial, the Radiation Therapy Oncology Group (RTOG) performed a study that evaluated 277 patients with lesions of the oral cavity, oropharynx, supraglottic larynx, and hypopharynx (KRAMER 1985; KRAMER et al. 1987). Preoperatively treated patients received 5000 cGy followed by surgery in approximately 4-6 weeks while the postoperatively treated group received 6000 cGy starting approximately 2-4 weeks after completion of surgery. The study found that more of the postoperative patients completed therapy within protocol guidelines (74% vs. 56%). The 4-year competing risk local/regional control was 65% for the postoperative group and 48% for the preoperative group (statistically significant at $p=0.04$). When one considers only the subgroup of 194 patients who completed the planned treatment per protocol guidelines, the local/regional control rates were 74% for the postoperative group compared to 56% for the preoperative group. The incidence of significant complications due to the *combined* treatment was 32% for the preoperatively treated group and 34% for the postoperatively treated group. There was also a difference in survival at 4 years being 33% on the preoperative arm and 38% on the postoperative arm. The statistical power of this difference was suggestive (but not definitive) at $p=0.10$. Considering again the subgroup of patients completing treatment as planned, the survival rates were 45% for the postoperative group compared to 40% for the preoperative group. As might be expected in this patient population, deaths from intercurrent disease including second primary tumors tended to obscure the effects of any local/regional control differences between the two treatment arms.

In general, there is little, if any, role for "debulking surgery" to be followed by postoperative radiotherapy. If gross tumor is left behind, then high dose definitive radiotherapy is required - exactly as needed in the primary treatment of the tumor. This generally means giving 6500-7500 cGy in 6½ to 8 weeks. Specific doses and fields will be discussed in subsequent chapters as will be the treatment of the clinically positive and negative necks.

A classic problem in the radiotherapeutic treatment of head and neck tumors relates to the junctioning between fields used to treat the primary tumor site and the upper neck and the field(s) used to treat the lower neck and the supraclavicular fossae. The former are usually parallel-opposed, right and left lateral fields while the latter is generally an anterior field. It is important to guard against the inadvertent overlap of the fields - particularly over the spinal cord. Techniques that avoid this are to use field blocks in the junction region as shown in Fig. 3-2. Figure 3-2a shows the use of a block at the posterior-inferior portion of the upper neck fields and Fig. 3-2b shows the use of a block at the upper-central portion of the anterior supraclavicular field. The former arrangement is advantageous when the primary tumor is located in the lower neck such as in the larynx or hypopharynx while the latter is advantageous when the primary tumor is located in the nasopharynx or oral cavity. This also has the advantage of protecting the larynx from the radiation and thereby reducing the risk of a transient laryngeal edema. Needless to say, one should always choose the blocking arrangement that involves shielding the region at least risk for tumor presence. It is recommended that the junction between the upper and lower neck fields be moved once or twice during the course of radiotherapy. However, there will occasionally be situations where either of the above blocking techniques would shield either known tumor or areas felt to be at high risk for postsurgical residual disease. One way around this problem is to use a half-beam block at the central axis for both fields and hence match the fields along a "zero-divergence" plane (DATTA et al. 1979). Another way is to use a calculated gap between the fields which usually works out to be approximately 0.5 cm (GILLIN and KLINE 1980). Again, as an added safety factor, it is recommended that at least 2 junction moves be done when either of these later two matching techniques is used.

3.3.3 Radiation Side-Effects

Adequate treatment of many head and neck cancers requires irradiating a considerable portion of the salivary glands. MOSSMAN et al. (1981) measured changes in parotid salivary function with radiotherapy and found a 50% decrease in saliva production and a 60% decrease in protein secretion by the gland after the first week of therapy. MOSSMAN

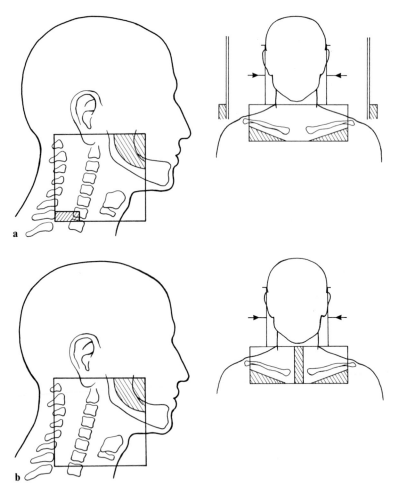

Fig. 3-2a, b. Blocking techniques to shield the spinal cord at the junction between the upper and lower head and neck fields. **a** shows the use of a small block at the posterior-inferior portion of the upper neck fields. **b** shows the use of a small block at the central-superior portion of the lower neck and supraclavicular field. The junction between the fields should also be moved once or twice during the course of radiotherapy

(1983) subsequently determined a clinical dose-response curve for the salivary glands. The loss of saliva was significant after 1000 cGy and the associated loss of taste was significant after 4000–4500 cGy when given in a conventional fractionation pattern. This work is reproduced in Fig. 3-3. The salivary dysfunction persists for years following radiotherapy and is associated with taste loss as indicated in Fig. 3-3. The most several affected taste qualities were "salt" and "bitter" (MOSSMAN et al. 1979) in contrast to chemotherapy which tends to affect mostly the "sour" and "sweet" taste sensations. The combined effects of chronic xerostomia and altered taste sensation often leads to significant weight loss

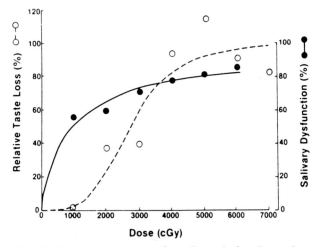

Fig. 3-3. Dose-response curves for salivary dysfunction and taste loss in patients receiving radiotherapy for head and neck malignancies using a conventional dose-fractionation scheme. Salivary dysfunction refers to the percentage decrease in flow rate compared to the pretreatment values and is shown as the closed circles and solid line. The open circles and dashed line show the dose response curve for taste loss. The abscissa shows the cumulative radiation dose. After MOSSMAN (1983)

during and after radiotherapy unless vigorous dietary counselling is undertaken (CHENCHARICK and MOSSMAN 1983). Because of the taste changes, there is a tendency for the patient to shift his caloric intake pattern to a higher percentage of carbohydrates.

The decrease in amount of saliva and changes in its chemical constituency causes a shift in the microflora inhabiting the oral cavity. This can cause a dramatic increase in the number of caries in the patient. Fortunately, an aggressive program of dental prophylaxis can mitigate this problem and it is highly recommended that each patient be seen by an experienced dentist prior to the onset of treatment. Fluoride gel treatments are effective in reducing the subsequent incidence of caries. The incidence of osteoradionecrosis of the mandible can be considerably reduced if the necessary repairs and extractions are done at this time rather than waiting until problems develop in a heavily irradiated field (BEDWINEK et al. 1976; MURRAY et al. 1980). An extensive review of the pathogenesis of osteoradionecrosis has been written by MARX and JOHNSON (1987). They also evaluated a data base of 536 patients with osteoradionecrosis and showed that its incidence is considerably reduced if one waits at least 2–3 weeks between prophylactic dental extractions and the initiation of radiotherapy. Their plot showing the incidence of this event as a function of the time delay is reproduced in Fig. 3-4.

Osteoradionecrosis can occur in spite of the above precautions. In some cases areas of devitalized bone will sequestrate and lesions will heal. Hyperbaric oxygen treatments are thought by some to expedite this by improving the oxygen delivery to regions of compromised vascularity (HART and MAINOUS 1976; MARX and JOHNSON 1987). Antibiotics are also sometimes used to aid the healing process. The incidence of osteoradionecrosis varies between 5–20% depending on the particular reported series. It depends upon the aggressiveness of the therapy, whether or not an implant was used in the treatment, the dental care given, and the length of patient followup. The incidence is considerably higher in dentulous patients than in edentulous ones (MORRISH et al. 1981). Osteoradionecrosis developed in 85% of dentulous patients and 50% of the edentulous patients who received more than 7500 cGy to the mandible and did not occur in patients who received less than 6500 cGy to the mandible (MORRISH et al. 1981). These workers felt there was increased risk associated with dental extractions after radiotherapy.

Soft tissue necrosis is another difficult manage-

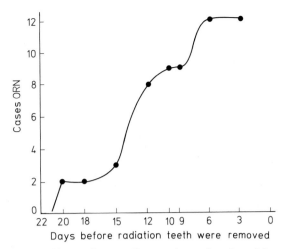

Fig. 3-4. Incidence of osteoradionecrosis as a function of the time between wounding (extractions, etc.) and the onset of radiotherapy. After MARX and JOHNSON (1987)

ment problem. Its incidence is related to total dose, overall time of treatment, and volume of tissue treated. The risk of it occurring is greater with interstitial implants because of the higher doses given to the central region. In a study of 278 patients BEUMER et al. (1972) noted a significant soft tissue necrosis in 18 cases (6.5%). Eleven of these patients had received implants or intraoral cones as part of their treatment. Fifteen cases healed with conservative medical management but 3 cases required a surgical intervention. The majority of cases occurred within one year of completing therapy. It is important to closely follow such cases since a local tumor recurrence often mimics this particular complication.

Patients receiving radiotherapy may experience a clinically significant candidiasis during treatment. This may be confused with a radiation mucositis. It usually responds well to oral (topical) antifungal preparations.

A few months following radiation treatments many patients develop a lymphedema in the upper neck and submental regions. This change often causes considerable consternation to the patient who frequently associates it with tumor recurrence. With passage of more time new lymphatic channels develop and the lymphedema resolves to be replaced by a firm to "woody" fibrosis. Proper design of radiation portals and the use of dose-shaping compensators can reduce this problem to some extent.

The specter of a "radiation-induced" second malignancy is often raised when various treatment options are discussed. There is no doubt that there is an appreciable incidence of second primary cancers in head and neck cancer patients but this likely relates more to their socioeconomic habits than the treatment given for their "first" tumor. In a classic paper SEYDEL (1975) reviewed the records of 1464 patients treated with definitve radiotherapy for carcinomas of the oral cavity and oropharynx. There were 611 5-year survivors and among these, were only 9 cases of second malignant tumors in the radiated tissues. This incidence was only 1.5%. Eight cancers were squamous cell in histology and one was a fibrosarcoma. The latency period ranges from 2–32 years with 7 of the lesions not occurring until more than 5 years from completion of treatment. PARKER and ENSTROM (1988) evaluated the records of 2853 patients treated at UCLA for first primary cancers of the head and neck region. With followup data ranging between 5–30 years, the incidence of head and neck second primaries was 2.2% for patients treated by surgery alone vs 2.9% for patients treated by either radiation alone or surgery with adjuvant radiotherapy. The data were evaluated for risk factors such as age, sex, and tumor site and it was concluded that there was no increased risk of a second malignancy associated with radiotherapy compared to surgery.

3.4 Chemotherapy

In general, local/regional tumor persistence or recurrence is the primary failure mode in head and neck cancer. STRONG (1983) evaluated the failure pattern in 798 patients treated primarily with surgery at the Memorial Sloan-Kettering Cancer Center and found that distant metastasis occurred in only 11.7% of the patients. The most common site developing distant metastases was the nasopharynx (39.5%) followed by the tonsil (18.6%), base of tongue (16%) and pharynx (15.9%). The Radiation Therapy Oncology Group (RTOG) conducted a trial that compared "split course" radiotherapy with "conventional fractionation" radiotherapy for patients with tumors arising in the nasopharynx, tonsillar fossa, or base of tongue. A total of 387 evaluable patients were entered. There were no essential differences between the treatment arms in regard to local/regional control or survival but the pattern of failure was the same as noted by STRONG (1983). First failure was local/regional alone in 41% of patients with nasopharyngeal primaries, 60% of patients with tonsillar primaries, and 63% of patients with base of tongue primaries. Distant metastases

were a component of first failure in 21% of patients with nasopharyngeal primaries, 11% of patients with tonsillar primaries, and 10% of patients with base of tongue primaries. While local/regional failure is the primary cause of cancer related death for patients with squamous cell tumors of the head and neck, the incidence of clinically apparent distant metastases would likely increase if better local/regional tumor control could be achieved. One autopsy study showed an incidence of distant metastases of 40–51% for various head and neck tumors (DENNINGTON et al. 1980). However, current interest is primarily to use chemotherapy in a *neoadjuvant* role in order to improve local/regional control rather than in the traditional *adjuvant* role in order to prevent the development of distant metastases. The issue becomes more complicated when radiotherapy is involved since some chemotherapeutic agents have radiosensitizing properties in regard to the "normal" tissues in the treatment fields.

Current interest in neoadjuvant trials centers on multi-agent drug regimes. Many pilot studies show drug efficacy in terms of tumor response but no conclusive benefit in either improved local/regional control or survival. Fortunately, there is renewed interest in large scale cooperative studies which will address the latter issues in meaningful ways. Poor patient compliance with the planned therapeutic programs is a major problem in carrying out such studies.

When several modalities are used in a planned treatment approach, a major question is how to best sequence them. Induction chemotherapy allows one to determine tumor response to the particular agents used but this may not be the optimal "first treatment". Using a cis-platinum/5-FU regimen, the RTOG performed a pilot study comparing the sequence chemotherapy/surgery/radiotherapy vs. surgery/chemotherapy/radiotherapy. There was no overall difference in local/regional control or survival but there was a problem with patients who achieved a clinical complete tumor response with induction chemotherapy refusing the planned surgery. All of these patients subsequently relapsed. Also, it is not clear whether tumor shrinkage with chemotherapy means that a less extensive surgical resection can be safely performed.

When combined with radiotherapy, chemotherapy agents can be given first in a neoadjuvant mode or concomitantly with radiotherapy in a sensitization mode. It is not clear that the latter preferentially sensitizes the tumor and thereby improves the therapeutic index. This is the subject of certain ongoing clinical trials.

Chemotherapeutic agents can be given either orally, intravenous push, intravenous infusion, or intra-arterially. The mode of delivery chosen depends on the agents used and the aims of clinician. Oral agents may be most suitable for maintenance where the aim is to reduce the incidence of distant metastases with a "low-morbidity" chemotherapeutic regimen. Intravenous delivery is suitable either for induction or maintenance but frequently requires hospitalizing the patient. A slow infusion of a radiosensitizing agent might be most effective during brachytherapy. Intra-arterial delivery of a drug is a way of dramatically increasing its concentration at the tumor site without causing extremely high (and toxic) levels throughout the body.

The current status of chemotherapy for squamous cell tumors of the head and neck will be reviewed by MORTIMER and GRIFFIN in a subsequent chapter of this book. However, its use should be regarded as experimental at the present time and restricted to formal protocol settings.

References

Barkely Jr HT, Fletcher GH (1977) The significance of residual disease after external irradiation of squamous cell carcinoma of the oropharynx. Radiology 124: 493–495

Bauer WC, Lesinski SG, Ogura J (1975) The significance of positive margins in hemi-laryngectomy specimens. Laryngoscope 85: 1–13

Bedwinek JM, Shukovsky LJ, Fletcher GH, Daley TE (1976) Osteonecrosis in patients treated with definitive radiotherapy for squamous cell carcinomas of the oral cavity and naso- and oropharynx. Radiology 119: 665–667

Beumer III J, Silverman Jr S, Benak SB (1972) Hard and soft tissue necrosis following radiotherapy for oral cancer. J Prosthet Dent 27: 640–644

Blakeslee D, Vaughan CW, Shapshay SM, Simpson GT, Strong MS (1984) Excisional biopsy in the selective management of T_1 glottic cancer: a three year followup study. Larnygoscope 94: 488–494

Bocca E, Pignatabo O, Oldini C (1983) Supraglottic laryngectomy: 30 years experience. Ann Otol Rhinol Laryngol 92: 14–18

Chencharick JO, Mossman KL (1983) Nutritional consequences of the radiotherapy of head and neck cancer. Cancer 51: 811–815

Datta R, Mira JG, Pomeroy TC, Datta S (1979) Dosimetry study of split beam technique using megavoltage beams and its clinical implications I.^{60} Co beam, head and neck tumors. Int J Radiat Oncol Biol Phys 5: 565–571

Dennington ML, Carter DR, Meyers AD (1980) Distant metastases in head and neck carcinoma. Laryngoscope 90: 196–201

Duranceau A, Jamieson G, Hurwitz AL, Jones RS, Postlethwait RW (1976) Alteration in esophageal motility after laryngectomy. Am J Surg 131: 34–35

Fazekas JT, Sommer C, Kramer S (1983) Tumor regression and other prognosticators in advanced head and neck cancers: a sequel to the RTOG methotrexate study. Int J Radiat Oncol Biol Phys 9: 957–964

Fletcher GH (1973) Clinical dose-response curves of human malignant epithelial tumors. Br J Radiol 46: 1–12

Fletcher GH (1984) Lucy Wortham James Lecture: Subclinical disease. Cancer 53: 1274–1284

Gillin MT, Kline RW (1980) Field separation between lateral and anterior fields on a 6 MV linear accelator. Int J Radiat Oncol Biol Phys 6: 233–237

Griffin TW, Davis R, Laramore GE, Hussey DH, Hendrickson FR, Rodriguez-Antunez A (1983) Fast neutron irradiation of metastatic cervical adenopathy: the results of a randomized RTOG study. Int J Radiat Oncol Biol Phys 9: 1267–1270

Harrison DFN (1979) Surgical management of hypopharyngeal carcinoma. Arch Otolaryngol 105: 149–152

Hart GM, Mainous EG (1976) The treatment of radiation necrosis with hyperbaric oxygen (OHP). Cancer 37: 2580–2585

Jackson CG, Glasscock ME, Harris PF (1982) Glomus tumors. Arch Otolaryngol 108: 401–406

Jenkins HA, Fisch U (1981). Glomus tumors of the temporal bone. Arch Otolaryngol 107: 209–214

Kashima HK, Kirkham WR, Andrews JR (1965) Postirradiation sialadentis: a study of the clinical features, histopathologic changes and serum enzyme variations following irradiation of human salivary glands. Am J Roentgenol 94: 271–291

Kramer S (1985) Surgery and radiation therapy in the management of locally advanced head and neck squamous cell carcinoma. In: Chretein PB, Johns ME, Shedd DP, Strong EW, Ward PH (eds) Head and Neck Cancer, Vol 1: BC Decker, Philadelphia pp 48–54

Kramer S, Gleber RD, Snow JB, Marcial VA, Lowry LD, Davis LW, Chandler R (1978) Combined radiation therapy and surgery in the management of advanced head and neck cancer: final report of the study 73-03 of the Radiation Therapy Oncology Group. Head Neck Surg 10: 19–30

Lewis JS (1975) Temporal bone resection: review of 100 cases. Arch Otolaryngol 101: 23–25

Logeman JA, Bytell DE (1979) Swallowing disorders in three types of head and neck surgical patients. Cancer 44: 1095–1105

Looser KG, Shah JP, Strong EW (1978) The significance of "positive" margins in surgically resected epidermoid carcinomas. Head Neck Surg 1: 107–111

Mantravadi RUP, Haas RE, Skolnick EM (1983) Postoperative radiotherapy for persistent tumor at the surgical margin in head and neck cancer. Laryngoscope 93: 1337–1340

Marx RE, Johnson RP (1987) Studies in the radiobiology of osteoradionecrosis and their clinical significance. Oral Surg Oral Med Oral Pathol 64: 379–390

Mohr RM, Quenelle DJ, Shumrick DA (1983) Verticofrontolateral laryngectomy. Arch Otolaryngol 109: 384–395

Morrish RB, Chan E, Silverman S, Meyer J, Fu KK, Greenspan D (1981) Osteonecrosis in patients irradiated for head and neck carcinoma. Cancer 47: 1980–1983

Mossman KL (1983) Quantitative radiation dose-response relationships for normal tissues in man II: response of the salivary glands during radiotherapy. Radiat Res 95: 392–398

Mossman KL, Choncherick JD, Scheer AC, Walker WP, Ornitz RD, Rogers CC, Hendin RI (1979) Radiation-induced changes in gustatory function – comparison of effects of neutron and photon irrradiation. Int J Radiat Oncol Biol Phys 5: 521–528

Mossman KL, Shatzman AR, Chencharick JD (1981) Effects of radiotherapy on human parotid saliva. Radiat Res 88: 403-412

Murray CG, Herson J, Daly TE, Zimmerman SO (1980) Radiation necrosis of the mandible: a 10-year study. Part I. factors influencing the onset of necrosis. Int J Radiat Oncol Biol Phys 6: 543-553

Parker RG, Enstrom JE (1988) Second primary cancers following initial treatment of patients with head and neck cancers. Int J Radiat Oncol Biol Phys 14: 561-564

Peters LJ, Withers HR, Fletcher GH (1980) Alternatives to radical neck dissection: the MD Anderson approach. Aust Radiol 24: 303-306

Rubin P, Cooper R, Phillips TL (1975) Radiation biology and Radiation Pathology Syllabus (SDT RT 1: Radiation Oncology). American College of Radiology, Chicago

Shah JP, Cendon RA, Farr HW (1976) Carcinoma of the oral cavity - factors affecting treatment failure at the primary site and neck. Am J Surg 132: 504-507

Sessions DG (1985) Composite resection and reconstruction with skin grafts for oral cavity and oropharyngeal cancer. In: Chretein PB, Johns ME, Shedd DP, Strong EW, Ward PH (eds.) Head and Neck Cancer Volume 1. BC Decker, Philadelphia pp 187-193

Sessions DG, Zill R, Schwartz SL (1979) Deglutition after conservation surgery of the larynx and hypopharynx. Otolaryngol Head Neck Surg 87: 779-796

Seydel HG (1975) The risk of tumor induction in man following medical irradiation for malignant neoplasm. Cancer 35: 1641-1645

Stell PM, Ramadan MF, George WD (1982) Postcricoid carcinoma: the place of visceral transposition. Clin Oncol 8: 17-20

Strong FW (1983) Sites of treatment failure in head and neck cancer. Cancer Treat Symposia 2: 5-20

4 Treatment of Nodes in the Clinically N_0 Neck

GEORGE E. LARAMORE

CONTENTS

4.1 General Overview

There are an estimated 300 lymph nodes located within the neck (HELLSTROM and HELLSTROM 1970) and squamous cell primaries have a definite propensity to spread to these areas. When these nodes are clinically positive and the primary planned treatment of the primary lesion is surgical, then there is little argument that a neck dissection of the involved side(s) is in order. Postoperative radiotherapy is then generally warranted because of the risk of occult disease in the contralateral neck and/or the retropharyngeal nodal group. The incidence of positive neck nodes at the time of presentation and their treatment will be discussed in a general overview chapter and the following site-specific chapters. Here we wish to focus on the general question of how to manage the patient with a documented head and neck primary and no clinical evidence of metastatic tumor in the cervical and supraclavicular lymph nodes.

The first question to address relates to the frequency of occult lymph node metastasis for tumors in various head and neck sites. This data can be obtained from reported series of N_0 patients treated with only surgical resection of the primary who subsequently fail in the neck, from series of patients with N_0 necks found to have occult disease after a "prophylactic" neck dissection and from patients whose primary alone was treated with radiotherapy without the fields covering the nodal site of failure. A representative sampling of this data is summarized in Table 4-1.

GEORGE E. LARAMORE, Ph.D., M.D., Department of Radiation Oncology, RC-08, University Hospital, University of Washington, Seattle, WA 98185, USA

Although the number in some cases are small – for example, most patients with nasopharyngeal carcinoma have their necks irradiated and HO's data is based upon 32 patients with T_1 primaries who did not – some interesting trends are apparent. For example, there is not much difference in the risk of

Table 4-1. Incidence of occult positive cervical nodes of a function of primary tumor site. Data is for both ipsilateral and contralateral necks

Site	Incidence (%)
Nasal cavity	
BOSCH et al. (1976)	5
Ethmoid sinus	
ROBIN and POWELL (1980)	13
Maxillary sinus	
PEZNER et al.	17
LEE and OGURA (1981)	16
Lip	
MODLIN (1950)	10
STRONG (1983)	8
Oral tongue	
MENDELSON et al. (1976)	20
STRONG (1983)	28
Floor of mouth	
HARROLD (1971)	33
STRONG (1983)	17
Tonsil	
STRONG (1983)	20
Base of tongue	
WHICKER et al. (1972)	48
STRONG (1983)	27
Nasopharynx[a]	
HO (1978)	19
Piriform sinus	
SHAH et al. (1976)	33
BILLER and LUCENTE (1977)	41
Supraglottic larynx	
BILLER and LUCENTE (1977)	25
STRONG (1983)	30
Glottic Larynx	
T_1: MITTAL et al. (1983)	2
LINDBERG (1983)	15

[a] T_1 only

Table 4-2. Incidence of clinically positive and occult neck nodal disease as a function of T-stage for squamous cell carcinoma arising in the floor of mouth. (After HARROLD 1971)

T-Stage		N_+ at Presentation (%)	N_0 Converting to N_+[a] (%)	Total (%)
T_1	(128)	19	35	54
T_2	(416)	32	23	55
T_3, T_4	(341)	40	6	46

[a] Refers to percentage of overall number of patients presenting with a given T-stage

developing disease in the untreated N_0 neck between sites such as nasopharynx and piriform sinus which have a high incidence of clinically positive nodes at the time of presentation (60–85%) and the oral tongue which has a much lower incidence of positive nodes at the time of presentation (13–36%). This is perhaps reflective of the tendency of lesions in the former regions to metastasize earlier rather than later and so both the primary and the nodal disease becomes clinically apparent at about the same time. The incidence of occult disease from maxillary sinus tumors is surprisingly high for a site where traditionally N_0 necks are not treated prophylactically. It is probably reasonable to treat the necks prophylactically when the risk of subsequent failure (untreated) is greater than about 15%.

The incidence of clinically apparent and occult disease in the cervical neck nodes is also a function of the stage of the primary tumor. Table 4-2 shows the incidence of nodal disease for floor-of-the-mouth primaries as a function of T-stage. The main point to note from this table is that although the percentage of N_+ nodes at presentation dramatically increases with increasing T-stage, the overall percentage of those patients who initially are N_0 and then convert to N_+ *decreases* with increasing T-stage. Hence, the overall incidence of clinically positive plus occult metastatic disease is relatively constant. This argues that it is more important to treat the clinically negative neck for a smaller primary than a larger one – a statement that at first appears paradoxical. However, it is in large part due to the increased survival of low T-stage N_0 patients and with increased survival comes increased risk of subsequent neck failure. Moreover, it calls into question the wisdom of treating early stage lesions with a radioactive implant alone.

4.2 Surgical Neck Dissection

Credit for the radical neck dissection is given to Crile (1906) who published a series on 132 patients. He stated that the key to the procedure was the excision of the internal jugular vein and its associated fibrous, adipose, and lymphatic tissue. The spinal accessory nerve was sacrificed in this procedure. This procedure was carried out without change for approximately 60 years. Then surgeons finally began to question whether it would not be possible in some instances to spare structures such as the spinal accessory nerve, the sternocleidomastoid muscle, and the internal jugular vein in order to have better function of the neck and shoulder. This has led to three somewhat different surgical procedures under the appelation "modified neck dissection".

The first is simply the standard neck dissection with the sparing of the spinal accessory nerve. The

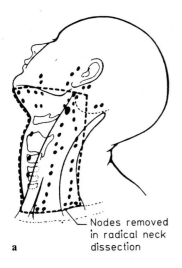

a   Nodes removed in radical neck dissection

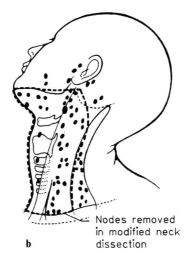

b   Nodes removed in modified neck dissection

Fig. 4-1a, b. The dotted outlines show the lymph nodes in the neck that are removed in a radical neck dissection (**a**) and a modified neck dissection (**b**). The lymph nodes at risk for metastatic cancer are also shown on the outlines. This figure is meant to be only illustrative as a given procedure may take or leave the nodes in a somewhat different manner

second modifies the classic "en bloc" approach by also preserving the sternocleidomastoid muscle. The third version also spares the internal jugular vein. The basic rationale for the conservative neck dissection is well described by BOCCA (1975) and a detailed description of the three basic variants of the procedure is given by LINGEMAN (1985).

An illustration of nodes in the neck removed in the "classical" radical neck dissection and in the modified neck dissection is shown in Fig. (4-1). The modified procedure tends to leave the nodes beneath the sternocleidomastoid muscle. Neither the modified nor the radical version of the neck dissection is a guarantee against a subsequent recurrence in the neck. LINGEMAN (1985) reports on 115 cases with N_0 necks treated with radical neck dissections with a 14% incidence of subsequent neck failures. He also discussed 235 cases with N_0 necks treated with a modified neck dissection with an 11% recurrence rate in the neck. However, many cases had tumor present at the primary site at the time of recurrence and so the failures may represent a subsequent reseeding of tumor into the regional lymphatics. He also does not mention whether or not microscopic nodal disease was initially present in the subgroup of patients that ultimately recurred.

Both the radical and modified neck dissections can cause appreciable patient morbidity. The most common consequences of a radical neck dissection include a dropping shoulder with limitation of arm abduction, disfigurement of the neck contour, chronic swelling and discoloration of the lower half of the face, painful neuromas, anesthesia, paresthesia, and dysphagia (BOCCA 1975). Patient with midline primary tumors would have both sides of the neck at equal risk for metastatic disease. A bilateral radical neck dissection gives rise to a much more severe cosmetic and functional deformity and in general should be avoided for the N_0 neck. If positive nodes are found in the surgical specimen then postoperative radiotherapy, while required to maximize tumor control, carries increased morbidity in the face of such an extensive procedure.

A modified neck dissection with sparing of the spinal accessary nerve may cause a transient problem with pain and limitation of shoulder girdle movement but this generally resolves. However, it does not remove the nodes along the spinal accessory chain. Early studies which evaluated surgically the spinal accessory nodal chain lying within the posterior triangle showed a very infrequent tumor involvement for the N_0 neck (McGAVRAN et al. 1961; SKOLNIK et al. 1967). However, a prospective study showed a higher frequency of nodal involvement in the superior portion of the spinal accessory chain where the XIth nerve is more intimately related to the internal jugular vein (SCHULLER et al. 1978). Hence, while a less morbid procedure, the modified neck dissection still might need to be followed by postoperative radiotherapy in order to adequately treat all of the nodal groups at risk. Thus, the procedure in itself is not a priori advantageous to the patient unless it is used as part of the approach to a surgical treatment of the primary lesion.

4.3 Radiation Therapy Treatment

A clinically N_0 neck may be assumed to be at risk for microscopic disease and sterilization of this requires a lower total dose of radiation than required to eradicate macroscopic concentrations of tumor cells. In his recent Lucy Wortham James Lecture, FLETCHER (1984) reviewed a tremendous amount of clinical data relating to the radiotherapeutic management of subclinical disease. He noted that modest doses of irradiation in the range of 4500–5000 cGy given in conventional fractionation patterns of 180–200 cGy per fraction for 5 days a week are sufficient to eradicate subclinical disease in cervical neck nodes in 90% of cases. Furthermore, doses of 3000–4000 cGy will eradicate such disease in 60–70% of cases. The effectiveness of this type of treatment is confirmed in additional clinical data summarized by COX (1985) which is reproduced in Table 4-3. While it is certainly not to be implied that all of the patients would have developed neck disease if not irradiated, comparison with Table 4-1 shows a probable benefit to radiotherapy in this setting.

LEBORGNE et al. (1987) reviewed the neck recurrence patterns of 50 patients with stages T_{1-3} N_0 squamous cell carcinoma of the oral tongue who had controlled primary disease. Twenty-five pa-

Table 4-3. Frequency of the development of clinically apparent lymph node metastases after radiotherapeutic treatment of the N_0 neck. (After COX 1985)

Primary site	Number of patients	Number cervical nodal metastases
Oral tongue, floor of mouth	32	1
Tonsil, base of tongue	29	0
Supraglottic larynx, hypopharynx	84	3
Total	145	4 (3%)

tients treated prior to 1974 had no elective neck treatment and 25 patients treated after 1974 had radiotherapy to all or a portion of the neck nodes at risk for microscopic metastatic disease. A dose of 4000–5000 cGy was delivered in 4–5 weeks. In the group with untreated necks, 40% of patients developed lymph node metastases while in the treated group, the rate of lymph node metastases was only 20%. However, it is important to note that in the later subgroup, there was only a 4% recurrence rate within the treated portion of the neck.

The treatment of subclinical disease in this manner causes very minimal patient morbidity. There can be a transient pharyngitis that generally resolves about 2 weeks after completion of therapy. There is little xerostomia unless the parotid glands are included in the fields for other clinical reasons. Late effects include skin dryness and desquamation and epilation of the beard.

Higher radiation doses are thought to be required (as discussed in Chapter 3) to treat subclinical disease in a previously operated field. Generally, 6000 cGy (conventional fractionation scheme) is used which can cause some increase in morbidity. Delays in initiating radiotherapy after surgery allow for the progression of microscopic residual disease to macroscopic focii and this can reduce the ultimate control rate. VIKRAM et al. (1980) found higher rates of local/regional tumor recurrence if initiation of postoperative radiotherapy was delayed more than 6 weeks following surgery.

The radiation fields used must cover the nodal groups shown in Fig. (4-1). Normally, such treatment is given in connection with treatment of the primary tumor and so details of the fields will be left to the following chapters. However, there may be some cases where a patient will be referred for treatment after the surgical resection of the primary lesion.

Prophylactic neck irradiation to the N_0 neck should be given if the risk factors as summarized in Table 4-1 and other literature so warrant. Normally, this will be the case for lesions of the nasopharynx, oral cavity, oropharynx, hypopharynx and supraglottic larynx. It is generally not the case for lesions of the nasal cavity, lip, ethmoid sinuses, and early lesions. Radiotherapy to the N_0 neck for lesions of the maxillary sinuses is not traditionally given but this should perhaps be reconsidered (PEZNER et al. 1979).

References

Biller HF, Lucente FE (1977) Conservation surgery of the head and neck. Semin Oncol 4: 365–373

Bocca E (1975) Conservative neck dissection. Laryngoscope 85: 1511–1515

Bosch A, Vallecillo L, Frias Z (1976) Cancer of the nasal cavity. Cancer 37: 1458–1463

Cox JD (1985) Management of clinically occult (N_0) cervical lymph node metastases by radiation therapy. In: Head and Neck Cancer, Vol 1 (eds) Chretein PB, Johns ME, Shedd DP, Strong EW, Ward PH (Decker, Philadelphia, 1985) pp 151–155

Crile SrG (1906) Excision of cancer of the head and neck with special reference to the plan of dissection based on 132 operations. JAMA 47: 1780–1786

Fletcher GH (1984) Lucy Wortham James. Lecture: subclinical disease. Cancer 53: 1274–1284

Harrold Jr CC (1971) Management of cancer of the floor of mouth. Am J Surg 122: 487–493

Hellstrom KE, Hellstrom I (1970) Immunologic defenses against cancer. Hosp Practice 5: 45–61

Ho JHC (1978) An epidemiologic and clinical study of nasopharyngeal carcinoma. Int J Radiat Oncol Biol Phys 7: 447–453

Leborgne F, Leborgne JH, Barlocci LA, Ortega B (1987) Elective neck irradiation in the treatment of cancer of the oral tongue. Int J Radiat Oncol Biol Phys 13: 1149–1153

Lee F, Ogura JH (1981) Maxillary sinus carcinoma. Laryngoscope 91: 133–139

Lindberg RD (1983) Sites of first failure in head and neck cancer. Cancer Treat Symp 2: 21–31

Lingeman RE (1985) Surgical Management of the N_0 neck. In: Head and Neck Cancer, Vol 1 (eds) Chretein PB, Johns ME, Shedd DP, Strong EW, Ward PH (Decker, Philadelphia, 1985) pp 145–148

McGavran MH, Bauer WC, Ogura JH (1961) The incidence of cervical lymph node metastases from epidermoid carcinoma of the larynx and their relationship to certain characteristics of the primary tumor. Cancer 14: 55–66

Mendelson BC, Woods JE, Beahrs OH (1976) Neck dissection in the treatment of carcinoma of the anterior two-thirds of the tongue. Surg Gynecol Obstet 143: 75–80

Mittal B, Rao DV, Marks JE, Perez CA (1983) Role of radiation in the management of early vocal cord carcinoma. Int J Radiat Oncol Biol Phys 9: 997–1002

Modlin J (1950) Neck Dissections in cancer of the lower lip: five year results in 179 patients. Surgery 28: 404–412

Pezner RD, Moss WT, Tong D, Blasko J, Griffin TW (1979) Cervical lymph node metastases in patients with squamous cell carcinoma of the maxillary antrum: the role of elective irradiation of the clinically negative neck. Int J Radiat Oncol Biol Phys 5: 1977–1980

Schuller DE, Platz CE, Krause CJ (1978) Spinal accessory lymph nodes: a prospective study of metastatic involvement. Laryngoscope 138: 439–450

Shah JP, Shaha AR, Spiro RH, Strong EW (1976) Carcinoma of the hypopharynx. Am J Surg 132: 439–443

Skolnik EM, Tenta LT, Wineinger DM, Tardy Jr ME (1967) Preservation of XI cranial nerve in neck dissections. Laryngoscope 77: 1304

Strong EW (1983) Sites of treatment failure in head and neck cancer. Cancer Treat Symp 2: 5–20

Vikram B, Strong EW, Shah J, Spiro RH (1980) Elective postoperative irradiation in stages III and IV epidermoid carcinoma of the head and neck. Am J Surg 140: 580–584

Whicker JH, DeSanto LW, Devine KD (1972) Surgical treatment of squamous cell carcinoma of the base of the tongue. Laryngoscope 91: 333–354

5 Treatment of Nodes in the Clinically N+ Neck

GEORGE E. LARAMORE

CONTENTS

5.1 General Overview

The incidence of clinically positive cervical neck nodes at the time of presentation varies both with the primary site and the patient population seen at a given institution. Patients from higher socioeconomic strata tend in general to present with earlier stage disease while institutions primarily drawing patients from lower socioeconomic strata tend to see positive nodes more frequently when the patients ultimately seek medical attention. Table 5-1 shows a representative sampling of the incidence of positive nodes at the time of presentation for the various primary sites from selected institutions. FLETCHER et al. (1980) specifically discuss the frequency with which particular nodal groups are involved for the various primary sites and this information will also be given in the site-specific chapters later in this book. This chapter is intended to present a concise overview of the problem and to discuss some general principles of treatment.

5.2 Surgery and Adjuvant Radiotherapy

Provided that the clinically-involved nodes are not fixed to the underlying structures and hence are technically resectable, it is likely that a neck dissection will be utilized as the main form of treatment of the involved nodes *if* surgery is also to be the

GEORGE E. LARAMORE, Ph.D., M.D., Department of Radiation Oncology, RC-08, University Hospital, University of Washington, Seattle, WA 98195, USA

Table 5-1. Incidence of clinically positive cervical neck nodes as a function of primary tumor site

Site incidence	%
Nasal cavity	
BOSCH et al. (1976)	13
ROBIN and POWELL (1980)	10
Ethmoid sinus	
ROBIN and POWELL (1980)	13
Maxillary sinus	
PEZNER et al. (1979)	21
ROBIN and POWELL (1980)	17
LEE and OGURA (1981)	7
Lip	
MODLIN (1950)	12
STRONG (1983)	3
Oral tongue	
MENDELSON et al. (1976)	13
FLETCHER et al. (1980)	35
STRONG (1983)	36
Floor of mouth	
HARROLD (1971)	38
FLETCHER et al. (1980)	31
STRONG (1983)	43
Tonsil	
FLETCHER et al. (1980)	76
STRONG (1983)	66
Base of tongue	
WHICKER et al. (1972)	55
FLETCHER et al. (1980)	78
STRONG (1983)	70
Nasopharynx	
HO (1978)	87
FLETCHER et al. (1980)	87
DICKSON (1981)	72
Piriform sinus	
SHAH et al. (1976)	65
BILLER and LUCENTE (1977)	59
FLETCHER et al. (1980)	75
Supraglottic larynx	
BILLER and LUCENTE (1977)	28
FLETCHER et al. (1980)	55
STRONG (1983)	49
Glottic larynx	
LINDBERG (1983)	12

main form of treatment for the primary tumor itself. Until recently this would have meant a classical radical neck dissection as described by CRILE (1906) but now it is more likely to mean a modification of this procedure as discussed in the preceding chapter. Even the classical radical neck dissection, if used as the only therapeutic procedure for the N_+ neck, is associated with a high local failure rate. Adjuvant radiotherapy is a means of reducing this failure rate.

STRONG et al. (1966) in a randomized study explored the utility of adding low-dose, preoperative radiotherapy to a classical, radical neck dissection. Their radiation therapy was 2000 cGy/5 fractions/5 days followed by immediate surgery. Thus, the time interval between radiation and surgery was likely too short to allow for significant "down-staging" in the pathological specimen. There were 100 patients in the control group with histologically positive nodes and they exhibited a local control rate in the neck of only 50%. The addition of low-dose, preoperative radiotherapy improved the control rate in the neck to 69% for the 81 patients in the combined treatment arm who had histologically positive nodes. This difference was statistically significant at the $p \leq 0.01$ level.

It is currently felt that higher doses of adjuvant radiotherapy will yield even better local control. In a retrospective study JESSE and FLETCHER (1977) considered the effect of doses of radiation between 5000 cGy and 6000 cGy given according to the particular clinical situation. Patients treated preoperatively received 5000 cGy, patients treated postoperatively for presumed microscopic disease after a clean resection received 5500 cGy, while patients at high risk for residual disease (e.g. gross tumor "peeled off" structures such as the carotid artery or paraspinous muscles) received 6000 cGy. In all cases the radiation was given in 200 cGy daily fractions for 5 days-a-week. Their local control results for various stages of neck disease is shown in Table 5-2. Note that the staging system they utilized

Table 5-2. Effect of adjuvant radiotherapy on lymph node control in the N_+ neck as a function of disease stage. After JESSE and FLETCHER (1977)

Nodal stage[a]	Surgery alone (%)	Surgery and adjuvant radiotherapy (%)
N_1	86	98
N_2	74	89
N_3	66	75

[a] M. D. Anderson staging system. See text for details of how it differs from the current AJC staging system.

Table 5-3. Local control rates in the neck for patients treated with surgery alone, with "low-dose" 2000 cGy preoperative irradiation and immediate surgery, or with surgery followed by 5000–6000 cGy postoperative irradiation given in a standard fractionation schema. (After VIKRAM et al. 1984)

	Surgery alone (%)	Low-dose preoperative radiotherapy and surgery (%)	Surgery and standard postoperative radiotherapy (%)
Single level Metastases	64	72	84
Multiple level Metastases	28	63	87

is *not* the AJC system given in Chapter 1 but differs in that fixed nodes are defined as N_3 regardless of size and nonfixed nodes greater than 6 cm are classified as N_2. They restricted their analysis to patients surviving at least 2 years with control of their primary tumors. The latter restrictions make it difficult to compare the figures in Table 5-2 with the results of STRONG et al. (1966) but the benefit of adjuvant radiotherapy is highly suggestive for each stage of disease.

VIKRAM et al. (1984) have reviewed the Memorial data and have concluded that the local control rate with postoperative radiation in the range of 5000–6000 cGy is better than low-dose preoperative irradiation for both high and low risk patients (risk being defined as the degree of tumor involvement in the nodes). Their results are summarized in Table 5-3. Note that the effect of the higher radiation doses is more pronounced for the higher risk patients.

The evidence is fairly strong that adjuvant radiotherapy should be used in node positive patients treated primarily with surgery. While 5000 cGy is probably adequate for microscopic disease, risk factors such as either close surgical margins (<5 mm) or extra-capsular nodal extention (CARTER et al. 1987) warrant a higher dose of at least 6000 cGy to the areas in question.

5.3 External Beam Radiotherapy

Definitive radiotherapy in the range of 6500 cGy has been reported as being able to control N_1 nodal disease approximately 90% of the time (SCHNEIDER et al. 1975). However, the control rates in other series are generally less than this.

FAZEKAS et al. (1983) have analyzed the results of an RTOG study testing the efficacy of adjuvant methotrexate with definitive radiotherapy for patients with inoperable head and neck cancer. There was no demonstrable benefit to the additon of methotrexate but information relevant to this chapter relates to an analysis of the clearance in the neck of 386 node-positive patients with either oral cavity or oropharyngeal primaries. Their results are summarized in Table 5-4. Due to patient numbers the observed decrease of nodal clearance with increasing N-stage is statistically significant only for the patients with oropharyngeal lesions. Moreover, the salvage surgery was generally attempted only for the patients who initially had the less advanced disease.

There is some evidence that tumor deposits in lymph nodes may have a greater proportion of hypoxic cells than similar size primaries (GUICHARD et al. 1979). If this is important clinically, then one would expect high linear energy transfer neutron irradiation to be better than conventional photon or electron irradiation in controlling nodal disease. This appeared to be the case in two neutron pilot studies (GRIFFIN et al. 1978; MAOR et al. 1981) and in an RTOG randomized study (GRIFFIN et al. 1983). The later study evaluated 199 patients with positive cervical adenopathy who received either mixed beam (neutron/photon) irradiation or conventional photon irradiaton for inoperable head and neck tumors. The percentages of patients remaining free of their cervical adenopathy for 2 years after therapy is shown in Table 5-5. Although clearly suboptimal, it is interesting to note that for patients with N_3 disease, the local control rate with mixed beam irradiation was almost double that with conventional photon irradiation. It would clearly be of interest to evaluate systematically the efficacy of hypoxic cell sensitizers for patients with advanced nodal disease. Note that because of different patient populations one cannot directly compare the results in Tables 5-4 and 5-5.

To maximize the chances of controlling clinically involved neck nodes, adequate doses of radiation must be delivered. Normally, this is done in conjunction with treatment of the primary tumor and so specific details of field design will be left to the chapters on the various primary sites. The following doses are recommended to the clinically involved nodes as a function of their size: 6600 cGy for nodes ≤ 2 cm, 7000 cGy for nodes between 2 and 4 cm, and 7500+ cGy for nodes greater than 4 cm.

The rate of tumor clearance at the nodal sites is not the same as at the primary sites. BATAINI et al. (1987) reviewed a group of 708 patients with tumors

Table 5-4. Nodal clearance rates as a function of N-stage for patients with oral cavity and oropharyngeal primaries. The clearance rates are shown for radiotherapy alone and with the addition of surgical salvage. (After FAZEKAS et al. 1983)

	Radiation (%)	Radiation and surgical salvage (%)
Oral cavity (103 patients)		
N_1	69	75
N_2	63	63
N_3	46	46
Oropharynx (283 patients)		
N_1	84	90
N_2	75	76
N_3	62	71

Table 5-5. Percentages of node-positive patients with control of nodal disease two years after completing therapy. (After GRIFFIN et al. 1983)

N-Stage	Mixed beam (%)	Photons (%)
N_1	78	55
N_2	39	39
N_3	24	13
Overall[a]	46	33

[a] Statistically significant at $p = 0.03$

of the oropharynx, hypopharynx, and larynx who had positive neck nodes and who received more than 5500 cGy (more than ⅔ of patients received doses greater than 7000 cGy). A total of 759 nodal groups were evaluated. The clearance rate at the end of treatment was greater at the primary site than for the nodal metastases (56% vs 37%, $p \leq 0.0001$) whereas they were equivalent at the two month followup point (76% vs 73%). The larger lymph nodes had the slowest clearance rates. It was also note that adenopathy from oropharyngeal primaries tended to regress more rapidly than adenopathy from laryngeal or hypopharyngeal primaries.

5.4 Other Approaches

Patients with N_3 neck disease present a difficult management problem in that they are often inoperable and the control rate with external beam radiotherapy alone is clearly unsatisfactory. Other approaches to the problem are the use of intraoperative interstitial implants and intraoperative electron beam radiotherapy. Both of these approaches are designed to treat high risk areas (such as where tumor is adherent to the deep neck structures) to higher radiation doses than can be safely delivered with external beam radiation alone.

GOFFINET et al. (1985) discuss 41 patients with N_3 nodal disease who were treated intraoperatively with permanent ^{125}I seed Vicryl suture implants. Thirteen of these patients were previously untreated and local control was achieved in 10/13 (77%). Thirty patients were treated for a neck failure following prior surgery and/or radiotherapy. Local control was achieved in 23/30 (77%) of cases. The radiation dose delivered was stated as approximately 15,500–16,000 cGy although the details of the isodose specification were not given in the paper. The rate of significant complications was 54% for the previously untreated patients and 20% for the previously treated patients (no typographical error).

HAMAKER et al. (1985) discuss the technique of intraoperative, electron-beam radiotherapy and report on a small series of 12 patients. Single fraction doses in the range of 1000–2000 cGy were typically given. Two patients died within one month and so the status of their treated disease is unknown. Five patients died 6–13 months after treatment and only one had uncontrolled disease in the treatment region. Five patients were still alive with apparently controlled disease at the time the report was written but follow-up times were quite short. External beam photon irradiation was given in addition to the intraoperative treatment. The overall rate of significant complication was about 25%.

Both of these techniques deserve further investigation in the context of carefully controlled protocol studies.

References

Bataini JP, Bernier J, Jaulerry C, Brunin F, Pontuert D, Lave C (1987) Impact of neck node responsiveness on the regional control probability in patients with oropharynx and pharyngolarynx cancers managed by definitive radiotherapy. Int J Radiat Oncol Biol Phys 13: 817–824

Biller HF, Lucente FE (1977) Conservation surgery of the head and neck. Semin Oncol 4: 365–373

Bosch A, Vallecillo L, Frias Z (1976) Cancer of the nasal cavity 37: 1458–1463

Carter RL, Bliss JM, Soo KC, O'Brien CJ (1987) Radical neck dissections for squamous carcinomas: pathological findings and their clinical implications with particular reference to transcapsular spread. Int J Radiat Oncol Biol Phys 13: 825–832

Crile GW (1906) Excision of cancer of the head and neck with special reference to the plan of dissection based on 132 operations. JAMA 47: 1780–1786

Dickson RI (1981) Nasopharyngeal carcinoma: an evaluation of 209 patients. Laryngoscope 91: 333–354

Fazekas JT, Sommer C, Kramer S (1983) Tumor regression and other prognostic factors in advanced head and neck cancers: a sequel to the RTOG methotrexate study. Int J Radiat Oncol Biol Phys 9: 957–964

Fletcher GH, Jesse RH, Lindberg RD, Westbrook KC (1980) Neck nodes. In: Textbook of Radiotherapy, 3rd edn. (ed) Fletcher GH. Lea & Febiger, Philadelphia, PA. pp 249–271

Goffinet DR, Paryani SB, Fee Jr WE (1985) Management of patients with N_3 cervical adenopathy and/or carotid artery involvement. In: Head and Neck Cancer, Vol. 1 (eds). Chretein PB, Johns ME, Shedd DP, Strong EW, Ward PH. Decker, Inc., Philadelphia, PA. pp 159–162

Griffin TW, Davis R, Laramore GE, Hussey DH, Hendrickson FR, Rodriguez-Antunez A (1983) Fast neutron irradiation of metastatic cervical adenopathy: the results of a randomized RTOG study. Int J Radiat Oncol Biol Phys 9: 1267–1270

Griffin TW, Laramore GE, Parker RG, Gerdes AJ, Hebard DW, Blasko JC, Groudine MT (1978) An evaluation of fast neutron beam teletherapy of metastatic cervical adenopathy from squamous cell carcinomas of the head and neck region. Cancer 42: 2517–2520

Guichard M, Courdi A, Fertil B, Malaise EP (1979) Radiosensitivity of lymph node metastases versus initial subcutaneous tumors in nude mice. Radiat Res 78: 278–285

Hamaker RC, Singer MI, Pugh N, Ross D, Garrett P (1985) Management of the N_3 neck: intraoperative radiation. In: Head and Neck Cancer, Vol. 1 (eds). Chretein PB, Johns ME, Shedd DP, Strong EW, Ward PH, Decker, Inc., Philadelphia, PA. pp 162–166

Ho JHC (1978) An epidemiologic and clinical study of nasopharyngeal carcinoma. Int J Radiat Oncol Biol Phys 4: 181–198

Jesse RH, Fletcher GH (1977) Treatment of the neck in patients with squamous cell carcinoma of the head and neck. Cancer 39: 868–872

Lee F, Ogura JH (1981) Maxillary sinus carcinoma. Laryngoscope 91: 133–139

Lindberg RD (1983) Sites of first failure in head and neck cancer. Cancer Treat Symp 2: 21–31

Maor MH, Hussey DH, Fletcher GH, Jesse RH (1981) Fast neutron therapy for locally advanced head and neck tumors. Int J Radiat Oncol Biol Phys 7: 155–163

Mendelson BC, Woods JE, Beahrs OH (1976) Neck dissection in the treatment of carcinoma of the anterior two-thirds of tongue. Surg Gynecol Obstet 143: 75–80

Modlin J (1950) Neck dissections in cancer of the lower lip: five-year results in 179 patients. Surgery 28: 404–412

Pezner RD, Moss WT, Tong D, Blasko J, Griffin TW (1979) Cervical lymph node metastases in patients with squamous cell carcinoma of the maxillary antrum: the role of elective irradiation of the clinically negative neck. Int J Radiat Oncol Biol Phys 5: 1977–1980

Robin PE, Powell DJ (1980) Regional node involvement and distant metastases in carcinoma of the nasal cavity and paranasal sinuses. J Laryngol Otol 94: 301–309

Schneider JJ, Fletcher GH, Barkley Jr HT (1975) Control by irradiation alone of nonfixed clinically positive nodes from squamous cell carcinoma of the oral cavity, oropharynx, supraglottic larynx and hypopharynx. Am J Roentgenol 123: 42–48

Shah JP, Shaha AR, Spiro RH, Strong EW (1976) Carcinoma of the hypopharynx. Am J Surg 132: 439–443

Strong EW (1983) Sites of treatment failure in head and neck cancer. Cancer Treat Symp 2: 5–20

Strong EW, Henschke UK, Nickson JJ, Frazell EL, Tollefsen HR, Hilaris BS (1966) Preoperative x-ray therapy as an adjunct to radical neck dissection. Cancer 19: 1509–1516

Vikram B, Strong EW, Shah JP, Spiro R (1984) Failure in the neck following multimodality treatment for advanced head and neck cancer. Head Neck Surg 6: 724–729

6 Oral Cavity

Leslye Ingersoll and Don R. Goffinet

CONTENTS

Leslye Ingersoll, M.D. and Don R. Goffinet, M.D., Stanford University School of Medicine, Stanford, CA 94305, USA

6.1 Introduction

The oral cavity, after the larynx, is the most common site of head and neck cancers (Silverberg and Lubera 1988). The structures included within the oral cavity are the lips, mobile tongue, floor of mouth, buccal area, hard palate, maxillary and mandibular gingiva and the corresponding alveolar ridges. The incidence of lip cancers is decreasing and may be due to occupational changes, increased public awareness of solar damage and frequent use of protective sunscreen agents. Early intraoral carcinomas are usually asymptomatic and may go undetected until moderately advanced. Most intraoral tumors arise in a horse-shoe shaped area involving the floor of mouth, retromolar trigone and ventrolateral tongue, an area less than 25% of the total mucosal surface. Pooled saliva containing carcinogens from tobacco products and the direct irritation of alcohol are felt to be important etiological factors in this high risk area.

In 1988, 30,000 individuals are expected to develop intraoral or oropharnygeal carcinomas, and nearly one-third will die because of neoplasms (Silverberg and Lubera 1988). Varying degrees of oral dysfunction and discomfort may occur, even in cured patients. Fortunately, patients appear to be presenting with earlier diagnoses due to better cancer education and the widespread availability of medical and dental care.

6.2 Anatomy

6.2.1 Lip

The lips are muscular folds covered by skin and mucous membranes. The vermilion border is the zone between skin and mucous membranes and has a reddish hue due to the presence of capillary loops close to the thin, overlying stratified squamous epithelium. Labial branches of facial arteries form an anastomotic ring within and about the lips. Sensory impulses from the upper lip are carried by the infra-orbital branch of the maxillary nerve (V2) while the mental branch of the mandibular nerve (V3) carries sensory impulses from the lower lip. Motor activity to the orbicularis oris muscle is supplied by CN VII.

6.2.2 Buccal Mucosa

The buccal mucosa is attached at its superior, inferior and posterior margins to the maxilla, mandible, and pterygoid plates, respectively. Lateral to the buccal mucosa are the buccinator muscles which interdigitate anteriorly with the orbicularis oris muscle. These muscles are partially covered by buccal fat pads which give the cheeks their rounded contour. Bilateral parotid (Stenson's) ducts open into the oral cavity through the buccal mucosa opposite the maxillary second molars. Clusters of mucosal salivary glands are located around the terminal aspects of these ducts. Arterial supply and motor activity to the buccinator muscles are the same as those for the orbicularis muscle of the lips. The long buccal nerve, a branch of the mandibular nerve, carries sensation from the buccal mucosa and skin of the cheek.

6.2.3 Gingiva

The gingiva is composed of fibrous tissue and mucosa attached to the underlying alveolar bony processes. It extends posteriorly to include the mandibular retromolar trigone or maxillary tuberosity. The pterygomandibular space, which is located postero-medially to the retromolar trigone, communicates with the lateral pharyngeal space. (Fig. 6-1) Tumors which invade this space may extend along the lateral pharyngeal wall to the oropharynx and upper neck. Sensory fibers of the infraorbital and greater palatine nerves innervate the maxillary gingiva while the long buccal and mental branches of the mandibular nerve carry sensation from the mandibular gingiva.

6.2.4 Floor of Mouth

The floor of mouth is U-shaped and composed of layers of epithelial, glandular and muscular tissues. It extends from the lingual gingiva to the oral tongue, posteriorly to the anterior tonsillar pillar,

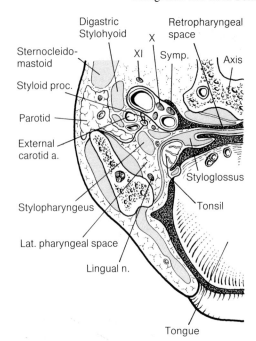

Fig. 6-1. Lateral pharyngeal space at level of parotid gland. (From Grant's Method of Anatomy. Printed with permission)

and inferiorly to the mylohyoid and digastric muscles. Beneath the mucosa are paired sublingual glands which are separated medially by the genioglossus and geniohyoid muscles. The mylohyoid muscles form a supporting sling in the floor of mouth. The deep lobe of each submandibular gland curves around the posterior aspect of this muscle while the majority of each gland lies externally to it. Each submandibular (Wharton's) duct is approximately 5 cm long and opens into the oral cavity in the anterior floor of mouth. Tissues in the floor of mouth are supplied by the lingual artery. Sensation is transmitted along the lingual nerve and motor activity is supplied by either the mylohyoid branch of the inferior alveolar nerve or motor branches of C-1.

6.2.5 Hard Palate

The hard palate forms the roof of the oral cavity. Deep to the mucosa are multiple small salivary glands. The anterior hard palate is supplied by the nasopalatine artery and nerve, while the majority of the hard palate is supplied by the greater palatine arteries and nerves, which enter the oral cavity through foramina located medially to the maxillary third molars.

6.2.6 Oral Tongue

The anterior or oral tongue is mobile and ends at the circumvallate papilla. The inferior surface and sides are smooth while the dorsum is roughened by multiple papillae containing taste buds. Mucous and serous glands heavily populate the tip and ventrolateral surfaces. A fibrous septum divides the tongue into halves and restricts branches of the paired lingual arteries from anastomosing except at the tip. The lingual nerve (from V3) is sensory to the oral tongue. The sense of taste is carried by the chorda tympani, a branch of the facial nerve. Motor activity to all intrinsic and most extrinsic muscles of the tongue is supplied by the hypoglossal nerve.

6.2.7 Lymphatics

Most lymphatic channels from the oral cavity drain directly into the submandibular and jugulodiagastric lymph nodes. (Fig. 6-2) Preauricular and parotid lymph nodes receive lymphatic channels from the upper lip. Lymphatic channels from the midportion of the lower lip and occasionally from the floor of mouth drain into submental lymph nodes. The oral tongue has lymphatics that bypass the submandibular and jugulodigastric lymph nodes and drain directly into lower cervical (jugulo-omohyoid) lymph nodes. Bilateral nodal involvement is more likely to occur with midline tumors. Contralateral involvement is rare. See Table 6-1 for the incidence of nodal involvement at diagnosis and subsequent involvement following treatment of the primary lesion for each anatomical site.

Table 6-1. Incidence of cervical nodal involvement at diagnosis and subsequent involvement following initial treatment of the primary tumor. Many series were not corrected for control of cancer at the primary site, therefore, both subclinical nodal involvement and metastatic nodal disease from uncontrolled primary tumors are reflected in these figures

Site	Incidence of nodal involvement at diagnosis (%)	Incidence of subsequent nodal involvement following treatment (%)	References
Lip	5–10	5–15	a, b, c, d, e
Oral tongue	23–36	20–50	a, f, g, h, i, j, k, m, n, o, p, q, r, s, t
Floor of mouth	30–42	23–30	a, u, h, dd, v, f, g, i, s
Buccal mucosa	8–44	9–37	a, w, x, y, z, aa, bb, g, i
Gingiva	15–48	14–19	a, w, x, y, z, aa, bb, g, i
Hard palate	15–25	20–25	aa, i

[a] Ash (1961); [b] Byers et al. (1978); [c] Gladstone and Kerr (1958); [d] Heller and Shah (1979); [e] Hornback and Shidnia (1978); [f] Lindberg (1972); [g] Jesse et al. (1970); [h] Fayos and Lampe (1967); [i] Mustard and Rosen (1963); [j] Mendelson et al. (1976); [k] Vermund et al. (1984); [l] Monaco et al. (1962); [m] Spiro and Strong (1971); [n] Whitehurst (1977); [o] Decroix and Ghossein (1981); [p] Fu et al. (1976); [q] Ildstad et al. (1983); [r] Schleuning and Summers (1972); [s] Teichgraeber and Clairmont (1984); [t] Marchetta and Sako (1975); [u] Aygun et al. (1984); [v] Harrold (1971); [w] Bloom and Spiro (1980); [x] Conley and Sadoyama (1973); [y] Mendenhall et al. (1980); [z] Vegers et al. (1979); [aa] Wang (1983); [bb] Lee and Wilson (1973); [cc] Landa and Zarem (1973); [dd] Love et al. (1977)

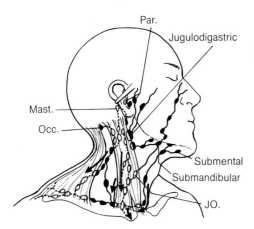

Fig. 6-2. Head and neck lymphatics. (From Grant's Method of Anatomy, 1980. Printed with permission)

6.3 Staging

Carcinomas arising in the oral cavity are staged according to the following American Joint Committee for Cancer Staging and End Results Reporting criteria:

T_1 tumor 2 cm or less in greatest diameter.

T_2 tumor greater than 2 cm but not greater than 4 cm in greatest diameter.

T_3 tumor greater than 4 cm in greatest diameter.

T_4 massive tumor greater than 4 cm in diameter with deep invasion of muscle, pterygoid, base of tongue, bone, cartilage or skin.

N_0 no clinically positive node.

N_1 single clinically positive homolateral node less than 3 cm in diameter.

N_{2a} single positive homolateral node 3–6 cm in diameter.

N_{2b} multiple clinically positive homolateral nodes, none greater than 6 cm in diameter.

N_{3a} clinically positive homolateral nodes, one or more greater than 6 cm in diameter.

N_{3b} bilateral clinically positive nodes.

N_{3c} contralateral clinically positive node(s) only.

M_0 no distant metastases.

M_1 distant metastases present.

Stage 1, $T_1 N_0 M_0$

Stage 2, $T_2 N_0 M_0$

Stage 3, $T_3 N_0 M_0$
            $T_{1-3} N_1 M_0$

Stage 4, $T_4 N_0 M_0$
            AnyT $N_{2-3} M_0$
            AnyT Any $N M_1$

6.4 Lip

6.4.1 Presentation

Tumors involving the lips are nearly always well differentiated squamous cell carcinomas. They occur much more frequently on the lower than upper lip and often present as painless ulcers or crusted lesions. A background of leukoplakia may be present for months to years before diagnosis. Erythroplakia is also a common feature.

Elderly males who have fair or ruddy complexions and have a history of prolonged sun exposure make up the largest population group. Local irritation from smoking and heavy consumption of alcohol are other etiological factors (BAKER and KRAUSE 1950; MOLNAR et al. 1974). Five per cent of patients have multiple lesions at diagnosis (BAKER et al. 1950) and approximately 5% develop additional cancers.

Basal cell carcinomas are rare and occur twice as frequently on the upper lip as the lower lip (WARD and HENDRICK 1950). Other unusual tumors are verrucous carcinomas, mucosal melanomas, and minor salivary gland tumors.

Advanced lesions may infiltrate the commissure, buccal mucosa or alveolar ridge. The incidence of lymph node involvement at diagnosis is 5–10% (BAKER et al. 1977; HENDRICKS et al. 1977; MAC-KAY and SELLER 1964; PETROVICH et al. 1987) and increases to 19% for commissure lesions (PETROVICH et al. 1987). The risk for lymph node metastasis increases with larger primary lesions and when muscle invasion has occurred. Clinically involved lymph nodes are frequently present at diagnosis in tumors with perineural invasion (BYERS et al. 1978; FRIERSON and COOPER 1986). Numbness from mental nerve involvement may be observed in advanced lesions. The lungs are the most frequent site for distant metastasis, which is a rare event.

6.4.2 Treatment

Primary radiotherapy is frequently selected for patients who have lesions which involve the upper lip, the commissure or one-third or more of the lower lip. Small T_1 cancers involving the lower lip are usually resected. Excision is the treatment of choice in young patients who will have many more years of sun exposure. Moderately advanced (T_3) lesions may be treated by surgery, irradiation, or both. Advanced tumors (T_4) with bony invasion or mental nerve involvement are best managed by resection and pre- or postoperative irradiation. Palliative radiotherapy is given to patients with advanced cancers who are unwilling to undergo resection or are poor surgical candidates. If cervical lymph nodes are uninvolved by metastases, the neck is not irradiated except in cases where the primary tumor is advanced, recurrent, or characterized by poorly differentiated histology or perineural invasion. Neck dissection is indicated in patients who have regional lymph node involvement, followed by postoperative irradiation.

Small, superficial lesions may be treated with either orthovoltage (100–200 Kv) or low energy electron beams to a total dose of 5000 to 5500 cGy in 4–5 weeks. A lead mask with a cutout over the treatment volume may be used to protect uninvolved skin. A lead shield between the lip and teeth limits the exit dose to oral structures, but may increase backscatter to the inner surface of the lip.

Since larger cancers may spread several centimeters beyond the clinically palpable or visible borders (HORNBACK and SHIDNIA 1978) they should be treated with wide radiation fields to higher doses (6000–7000 cGy). Mixed photon and electron beams or interstitial implantation techniques may be required to decrease the radiation dose to normal structures. Fraction sizes of less than 250 cGy per day are best for preservation of function and obtaining a good cosmetic result.

Moist desquamation of the irradiated tissue is nearly always present at the completion of therapy. This acute reaction usually heals within 2–8 weeks but may take longer for larger lesions. Less satisfactory cosmetic results, including mucosal and soft tissue atrophy and telangiectasia, may also occur. The risk of soft tissue necrosis or osteoradionecrosis increase substantially with doses higher than 6500 cGy.

6.4.3 Results

Carcinomas of the lip are among the most curable head and neck tumors because of indolent growth patterns and early detection and treatment. Cure rates vary according to size of the primary lesion, nodal status, and histology. Generally, the 5 year determinate survival rate for small carcinomas of the lip is 90% or greater (BAKER et al. 1950; HELLER and SHAH 1979; JORGENSEN et al. 1973; MACKAY and SELLER 1964; PETROVICH et al. 1987). Radiation therapy or surgical resection are equally effective. Baker and Krause (BAKER et al. 1950), in a retrospective study of 300 patients treated with curative intent, found that the 5 year determinate survival for patients who had small tumors was 95.2% for those treated with radiation therapy and 95.3% for those treated surgically. Five year determinate survival rates decreased to 70-80% (BAKER et al. 1950; GLADSTONE and KERR 1958; HELLER and SHAH 1979) for patients with tumors larger than 3 cm and 25-50% (BAKER et al. 1950; GLADSTONE and KERR 1958; MACKAY and SELLER 1964) for T_4 lesions.

The incidence of cervical lymph node involvement increases as the size of the primary tumor increases (BROWN et al. 1976; HELLER and SHAH 1979; JORGENSEN et al. 1973). Petrovich, et al. (1987) in a review of 250 patients, noted that only 5% of patients with T_1 and T_2 tumors, but 67% of patients with more advanced lesions had clinical evidence of nodal metastasis at presentation. The overall curability of patients with lymph node involvement at diagnosis is 40-50% (JORGENSEN et al. 1973; MACKAY and SELLER 1964; MAHONEY 1969; MOLNAR et al. 1974; PETROVICH et al. 1987).

Low grade tumors are less likely to recur or metastasize than less well differentiated neoplasms. Frierson and Cooper (FRIERSON and COOPER 1986) reviewed 187 squamous cell carcinomas of the lower lip and found that 2% of grade II, 34% of grade III, and 92% of grade IV tumors had metastasized by the time of diagnosis. Perineural invasion, a sign of aggressive growth, is associated with an 80% risk of lymph node metastasis and only 35% five year survival rates (BYERS et al. 1978).

Recurrence rates for squamous cell carcinomas of the lip are similar for treatment either by radiation therapy or excision (Table 6-2). MCKAY and

Table-6-2. The incidence of local regional failure following initial treatment to the lip for squamous cell carcinoma. Note that surgical excision or radiation therapy are equally effective in limited and moderately advanced lip carcinomas

Author	Treatment	Size	No of Cases	Local regional failure (%)
BAKER and KRAUSE (1950)	47% XRT 53% Surgery	<1 CM 1-3 CM >3 CM deep	87 160 30 15	11[a] 9 21 91
HENDRICKS et al. (1977)	Surgery	<1 CM 1-3 CM >3 CM	340 247 24	5[a] 4 17
PETROVICH et al. (1979, 1987)	XRT	Stage I Stage II Stage III Stage IV	173 48 10 19	6 6 10 53

[a] Lip recurrences only

SELLER (1964) reviewed 2854 cases, 92% of whom were initially treated by radiation therapy. The minimum follow up was 5 years. The primary lesion was controlled by initial treatment in 84% of cases. An additional 8% were salvaged by further therapy, making the overall control rate 92%. Other authors, (PETROVICH et al. 1987; PIGNEUX et al. 1979) obtained a 94% local control rate in patients treated by radiation therapy who had stage I and II cancers. Twenty-three of the 250 evaluable patients had clinically involved lymph nodes at presentation, 18 (80%) of whom had N_2 and N_3 neck node staging. Fifty percent of these 23 patients had their neoplasms controlled by radiotherapy alone.

Approximately 50% of patients who develop local and/or regional recurrences following initial treatment are salvaged by subsequent surgery or radiation therapy (HELLER and SHAH 1979; PETROVICH et al. 1979). Heller et al. (HELLER and SHAH 1979) determined that the 5 year survival rate is 80% in patients who recur in the lip only, 50% in those who subsequently develop cervical lymph node metastasis, and 25% in patients who fail both locally and regionally.

Those who die from carcinoma of the lip usually do so within 24 months following treatment (MACKAY and SELLER 1964; PETROVICH et al. 1987). Death frequently occurs from failure to control local-regional disease. Some advanced tumors have been observed to involve the contents of the middle cranial fossa by spreading along nerves V2 or V3.

6.5 Oral Tongue

6.5.1 Presentation

Most neoplasms which involve the oral tongue are squamous cell carcinomas, while rhabdomyosarcomas, minor salivary gland and verrucous carcinomas occur rarely. Most are located along the middle or posterior aspects of the lateral tongue surfaces. The next most common site of involvement is the undersurface of the tongue. Dorsal tongue squamous carcinomas, while uncommon, are frequently associated with chronic atrophic glossitis and leukoplakia (FRAZELL and LUCAS 1962) and may be confused with granular cell myoblastoma, a benign neoplasm. Tumors arising from the tip of the tongue are rare.

Squamous cell carcinomas of the oral tongue usually arise in elderly individuals. While the majority of patients report long periods of tobacco use and regular alcoholic consumption, a small fraction of patients have never used these products (WHITE and BYERS 1980). They tend to be younger and frequently have aggressive carcinomas (SON and KAPP 1985). The incidence of oral tongue squamous carcinomas is increasing in women, correlating with an increased use of tobacco products and alcoholic beverages by females (MENDELSON et al. 1976; STRONG 1979; ILDSTAD et al. 1983).

Early squamous cell carcinomas of the oral tongue may be asymptomatic. Despite the tongue's well-developed tactile sense, pain may be a complaint only with more advanced or ulcerated lesions. Frequently, early carcinomas are not easily identified. The most common mucosal abnormality is erythroplakia (MASHBERG and MEYERS 1976) which may be a subtle finding. These lesions are often better visualized after the mucosa has been dried by a gauze sponge. Examination of the oral tongue must include the use of adequate light for a careful inspection and palpation of all surfaces of the organ, as well as a determination of tongue mobility.

When symptomatic, most patients report a tender tongue mass. Advanced lesions impair tongue mobility, leading to speech and swallowing difficulties. Less frequent presenting symptoms include weight loss, ear pain and neck mass.

Invasive squamous cell carcinomas tend to spread along the interdigitating tongue muscle planes and have indistinct borders. When moderately advanced, adjacent structures such as the floor of mouth and base of tongue may become involved.

This finding has been noted in approximately 25% of patients at presentation (CALLERY et al. 1984). Occasionally, advanced lesions in the posterior aspect of the oral tongue are palpable as a neck mass near the mandibular angle if the tumor extends laterally beyond the posterior aspect of the mylohyoid muscle.

Squamous carcinomas of the oral tongue have been associated with relatively high rates of lymph node involvement at diagnosis; therefore, a thorough understanding of the tongue's lymphatic drainage is helpful in managing these tumors successfully. Beneath the dorsum of the tongue is a superficial lymphatic plexus which drains to both sides and collects into lymphatic vessels which also cross the midline. Fewer crossings occur at the lateral tongue surface so that lymphatic drainage from this site is nearly always ipsilateral. In general, anterior lymphatic vessels drain into lymph nodes located in the submental and submandibular areas, while middle and posterior lymphatic vessels drain into more posterosuperiorly located lymph nodes (Fig. 6-3). Lymphatics from the tip of the tongue generally drain into the submental and submandibular lymph nodes, while lymphatics from the middle third are connected to the jugulocarotid and jugulodigastric lymph nodes. Less frequently the submandibular and jugulo-omohyoid nodes may be involved. Lymphatics from the posterior third of

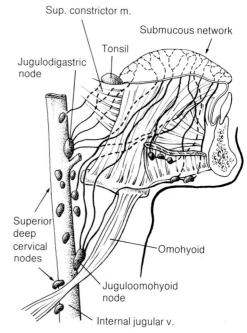

Fig. 6-3. Tongue lymphatics. (From Grant's Method of Anatomy, 1980. Printed with permission)

the tongue drain into the jugulodigastric, pharyngeal and jugulo-carotid nodes.

The incidence of clinically involved lymph nodes at diagnosis is 25–35%. (ASH 1961; LINDBERG 1972; JESSE et al. 1970; FAYOS and LAMPE 1972; MUSTARD and ROSEN 1963; VERMUND et al. 1984; MONACO et al. 1962; SPIRO and STRONG 1974; DECROIX and GHOSSEIN 1981; FU et al. 1976; TEICHGRAEBER and CLAIRMONT 1984). Since most oral tongue cancers are located laterally, the incidence of bilateral and contralateral nodal involvement at presentation is less than 10% (DECROIX and GHOSSEIN 1981; NORTHROP et al. 1972; SPIRO and STRONG 1971; STRONG 1979; FLAMANT et al. 1964). In general, 5–20% of patients with T_1, 30–40% with T_2, and 50% or more with advanced tumors have nodal metastases at the time of presentation. (BRADFIELD and SCRUGGS 1983; DECROIX and GHOSSEIN 1981; MENDELSON et al. 1976; MONACO et al. 1962; SPIRO and STRONG 1971; DECROIX and GHOSSEIN 1981).

When only the primary site is treated, an additional 25–50% of patients subsequently develop metastatic cervical adenopathy (ASH 1961; LINDBERG 1972; JESSE et al. 1970; MUSTARD and ROSEN 1963; MENDELSON et al. 1976; VERMUND et al. 1984; SPIRO and STRONG 1971; SPIRO and STRONG 1974; WHITEHURST and DROULIAS 1977; FU et al. 1976; ILDSTAD et al. 1983; SCHLEUNING and SUMMERS 1972; LEE and LITTON 1972; MARCHETTA and SAKO 1975). This conversion from a clinically negative to positive neck may occur despite successful control of the primary tongue lesion and is attributed to the presence of subclinical nodal metastases at the time of treatment. Decroix and Ghossein (DECROIX and GHOSSEIN 1981), in a review of 244 patients clinically staged $T_x N_0$ who underwent elective neck dissection, found that the incidence of occult lymph node involvement was 34%. Other reviews have reported the frequency of occult nodal involvement to be between 20–50% (BRADFIELD and SCRUGGS 1983; MENDELSON et al. 1976; ILDSTAD et al. 1983; LEE and LITTON 1972; TEICHGRAEBER and CLAIRMONT 1984; WHITE and BYERS 1980; CARTER et al. 1985). As the size of the primary tongue lesion increases, the incidence of subclinical nodal metastases also increases from 29% for $T_1 N_0$ to 50% for $T_2 N_0$ and 77% for $T_3 N_0$ lesions as determined by Spiro and Strong (SPIRO and STRONG 1971), who reviewed 185 patients who underwent only partial glossectomy as definitive treatment. Although these percentages were not corrected for cancer control at the primary site, this study illustrates that therapy directed to the primary neoplasm only is inadequate in many situations when metastatic adenopathy is

not clinically apparent. Decroix and Ghossein (DECROIX and GHOSSEIN 1981) found that the incidence of occult nodal metastases in the above mentioned 244 patients was 18% for $T_1 N_0$, 39% for $T_2 N_0$, and 46% for $T_3 N_0$ clinically staged patients.

A second primary cancer occurs in 10–20% of patients treated for squamous cell carcinoma of the oral tongue, usually in the upper aerodigestive tract. (BRADFIELD and SCRUGGS 1983; FRAZELL and LUCAS 1962; CALLERY et al. 1984; DECROIX and GHOSSEIN 1981; FU et al. 1976; ILDSTAD et al. 1983; MARKS et al. 1981). Distant metastases, usually to lung, bone, and liver, occur more frequently in patients who have recurrent neoplasms or uncontrolled neck node metastases rather than in patients whose primary cancers are initially controlled. Deaths are usually due to local-regional failure, although many patients with advanced cancers also succumb to distant metastases.

6.5.2 Treatment

The optimal treatment for squamous cell carcinoma of the oral tongue is dependent upon such factors as tumor location, size and extension; status of cervical lymph nodes; and the patient's reliability and vocational needs. Stage I and early stage II cancers may be treated by radiation therapy or surgery with equally good results (STRONG 1979; SPIRO 1985; FRAZELL 1971; ILDSTAD et al. 1983; FAYOS and LAMPE 1967; MARKS et al. 1981; SOUTHWICK 1973; WHITE and BYERS 1980). (Table 6-3) Partial glossectomy is the treatment of choice for small lesions involving the dorsal surface or tip of tongue. Patients who require preservation of normal articulation and speech patterns for occupational reasons may be treated by radiation therapy. Because of the high incidence of occult nodal metastases, the ipsilateral neck lymph nodes are electively treated in all but the few patients with small, well-circumscribed, superficial tumors. Any patient who requires hemiglossectomy and/or has histopathological evidence of nodal metastasis should receive postoperative external beam radiation therapy. Optimal treatment for patients with stage III or IV cancer is a mandibular sparing surgical resection, when possible, combined with postoperative radiation therapy. Palliative radiation therapy is given to those who are poor surgical candidates with advanced disease.

Prior to beginning radiation therapy, a careful dental evaluation must be made, so that the teeth may be cleaned and restored as required. Routine pre-irradiation extraction of all teeth is no longer

Table 6-3. The incidence of local-regional recurrence of squamous cell carcinoma of the oral tongue

Study	Treatment	No of Patients	Stage	Recurrence		
				Primary	P+N	Neck
DECROIX and GHOSSEIN (1981)	Interstitial	88	T_1N_0	9 (10)%	3 (3%)	9 (10%)
	Implant ± EXT	6	T_1N_+	1	–	1
	Beam XRT	199	T_2N_0	25 (13%)	15 (8%)	20 (10%)
	Neck-surgical	89	T_2N_+	13 (15%)	11 (12%)	9 (10%)
	Dissection	96	T_3N_0	19 (20%)	12 (13%)	11 (11%)
		122	T_3N_+	16 (13%)	17 (14%)	13 (11%)
WHITEHURST (1981)	Surgical resection	82	T_1N_0	8/82 (10%)	7/82 (8.5%)	13/82 (16%)
		28	T_2N_0	4/28 (14%)	4/28 (14%)	12/28 (43%)
		14	T_3N_0	0/14 (0%)	2/14 (14%)	6/14 (43%)
		13	T_XN_+	3/13 (23%)	2/13 (16%)	3/13 (23%)
ILDSTAD et al. (1983)	Surgical resection	29	I	4/29 (14%)	5/29 (17%)	4/29 (14%)
		12	II	0/2	1/12 (8%)	3/12 (25%)
		2	III	0/2	0/2	1/2
		2	IV	1/2	0/2	0/2
	Radiation therapy	11	I	1/11 (9%)	2/11 (18%)	4/11 (36%)
		23	II	5/23 (22%)	6/23 (26%)	4/23 (17%)
		10	III	2/10 (20%)	3/10 (30%)	3/10 (30%)
		14	IV	1/14 (7%)	9/14 (64%)	1/14 (7%)
LEIPZIG (1982)	Surgical resection	22	I	2/22 (9%)		8/22 (36%)
		16	II	1/16 (6%)		7/16 (44%)
		13	III + IV	8/13 (62%)		1/13 (8%)
	Radiation therapy	8	I	3/8 (37.5%)		2/8 (25%)
		14	II	8/14 (57%)		1/14 (7%)
		31	III + IV	22/31 (71%)		5/31 (16%)
	Combined	1	II			
		13	III + IV	2/13 (15%)		3/13 (23%)
WHITE (1980)	Surgical resection	41	T_1	3/41 (7%)		7/41 (17%)
		26	T_2	1/26 (4%)		5/26 (19%)
		14	T_3-T_4	3/14 (21%)		4/14 (29%)
	Radiation therapy	8	T_1	0/8		1/8 (12%)
		38	T_2	9/38 (24%)		14/38 (37%)
		17	T_3-T_4	12/17 (70%)		9/17 (56%)

recommended, but non-restorable teeth should be removed 10–14 days prior to the onset of the radiotherapy course. The use of prophylactic fluoride oral rinses or dental carriers during and after irradiation is mandatory in non-edentulous patients. Dental extractions in irradiated patients should be avoided if possible, but if required must be accompanied by careful mucosal coverage of the mandible and the use of prophylactic antibiotics (BEUMER et al. 1983; DRIEZEN et al. 1977).

Treatment of the clinically negative neck in patients with squamous cell carcinoma of the oral tongue has been a source of debate for many years. Elective neck therapy should be considered for several reasons: 1) There is a significant error in clinically evaluating cervical lymph nodes, 2) there is a risk of conversion from N_0 to N_+ when therapy

is limited to the primary tongue lesion, and 3) the poor survival of patients who subsequently develop regional lymph node involvement. The 5 year survival rate for patients who subsequently develop nodal metastasis is generally less than 40% (MENDELSON et al. 1976; VERMUND et al. 1984; FRAZELL and LUCAS 1962; STRONG 1979). Opponents of elective therapy of the neck claim that only a small fraction of patients with early lesions who are treated actually benefit from this treatment (JESSE et al. 1970). Also, there is no clear evidence that elective neck dissection improves survival (MENDELSON et al. 1976; VANDENBROUCK et al. 1980). Elective neck irradiation, however, does reduce the incidence of subsequent nodal metastases in the treated neck to less than 10% (Table 6-4). Radiation therapy has also proved beneficial in reducing the incidence of re-

Table 6-4. The incidence of cervical nodal metastases after elective neck irradiation vs. no elective treatment, partial or low dose neck irradiation for squamous cell carcinoma of the tongue

	Elective neck irradiation		Partial/ low dose/or no elective neck irradiation	
	Incidence	(%)	Incidence	(%)
MILLION (1974) $T_x N_0$	0/3	0	4/14	29
GILBERT et al. (1975) $T_x N_0$	0/34	0	7/18[a]	38
			2/6[b]	33
NORTHROP et al. (1972) $T_x N_0$	2/22[d]	9	8/30[d]	27
HORIUCHI et al. (1982) $T_x N_0$	1/21	5	6/16	38
MEOZ et al. (1982) $T_x N_0$	4/24	17	27/76[a]	36
			9/27[b]	33
			8/19[c]	42

[a] No radiation

[b] Low dose, 2000 cGy or less

[c] Ipsilateral neck irradiation to 5000 cGy, marginal miss because of inadequate coverage of high internal jugular lymph nodes

[d] Incidence of contralateral nodal involvement

currence in the dissected (DECROIX and GHOSSEIN 1981; NORTHROP et al. 1972; STRONG 1969) and contralateral (NORTHROP et al. 1972) neck. At Memorial Hospital in New York City, patients with advanced cancers who received post operative radiation therapy tended to live longer than patients who were treated by surgery alone (CALLERY et al. 1984).

External beam irradiation is usually delivered to the tongue through lateral opposed fields. The tongue may be depressed by a bite block composed of dental mold material on a tongue blade. Cotton rolls interposed between tongue and teeth, and teeth and buccal mucosa decrease mucosal absorption of electron scatter from dental fillings. Cerrobend or lead blocks are constructed at the treatment planning session. As much parotid gland as possible is excluded from the field. Exclusion of a small strip of skin and subcutaneous tissues in the submental area decreases the risk of persistent neck edema. The entire upper aspect of the sternoclei-

domastoid muscle is included in the field to adequately irradiate posterior subdigastric lymph nodes in the internal jugular chain. In a study by Meoz, et al. at the M.D. Anderson Hospital (MEOZ et al. 1982), this area was a frequent site of neck failure when it was excluded from the initial treatment volume. The authors suggest that the vertebral bodies be used as anatomical landmarks to ensure adequate coverage of these lymph nodes. A lower anterior neck, or supraclavicular field, treated to a depth of 3 cm with a midline bar is matched to the lateral opposed fields. Forty-five hundred to 5000 cGy is given over 5 weeks followed by a 2500–3000 cGy, removable 192 Iridium afterloading interstitial implantation boost to the primary tongue lesion. Maximum spinal cord dose is limited to 4000 cGy.

Postoperative irradiation may be used in conjunction with surgery for advanced cancers. Five thousand cGy over 5 weeks is delivered to the tumor bed and bilateral necks in conjunction with an anterior supraclavicular field with midline bar. The tumor bed is boosted with external beam irradiation with an additional 1000–2000 cGy if the surgical margins are close or positive. Again, the spinal cord is protected after a dose of 4000–4500 cGy.

6.5.3 Intra-Oral Cone Therapy

Intraoral cone radiation therapy may be used in place of an interstitial radioisotope implant boost or external beam radiation therapy in selected patients with small, well differentiated, superficial lesions. Edentulous patients are preferable because of greater accessibility in cone placement. Patient cooperation must be assured. The intraoral cone remains in constant contact with the oral mucosa during treatment. The physician checks the correctness of cone placement daily by visualizing the field through a periscope attached to the treatment cone. Tumor margins should be tattooed either before or soon after initiation of treatment to assure adequate daily localization by the physician.

Other oral cavity sites have been treated entirely by IOC therapy. Patients must be carefully selected as follows: 1) the tumor must be located in a site accessible to cone placement; 2) tumor size should not exceed 3 cm in greatest dimension; 3) no deep invasion of underlying tissues; 4) no regional or distant metastasis; 5) cooperative patient capable of remaining still during entire treatment time (GRIFFIN et al. 1977). Any lesion with 15% or greater incidence of occult nodal metastasis should be boosted rather than treated entirely by IOC therapy. The above guidelines apply to patients with selected oral tongue or T_1-T_2 floor of mouth cancers. Fractions of 200-300 cGy, using either 100-250 kVp x-rays or 6-9 MeV electrons, are given daily. Boost doses vary between 1000-2000 cGy following a 4500-5000 cGy external beam radiotherapy course to the primary site and first echelon lymph nodes. A dose range of 5000-7000 cGy is used when IOC therapy is used alone.

Excellent results are obtainable using IOC therapy when applied to properly selected patients. Acute treatment complications such as soft tissue necrosis occur in 5-15% of cases (GRIFFIN et al. 1977; WANG et al. 1983). Healing usually occurs spontaneously when supportive care is given. Local control rates of 90-100% have been obtained (GRIFFIN et al. 1977; WANG et al. 1983).

6.5.4 Results

The poor overall survival rate of patients with squamous cell carcinoma of the oral tongue has remained the same over the past 40 years (STRONG 1979; CALLERY et al.1984; ILDSTAD et al.1983; LEIPZIG et al.1982; LEIPZIG and HOKANSON 1982). Although improvements in treatment have resulted in better local and regional control, a survival benefit has not been appreciated. Many patients with advanced head and neck tumors are still dying of distant metastases as the first site of relapse (VIKRAM et al. 1984), and both second primary neoplasms and intercurrent deaths occur frequently in this patient population. The use of adjuvant chemotherapy in these patients is being evaluated in prospective clinical trials.

One of the most important prognostic factors in oral tongue cancer is the status of the cervical lymph nodes. As the tumor size increases the incidence of both occult and clinically positive nodal metastases increases. In general, patients who convert from NO to N+ have similar survival rates as those who present with clinically positive nodes (MONACO et al. 1962; FRAZELL and LUCAS 1962). The survival of patients who remain N_0 is 2-3 times better than the survival of patients who develop cervical nodal metastasis (VERMUND et al. 1984; FRAZELL et al. 1962).

The small increase in overall survival in the past decade from the usually reported figure of 50% to 60% has generally been attributed to more patients presenting with earlier stage cancers (MENDELSON et al. 1976). Five year determinate survival rates are approximately 70-80% for stage I, 50-60% for stage II, and 25-35% for stage III disease (WANG 1983; O'BRIEN et al. 1986; MONACO et al. 1962; SPIRO and STRONG 1974; DECROIX and GHOSSEIN 1981).

Patients who have smaller cancers and relapse after initial therapy usually do so in the untreated neck (FU et al. 1976; ILDSTAD et al. 1983; WHITE 1980). Surgical salvage of local radiation failures is successful in 50-60% of patients (ILDSTAD et al. 1983; LEIPZIG et al. 1982; WHITE and BYERS 1980). Patients who have advanced neoplasms may relapse in the primary site, the neck, or both sites. For those who fail after receiving combined modality therapy, very few are successfully salvaged (WHITEHURST and DROULIAS 1977; FU et al. 1976; ILDSTAD et al. 1983; LEIPZIG et al. 1982). Most recurrences appear within 2 years of treatment, although a few authors have noted occasional recurrences of small tumors after the second year of follow up (MC QUARRIE 1986; DECROIX and GHOSSEIN 1981; MARKS et al. 1981; CARTER et al. 1985).

Local control rates for patients who receive primary radiation therapy are better when interstitial implantation is used for all or part of the treatment (WALLNER et al. 1986; GILBERT et al. 1975; DECROIX and GHOSSEIN 1981; FU et al. 1976; VERMUND et al. 1984). Approximately 25% of patients treated with high dose radiotherapy will develop a radiation complication, usually soft tissue necrosis involving the tongue surface or floor of mouth (BRADFIELD and SCRUGGS 1983; DECROIX and GHOSSEIN 1981; MARKS et al. 1981). Osteoradionecrosis occurs less frequently and orocutaneous fistulae are rare. Most occur within one year following treatment; however osteoradionecrosis has been observed as late as four or more years following therapy (FU et al. 1976; FAYOS and LAMPE 1967). Nearly all complications are managed successfully without surgical intervention. Intractable pain may be present until the soft tissue ulceration heals. Hyperbaric oxygen therapy given daily for two hours over 60 days may shorten healing time in difficult cases (DAVIS et al. 1979). A biopsy should be obtained to distinguish between radiation necrosis and recurrent tumor when the diagnosis is in doubt.

Patients with persistent post-treatment oral leukoplakia may be helped by the use of 13-cis-retinoic acid (1-2 mg/kg) per day. In a randomized study, 67% of patients who were given the drug had objective decreases in the amount of leukoplakia. However, most patients relapsed after discontinuing the drug. Cheilitis and facial skin dryness are common side effect (HONG et al. 1986).

6.6 Floor of Mouth

6.6.1 Presentation

Nearly all neoplasms arising from the floor of mouth are squamous cell carcinomas. Malignant salivary gland tumors and mucosal melanomas comprise the remaining cases. The use of tobacco products and alcohol are important etiological factors in the formation of squamous cell carcinomas at this site. Ethanol acts as a direct irritant to the thin, atrophic floor of mouth epithelium while carcinogens derived from tobacco smoke collect in pooled saliva in this area. The majority of patients are men, usually 55-60 years of age.

Most squamous cell carcinomas originate in the anterolateral and midline floor of mouth. Although the majority of early lesions are asymptomatic, approximately 25% of patients present with localized pain (HARDINGHAM et al. 1977). As lesions advance, other symptoms such as worsening pain, bleeding, ill-fitting dentures or loose teeth, neck mass, dysphagia, otalgia and speech alterations from root of tongue involvement may occur. Invasion of adjacent structures has been noted in as many as 75% of cases at presentation (HARROLD 1971). One or both sublingual glands are the most frequently involved adjacent sites, followed by tongue and gingival extension. Periosteal invasion occurs early when the tumor is close to the mandible; however actual cortical bone invasion is a late event. Bimanual examination may help in determining the degree of tumor fixation to the mandible and the extent of soft tissue induration. Dental radiographs, including occlusal views, are necessary to assess the extent of bony involvement.

Large cancers which penetrate the mylohyoid muscle may emerge in the neck near the mandibular angle after extending beyond the posterior border of the muscle. MRI scans appear most useful in differentiating tumor extension from nodal or submandibular glandular involvement. One or both of the submandibular ducts may become obstructed by tumor or edema, leading to painful glandular enlargement. Direct glandular massage may be helpful in confirming salivary obstruction. When needed, fine needle aspiration biopsy may be usefil in making the distinction between an enlarged gland vs. lymph node metastasis.

The overall incidence of clinically involved lymph nodes at diagnosis is 30-40% (ASH 1961; AYGUN et al. 1984; FAYOS 1972; FU et al. 1976; HARROLD 1971; LINDBERG 1972; JESSE et al. 1970).

Another 20-30% of patients subsequently develop nodal metastases following treatment of the primary tumor (ASH 1961; FAYOS 1972; FU et al. 1976; HARROLD 1971; JESSE et al. 1970). As tumor size increases, the risk of nodal metastasis also rises. Generally, the incidence of lymph node metastases for T_1 lesions is less than 10%, 30% for T_2, and 50-75% for T_3 and T_4 neoplasms (WANG 1983; WALLNER et al. 1986; FU et al. 1976; GUILLAMONDEGUI et al. 1980). As many as 20-25% of patients either present with or subsequently develop bilateral enlarged cervical lymph nodes. Bilateral adenopathy is possible with primary tumors in this location, since most floor of mouth tumors approach or cross the midline (WANG 1983; HARROLD 1971). In a review by Harrold (HARROLD 1971) of 224 patients who had pathologically confirmed nodal metastases following neck dissection, 53% had involvement of the first echelon lymph nodes in the submandibular and jugulodigastric regions, 37% had middle and lower nodal involvement as well, and only 10% had skip metastases to middle and lower cervical lymph nodes.

Approximately one-fourth to one-third of patients either present with or subsequently develop a second primary tumor, many of which involve the upper aerodigestive tract (FU et al. 1976; GILBERT et al. 1975; MARKS et al. 1983; NAKISSA et al. 1978; YCO and CRUIZKSHAUK 1986). The reported incidence of distant metastases is less than 10% for limited stage and 26% for stage IV cancers (FLYNN et al. 1973; FU et al. 1976; ILDSTAD et al. 1983). Since many patients are lost to follow up and few autopsies are performed, these figures may significantly underestimate the true incidence of distant metastases. The most frequent sites of involvement are lung, liver, and bone (FU et al. 1976; GILBERT et al. 1975; NAKISSA et al. 1978).

6.6.2 Treatment

Multiple factors affect the choice of therapy for patients with squamous cell carcinoma of the floor of mouth including location, depth of invasion and size of the primary tumor, degree of local extension, status of the cervical lymph nodes, patient performance status, operative risk and the potential for post-treatment sialorrhea, swallowing difficulties or mandibular injury (after surgery and radiation therapy respectively). Similar local control rates for stage I and II tumors can be achieved using either radiation therapy or surgery alone (FLYNN et al. 1973; ILDSTAD et al. 1983; NAKISSA et al. 1978;

PANJE et al. 1980). Patients are best managed surgically when periosteal involvement is suspected. Posterior floor of mouth tumors without periosteal involvement and T2 tumors which involve the under surface of the tongue may be treated by radiation therapy to preserve function. In general, alcoholics and heavy smokers tolerate acute and late tissue radiation reactions poorly. When patient compliance is in doubt, the best approach is resection.

Patients with $T_3 N_0$ lesions who are treated by radiation therapy alone with curative intent require high dose treatment, which is frequently associated with unacceptable complication rates and poorer local control rates than when surgery or combined modality therapy is used (WALLNER et al. 1986; GILBERT et al. 1975; ILDSTAD et al. 1983; PANJE et al. 1980). Therefore, combined modality therapy is the treatment of choice for patients with stage III and IV neoplasms. Patients with locally advanced cancers who are poor surgical candidates may be treated by palliative radiation therapy alone or with combined chemotherapy, in the setting of a clinical trial.

The value of elective neck irradiation has been substantiated in a number of studies (MENDENHALL et al. 1980; GILBERT et al. 1975; MENDENHALL et al. 1981; MILLION 1974; NAKISSA et al. 1978; GOFFINET et al. 1975; FLETCHER 1972; SCHNEIDER et al. 1975). Of those patients who have squamous cell carcinoma of the floor of mouth staged $T_X N_0$ at diagnosis, 20–40% will have occult carcinoma in nodes removed at elective neck dissection or will subsequently develop clinical evidence of nodal metastasis if the neck is not electively treated (CRISSMAN et al. 1980; GILBERT et al. 1975; HARROLD 1971; MILLION 1974; SPIRO et al. 1986; GOFFINET et al. 1975). Subsequent neck treatment fails in one-fourth to one-third of the patients whose primary tumor remains controlled (FLYNN et al. 1973; ILDSTAD et al. 1983; MARCUS et al. 1980; CAMPOS et al. 1977; JESSE 1977). Elective neck irradiation has proved to be an effective means of preventing subclinical disease from appearing in the neck (GILBERT et al. 1975; MENDENHALL et al. 1981; MILLION 1974; GOFFINET et al. 1975).

The addition of a supplemental anterior lower neck radiation field appears to have little effect in further decreasing the frequency of late cervical lymph node metastases. Its use, however, is associated with negligible morbidity and is recommended for moderately advanced tumors or any lesion with evidence of perineural involvement.

Large lateral opposed fields are used to treat the primary tumor and first echelon lymph nodes in the upper neck. The tumor volume is localized by a barium soaked cottonball or its equivalent and a bite block is placed to retract the tongue when it is not involved or depress the tongue when the tumor extends onto it. Cerrobend or lead blocks are designed to extend from the base of skull to thyroid notch, and include the horizontal mandibular ramus and upper sternocleidomastoid muscle. As much parotid gland as possible is excluded from the field. A lower anterior neck field, with a midline bar, is treated to a depth of 3 cm and matched to the upper opposed lateral fields. Dosimetry planning assures a homogeneous dose to the tumor volume. Forty-five hundred to 5000 cGy by external beam radiotherapy is given over 5 weeks followed by a 2500–3000 cGy 192 Iridium interstitial implantation boost to the primary floor of mouth tumor. Not all floor of mouth tumors are suitable for implantation. Lesions 4 cm or larger and those with gingival extension are relative and absolute contraindications, respectively. Large tori may also interfere with proper placement of the afterloading catheters. The risk of soft tissue ulceration and/or osteoradionecrosis are approximately 10–15% (PEREZ et al. 1966; AYGUN et al. 1984; FAYOS 1972; FLYNN et al. 1973; FU et al. 1976; HARROLD 1971; MARKS et al. 1983).

Intraoral cone irradiation (IOC) may be substituted for interstitial implantation in patients who are edentulous and have small, accessible, superficial lesions. In some early, well localized T_1 floor of mouth carcinomas with no evidence of periosteal involvement, IOC therapy or brachytherapy alone may be used to delivered total doses of 5000–6000 cGy to the tumor volume.

Patients treated by combined modality therapy receive 5000 cGy to the primary floor of mouth lesion and bilateral necks either pre- or postoperatively. Small field boost irradiation is given for close or positive surgical margins as well as for extracapsular nodal involvement. A lower anterior neck field is also treated to 5000 cGy over five weeks. The spinal cord is protected after it has received a total irradiation dose of approximately 4000 cGy.

Patients with clinically staged N_{1-2} necks may be successfully treated with radiation therapy alone; however, neck dissection is recommended if a cervical mass is still present 4 weeks or more after the radiation course has been completed.

6.6.3 Results

Survival results for patients who receive radiation therapy, surgery, or both for treatment of squamous cell carcinoma of the floor of mouth vary according to the stage of the cancer. Five year determinant survival rates are generally 70-80% for stage I, 50-70% for stage II, 25-40% for stage III, and less than 15% for stage IV tumors (WALLNER et al. 1986; FLYNN et al. 1973; FU et al. 1976; HARROLD 1971; ILDSTAD et al. 1983).

The most important prognostic factor affecting survival is clinical stage at presentation. Locally advanced cancer, manifested by a large primary tumor and/or the presence of nodal involvement, is associated with a less favorable response to aggressive therapy and, ultimately, poor survival. Tumor thickness is also an important prognostic factor in predicting treatment failure and survival. MOHIT-TABATUBAI et al. (MOHIT-TABATUBAI et al. 1986), in a review of 248 surgically treated patients who were clinically staged $T_X N_0$, found a strong correlation between tumor thickness and the subsequent development of cervical lymph node metastases. A thickness of 3.5 mm or greater was associated with a 60% risk for subsequent relapse in nodal sites. A similar review (SPIRO et al. 1986) noted that cancer related deaths were unusual in patients with oral neoplasm 2 mm or less in thickness, regardless of tumor stage.

Major causes of treatment failure are inability to control the primary tumor and cervical nodes (FLYNN et al. 1973; FU et al. 1976; HARROLD 1971; ILDSTAD et al. 1983). Most recurrences are detected within two years of treatment. Superficial cancers, when treated by local excision alone, may have unacceptably high local recurrence rates (MARKS et al. 1983; PANJE et al. 1980). When more extensive surgical procedures are performed, the 2 and 5 year local-regional control rates for stage I and II neoplasms are similar to the rates obtained by radiation therapy. (FLYNN et al. 1973; FU et al. 1976; ILDSTAD et al. 1983; NAKISSA et al. 1978; PANJE et al. 1980). For advanced cancers, combined modality therapy has been associated with improved local control over that obtained by surgery or radiation therapy alone (FLYNN et al. 1973; FU et al. 1976; ILDSTAD et al. 1983).

Local control rates for patients with stage I and II carcinomas are improved when interstitial implantation is included as part or all of the therapy (WALLNER et al. 1986; CHU and FLETCHER 1973; GILBERT et al. 1975). Care must be taken to select patients suitable for brachytherapy. Floor of mouth tissues have limited tolerance to high dose radiotherapy and interstitial implantation is contraindicated when the tumor extends onto the gingiva and mandible. The risks of soft tissue ulceration and osteoradionecrosis are increased when radiation doses to the floor of mouth and mandible exceed 6600-7000 cGy. Complication rates as high as 40% have been reported after such radiation doses have been delivered (MARKS et al.1983).

6.7 Buccal Mucosa

6.7.1 Presentation

Buccal mucosal cancers are relatively rare and occur predominately in elderly men who smoke or chew tobacco, although such neoplasms are occasionally seen today in young male snuff users. The median age at diagnosis is 65 years (BLOOM and SPIRO 1980). Nearly all of these malignancies are low grade squamous cell carcinomas and multiple biopsies may be required to establish the diagnosis. The buccal mucosa is the most frequent head and neck site of involvement by verrucous squamous cell carcinomas. Other neoplasms involving this site include sarcomas, plasmacytomas and minor salivary gland tumors.

Tumor characteristics (squamous cell carcinoma) vary from ulcerative lesions to discrete exophytic growths. A common site of involvement is the mucosa opposite the occlusal surfaces of the posterior teeth, an area of chronic irritation. Leukoplakia is frequently present and may be extensive. Occasionally, multiple lesions are present. Pain is an unusual occurrence until the lesion becomes large and invades the sensory nerves. Lateral extension into the buccal fat pad is common and advanced lesions may ultimately involve the facial skin. Obstruction of Stenson's duct leads to parotid enlargement. Inferior extension onto the mandibular gingiva and posterior growth into the pterygoid region occur in advanced cases. Involvement of the pterygoid and/ or masseter muscle may lead to trismus. Since the diagnosis may be delayed until lesions are large, the incidence of lymph node involvement at the time of diagnosis is approximately 40% (BLOOM and SPIRO 1980; CONLEY and SADOYAMA 1973; VEGERS et al. 1979). Distant metastasis, usually to lungs, may occur in as many as 20% of cases (CONLEY and SADOYAMA 1973).

6.7.2 Treatment

Small, well-defined superficial tumors are usually resected unless the lesion is located close to or involves the oral commissure, in which case radiation therapy may be used to preserve function and cosmesis. Larger (T_2) lesions may require a skin graft for primary closure after an intra-oral resection. These cancers may also be treated by radiation therapy. Control of deeply infiltrating tumors associated with significant muscular invasion is poor when radiotherapy alone is used. Stage III and IV neoplasms are best managed by resection, in combination with postoperative irradiation. If the patient is a poor surgical candidate, radiation therapy alone is an appropriate alternative treatment.

In order to spare normal contralateral oral tissues, radiotherapy is given by ipsilateral or anterior and lateral wedged pair external beam techniques. The initial treatment volume is generous since marginal failures have been reported. First echelon lymph nodes in the submandibular and jugulodiagastric regions are included in the initial treatment volume and a lower anterior neck field is included when the primary tumor is large. A dose of 5000 cGy is given to the tumor volume over 5 weeks via external beam irradiation, followed by a small field boost to the primary tumor for a total dose of 6500–7000 cGy. Although the buccal mucosa is quite tolerant to high dose irradiation, adjacent osseous structures should be protected during the boost irradiation if possible. Two thousand to 2500 cGy may also be given using electron beam or interstitial implantation techniques. Intraoral cone therapy is suitable for edentulous patients with small, well-localized tumors. If the lesion is limited to the gingivobuccal sulcus, a dental mold implant boost may be appropriate.

6.7.3 Results

The most significant prognostic factor affecting survival is the presence of nodal metastasis. Bloom et al. (BLOOM and SPIRO 1980) in a review of 121 patients found that the 5 year survival rate for patients without nodal involvement was 72% compared to 38% for those who had lymph node involvement at diagnosis.

Overall 5 year cure rates are 35–60%, regardless of treatment (ASH 1961; BLOOM and SPIRO 1980; CONLEY and SADOYAMA 1973; VEGERS et al. 1979). Ash (ASH 1961) reported that radiation therapy initially controlled the primary tumor in 53% of

223 patients who had early lesions and 25% of 175 patients with advanced cancers. For those who failed initial therapy, subsequent treatment salvaged 43% of patients with early lesions and 25% of those with advanced neoplasms.

The risk of local recurrence increases with tumor stage. MacComb, et al. (MACCOMB 1967) analyzed 115 patients treated by surgery, radiation therapy, or both, at the M.D. Anderson Hospital between 1947–1962. The local recurrence rate was 10% for stage I, 12% for stage II and III, and 38% for stage IV tumors.

6.8 Verrucous Carcinomas

The term "verrucous carcinoma" was first used by Ackerman in 1948 to describe a well-differentiated keratinizing variant of squamous carcinoma. Oral verrucous carcinomas are usually observed in elderly men who have a long history of tobacco use. The tumor is an exophytic, warty mass, nearly always associated with extensive leukoplakia. The diagnosis of malignancy is based upon the invasive quality of the deep margin, which pushes rather than infiltrates adjacent tissues. Biopsies of the full tumor thickness are required for accurate histopathological diagnosis. Superficial biopsies are frequently misinterpreted as benign proliferation.

Nearly 50% of all oral verrucous tumors involve the buccal mucosa (MACDONALD et al. 1982). The next most frequent site is the gingiva. Occasionally, more than one lesion may be present at diagnosis. Large buccal and bulky gingival tumors may become fixed to the periosteum where bony invasion and extensive destruction eventually occur. These tumors rarely metastasize either to regional lymph nodes or distantly. Reactive lymph node enlargement has been noted in some patients and is felt to be the result of an inflammatory process caused by or associated with the tumor.

The use of radiation therapy in the treatment of verrucous carcinomas is controversial; therefore, resection has generally been recommended for such patients. A relatively high rate of local recurrence has been observed following radiation therapy of verrucous carcinomas and several cases of anaplastic transformation to a metastasizing, usually fatal lesion have been reported. This phenomenon occurred within months after the completion of radiation therapy. MacDonald (MACDONALD et al. 1982) in a 1982 literature review concluded that only 4 properly documented cases of anaplastic transfor-

Table 6-5. Comparison of treatment results by stage for verrucous carcinoma of the oral cavity

Treatment	Author	Control	T_1	T_2	T_3	T_4
Surgery	MEDINA et al. (1984)	Initial control	23/28 (82%)	33/38 (87%)	10/14 (71%)	4/6 (67%)
		Surgical salvage	5/5	3/5	2/4	1/2
		Overall control	28/28 (100%)	36/38 (95%)	12/14 (86%)	5/6 (83%)
XRT	MEDINA et al. (1984)	Initial control	1/1 (100%)	2/2 (100%)	4/5 (80%)	0/4 (0%)
		Surgical salvage			1/1	2/4
		Overall control			5/5 (100%)	2/4 (50%)
	MEMULA et al. (1980)	Initial control	1/1 (100%)	11/17 (60%)	3/5 (60%)[a]	4/9 (44%)
		Surgical salvage		6/6	–	
		Overall control		17/17 (100%)		
	SCHWADE et al. (1986)	Initial control	0/1[b]	3/3 (100%)	2/3 (67%)[c]	
		Surgical salvage	–			
		Overall control	–			

[a] Additional irradiation given in 1 case
[b] Recurrence 8 yrs after initial treatment
[c] 1 PT had partial regression @ 4 months after Tx when he expired of an intercurrent illness
   1 PT had complete regression @ 9 months after Tx when he expired of an intercurrent illness

mation following radiation therapy have been recorded. Three of the four cases were reported by Kraus and Perez-Mesa (KRAUS and PEREZ-MESA 1966) and Perez (PEREZ et al. 1966) in 1966. All 3 of these patients had tumors larger than 4 cm in diameter.

It is possible that large verrucous lesions contain clones of less differentiated cells which, when stimulated, give rise to less differentiated tumors. This speculation has been confirmed in a review by Medina (MEDINA et al. 1984) of 104 patients treated at the M.D. Anderson Hospital. He noted a tendency of verrucous carcinomas of recur as less differentiated squamous carcinomas regardless of treatment. Included in this series were 20 surgically treated patients who were felt to have hybrid tumors characterized by foci of less differentiated squamous carcinoma within the surgical specimens. Despite similar clinical characteristics, the hybrid tumors recurred more frequently than the pure verrucous carcinomas (30% vs. 18%) and all but one recurrence appeared more aggressive histopathologically. A transformation process, then, may represent an uncommon event in the natural history of this tumor. Since the initial reports by Kraus and Perez concerning radiation-induced anaplastic transformation in 1966, nearly 75 patients have been treated with radiation therapy at several institutions and not a single case of anaplastic transformation has been observed. (BURNS et al. 1980; MEDINA et al. 1984; MEMULA et al. 1980; SCHWADE et al. 1976).

Fairly high local failure rates have been reported; however, few of the early studies analyzed local re-

currence according to stage and a disproportionately large percentage of patients treated by radiation therapy had extensive lesions at the time of diagnosis. Recent reviews have included TNM staging data (Table 6-5). While the numbers of patients treated with curative intent by radiation therapy are limited, it appears that similar results are obtained in patients who have limited or moderately advanced cancers, whether surgery or radiation therapy is used.

6.9 Gingiva and Hard Palate

6.9.1 Presentation

The most frequent presenting symptom of gingival cancers is pain associated with an ulcerative lesion which bleeds easily when traumatized. The majority of tumors are squamous cell carcinomas. Verrucous carcinomas and mucosal melanomas occur rarely. Minor salivary gland tumors occur in the hard palate, but not in the gingiva, since glandular tissue is not present in the alveolar ridge mucosa. Extensive leukoplakic involvement occurs in nearly 25% of cases (BYERS et al. 1981). Slightly more than one-half of the patients report no smoking history or use of ethanol (BYERS et al. 1981). The average age at diagnosis is 63 years (BYERS et al. 1981).

The posterior mandibular region is the most frequent site of gingival squamous cell carcinomas. Bone involvement occurs early and is pathologically identified in 36–56% of patients (BYERS et al.

1981; SWEARINGEN et al. 1966; WHITEHOUSE 1976). Large lesions extend to adjacent structures such as the buccal mucosa, floor of mouth, or hard palate. Invasion of the maxillary antrum is a late finding for maxillary alveolar ridge squamous cell carcinomas unless direct invasion occurs via the sockets of recently extracted teeth. Lymph node involvement at diagnosis occurs in approximately 35% of patients (ASH 1961; LANDA and ZAREM 1973; LEE and WILSON 1973).

Neoplasms arising from the retromolar trigone may be associated with local pain or otalgia. Early involvement of the anterior tonsillar pillars, soft palate, gingiva, or buccal mucosa are also noted. Invasion into the pterygomandibular space may lead to parasthesias from inferior alveolar nerve invasion, otalgia from lingual nerve involvement, or trismus from pterygoid muscle invasion. Bone invasion occurs in only 15% of cases (WILLIN et al. 1975) because a tendinous band of tissue, the pterygomandibular raphe, separates the mucosa from the ascending mandibular ramus and impedes penetration. The median age at diagnosis is 62 years and nearly all patients are heavy smokers (WILLIN et al. 1975). Fifty per cent are admitted alcoholics (WILLIN et al. 1975). Lymph node involvement at diagnosis has been reported to be 30–40% (BAKER and FLETCHER 1977; BYERS et al. 1984).

The hard palate is the most frequently involved oral cavity site for malignant minor salivary gland tumors, which usually occur as an asymptomatic lump or irregularity in the palatal contour. Both sexes are affected equally, but patients with these malignancies are usually younger than those with squamous cell carcinomas (ILDSTAD et al. 1983). The incidence of lymph node involvement at diagnosis varies according to histology. Adenoid cystic is the most common variant of malignant salivary gland tumors; it rarely metastasizes to cervical lymph nodes (<15%) (SPIRO et al. 1973).

Squamous cell carcinomas of the hard palate, which occur less frequently than malignant salivary gland tumors, often present as non-healing ulcerative lesions. The majority of patients are males, 60 years of age or older (RATZER et al. 1970). The incidence of lymph node involvement at the time of diagnosis is 15–20% (WANG 1983). Large lesions may extend onto the gingiva, hard palate, tonsillar pillars, and buccal mucosa. Some tumors extend along the greater palatine nerve to the pterygomandibular fossa and gain access to the CNS through the foramen rotundum.

Intra-alveolar tumors may be either primary malignancies arising from the alveolar ridge structures or metastases from such primary sites as the prostate, breast, or lung. They all present as submucosal masses and are frequently associated with dental pain, numbness, or loose teeth.

Primary intra-alveolar tumors are rare and include ameloblastomas, osteogenic sarcomas, and other sarcomas. Ameloblastomas are epithelial tumors which appear histologically benign, but behave as low grade malignancies and cause local osseous destruction. They frequently recur following inadequate resection. Osteogenic sarcomas arising from the mandible have better 5 year survival rates than similar tumors arising from the long bones (LOOSER and KUEHN 1976). Most mandibular intra-alveolar neoplasms arise from the posterior alveolar ridge (RATZER et al. 1970).

6.9.2 Treatment-Gingiva

Most T_1 and nearly all T_2 gingival neoplasms should be resected. However, radiation therapy may be considered for superficial, small neoplasms without bone erosion. Mandible roentgenograms, including occlusal views, must be obtained and carefully reviewed to differentiate between smooth erosive defects caused by the margin of slowly growing tumors and frank neoplastic bone invasion with loss of cortical continuity. The latter is rarely curable by radiation therapy alone. Stage III and IV lesions are best managed by resection followed by 5000–6000 cGy postoperative irradiation, depending on the status of the surgical margins.

Anterior tumors are treated by parallel opposed lateral fields. Posterior lesions are usually treated by anterior and lateral wedge pair photon or mixed photon and electron beam fields. Care is taken to include adequate margins since extensive tumor spread within the subperiosteal lymphatic plexus may occur. Forty-five hundred to 5000 cGy are given to a large volume which includes the first echelon lymph nodes, followed by a 1500–2000 cGy reduced field boost to the primary lesion, when treating by radiation therapy alone. When feasible, intraoral cone therapy may be used for all or part of the treatment. Brachytherapy is limited to dental mold or gingival looping techniques since interstitial sources placed through the gingival mucosa may lead to mandibular exposure or osteoradionecrosis.

6.9.3 Treatment-Retromolar Trigone

Local control rates for Stage I and II squamous cell carcinomas are equal with either resection or radiation therapy (BYERS et al. 1984). Surgery is preferred for stage III and IV lesions except when the soft palate is extensively involved. If the soft palate is resected, a palatal obturator is required to prevent an unacceptable functional defect. High radiation doses are required for curative treatment by radiation therapy alone; usually 6500–7000 cGy over 6 to 7 weeks. A series of reduced fields using combination photon and electron beams minimizes the irradiation dose to normal tissue. The submandibular and jugulodigastric lymph nodes are included in the treatment volume. The lower neck is treated to 5000 cGy using a matched anterior field, calculated to a depth of 3 cm. Again, the spinal cord receives no more than 4000–4500 cGy during the treatment course. Contralateral nodal involvement at diagnosis is rare but has occurred following initial treatment (BYERS et al. 1984). Postoperative irradiation is required for stage III and IV neoplasms.

6.9.4 Treatment – Hard Palate

Squamous cell carcinomas of the hard palate are nearly always managed surgically since bone involvement occurs early. Selected early lesions may be treated with radiation therapy for curative intent with good results (WANG 1983). Postoperative irradiation is used when the surgical margins are either close or involved. The necks are treated when cervical lymph nodes are involved or the tumor is advanced.

The entire palate and pterygopalatine fossa are included in the initial treatment volume. Parallel lateral opposed fields extend from the base of skull to upper neck. Prescribed doses are 5000 cGy to the initial volume followed by 1500–2000 cGy boost to the surgical bed or primary lesion. (Spinal cord radiation dose: <4000 cGy). When feasible, intraoral cone therapy should be considered for the boost treatment.

Malignant minor salivary gland tumors are usually resected. Postoperative irradiation should be included, since a high local recurrence rate has been noted following surgery alone. Combined therapy has resulted in better local control than either surgery or radiation therapy alone (SIMPSON et al. 1986, SIMPSON et al. 1984) and has provided longer disease free survival.

6.9.5 Treatment – Intra-alveolar Tumors

Ameloblastomas were considered radioresistant until the modern era of megavoltage irradiation. Prescribed doses of 4500 cGy in 4 weeks have been curative when given as initial treatment or postoperatively for involved margins, but should be avoided in young patients to decrease the risk of a late radiation induced cancer. (ATKINSON et al. 1984). Radiation therapy has also been used for local recurrences but should be avoided in young patients. The entire hemimandible is treated, usually via anterior and lateral wedged portals. Successful therapy of maxillary gingival tumors requires careful planning to minimize radiation doses to the orbital contents while still irradiating the orbital floor. Postoperative treatment of sarcomas requires radiation doses of 5500–6600 cGy. The fields are designed according to the particular anatomic site and extent of involvement.

6.9.6 Results

The 3 and 5 year survival rates for squamous cell carcinomas of the gingiva, retromolar trigone, or hard palate range from 20–58% (WANG 1983; LOVE et al. 1977; BYERS et al. 1984; KONRAD et al. 1978). Special attention must be paid to the presence or absence of bony invasion, lymph node involvement, or extension to adjacent structures. Local recurrence rates for advanced tumors may be as high as 50% following either surgical resection or primary radiotherapy (BYERS et al. 1981; LOVE et al. 1977; BYERS et al. 1984; FOYOS 1973). Only a few patients with local/regional recurrences are successfully salvaged.

6.10 Brachytherapy – Oral Cavity

Interstitial implantation of accessible oral lesions is not a new technique. Early in the practice of therapeutic radiology radium-226 needles were used for temporary implantation of oral tongue and floor of mouth cancers. Radon-222 seeds were also inserted permanently into primary and recurrent tumors of the oral cavity and oropharynx. Proper placement of the radium-226 sources was difficult and often resulted in excessive radiation doses to radiologists and nursing personnel. Safe implants required haste in performing the procedures, which often resulted in poor source position and under-or overdoses of tumor and normal tissue volumes.

In the last two decades, the use of afterloading techniques and the availability of new isotopes combined with computerized dosimetry, has rejuvenated the practice of brachytherapy and made such procedures easier to perform with greater accuracy (NEBLETT et al. 1985). The most commonly used isotope for permanent implantation in the United States at present is iridium-192, with a half life of 74.2 days, and a gamma ray energy of approximately 340 KV. Permanent implants are usually performed with iodine-125 seeds, which have a low gamma ray energy (approximately 30 KV) and a long half life, 60 days. Gold-198 seeds (410 KV, 2.7 day half life) are less commonly used today, primarily due to the high radiation dose which the radiotherapist receives at the time of seed insertion.

6.11 Removable Implants – Oral Cavity

Most reviews of the treatment of oral tongue cancers reveal that improved local control is obtained when interstitial irradiation is used, either alone for small, superficial tumors, or combined with external beam irradiation. (GILBERT et al. 1975; FU et al. 1976; HORIUCHI et al. 1982; PUTHAWALA et al. 1981; PIERQUIN et al. 1971; SYED et al. 1977). To perform an adequate implant, the afterloading tubes may be placed in the tongue either in the form of regularly spaced loops or in multiple rows of blind end catheters, with isotope afterloading taking place through the submental open end of the tubes. It is extremely important that the tumor volume be adequately covered by the implant. Since oral squamous carcinomas may invade widely through the interdigitating tongue muscles, the minimum implant volume should encompass the tumor with at least 2 cm margins, similar to the amount of tissue removed by a hemiglossectomy (Fig. 6-4).

In general, 2-3 weeks after a 4000-5000 cGy fractioned external beam radiation course, the loop or multiple blind end parallel row implant is performed. An additional 2500-3000 cGy are delivered to the periphery of the desired implant volume in two to three days, at which time the implant is removed. Great care must be taken to avoid the lingual artery and the mandible. Keeping the latter structure in the low dose volume reduces the risk of subsequent osteoradionecrosis. In recent years, high intensity iodine-125 sources have been used as a iridium-192 substitute, and with this low energy gamma emitting isotope, it is feasible to provide intraoral shielding for the mandible and other sensitive structures, to minimize the risk of subsequent soft tissue and bone necrosis.

Superficial T_1 cancers of the floor of mouth, which have a low risk of metastasizing to the submental and submandibular lymph nodes may also be treated by interstitial implantation alone. However, larger tumors may require combined external beam and interstitial irradiation, as noted previously for oral tongue cancers (Fig. 6-5). For interstitial implantation of the floor of mouth to be successful without undue risk of soft tissue or mandibular necrosis, the neoplasm should be relatively superficial or have responded well to a prior planned course of external beam irradiation, should not invade the adjacent alveolar ridge, and be unattached to the mandibular periosteum. In general, multiple blind end tubes are preferable to loops in the floor of mouth, since "hot spots" near the mandibular periosteum may be more easily avoided by the former technique. Either iridium-192 or iodine-125 high intensity sources may be used for such implants, but if the latter are chosen, the adjacent mandible may be protected by shielding to prevent excessive radiation doses to this structure.

Interstitial implantation is difficult for lesions of the hard palate and the maxillary and mandibular alveolar ridges. If interstitial irradiation is to be considered for an alveolar ridge neoplasm, techniques should be used in which the sources loop over the ridge and are secured into the soft tissues on either side, so as to minimize the risk of bone exposure. Carcinomas of the lip, buccal area and occasionally the retromolar trigone are accessible to implantation techniques. Removable afterloading sources may be introduced into these areas. It is often difficult to insert sources and tubes into the buccal area with adequate spacing, so most patients, at present, have resection and postoperative radiation for these cancers. However, lesions of the vermilion and external border of the lip are readily amenable to afterloading implantation as primary therapy or as a boost after a planned external beam radiation course.

Cervical lymph node metastases, either at the time of diagnosis or after postsurgical and/or post irradiation failure, may be treated by resection and iodine-125 seed implantation, usually via an absorbable suture carrier (PALOS et al. 1980). These implants are preplanned in a manner similar to removable implants, so that the spacing and symmetry of the sources is known prior to the implant procedure (SANDOR et al. 1979). The tumor

Fig. 6-4 a, b. Localizing 192-Ir implant radiographs, 40 year old woman with $T_2 N_0$ squamous carcinoma of lateral oral tongue. She received a pre-implant radiation dose of 5000 rads to the tongue and cervical lymph nodes in 5 weeks, (200 per day, 5 fractions per week – 4 MeV Linc), followed 3 weeks later by 192-Ir seed tongue implantation. Through a submental approach, 5 trocar pairs were inserted into the oral tongue, (15 mm separation between pairs, 20–25 mm between trocars); hollow nylon tubes were then positioned in their place, forming afterloading loops. A blind end trocar was then positioned in the anterior tongue which allowed irradiation of the entire hemi tongue from the circumvallate papillae to the tip (**a**). The 192-Ir seeds were afterloaded on the day of implantation and 1800 rads were delivered to a 68 cc tongue volume in 53 hrs (**b**) at which time the implant was removed. The patient has remained without evidence of disease for 18 months and has normal tongue function

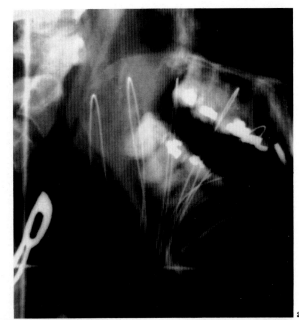

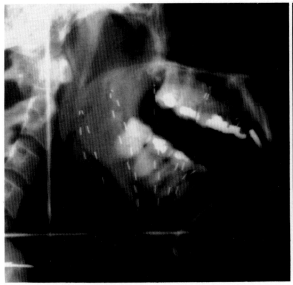

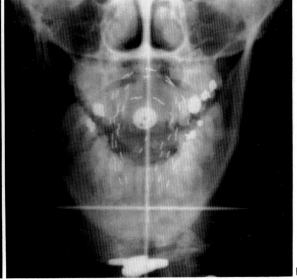

mass is resected as completely as possible and the sterile iodine seed containing Vicryl absorbable sutures are sewn into place with regular spacing across the carotid sheath when this structure is involved by the tumor. Placement is done prior to wound closure. Local control rates of approximately 80% may be obtained by this technique (FEE et al. 1983; GOFFINET et al. 1985; VIKRAM et al. 1983). If myocutaneous or other thick flaps are used, the primary risks of skin ulceration or necrosis from this procedure may be avoided.

Cervical lymph node masses have also been successfully implanted either percutaneously or during a neck dissection by afterloading iridium-192 seed techniques. These removable cervical implants also produce high local control rates.

6.12 Hyperthermia

The final radiotherapeutic option is interstitial microwave or radiofrequency-induced hyperthermia. Radiofrequency heating requires the use of hollow stainless steel needles or modified catheters inserted into the tumor volume under anesthesia. A hyper-

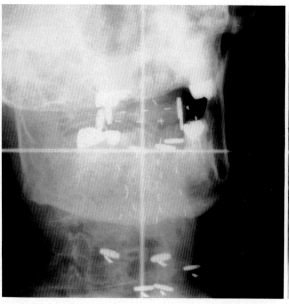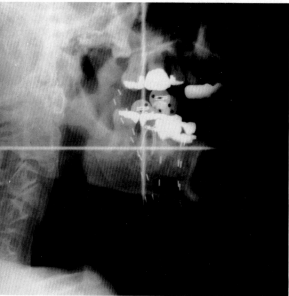

Fig. 6-5. Localizing radiographs, 56 year old male with a T_1N_0 squamous cell carcinoma of the anterior floor of mouth, post excisional biopsy. Prior to the initiation of a 5000 rad external beam radiation course to the primary site and regional lymph nodes, 3 blind end afterloading catheters were inserted submentally, into the anterior floor of mouth, using the trocar technique. These catheters were positioned at least 5 mm from the inner table of the mandible. A more posteriorly placed loop treated the oral tongue posterior to the frenulum. Two additional transverse catheters were inserted more anteriorly into the mobile tongue to ensure adequate coverage of this potential area of tumor extension. 2595 rads were delivered to a 37 cc volume in 86.5 hrs, at which time the implant was removed. The patient remains well, without side effects, 7 years after implantation

thermia session for 45 minutes is usually given before the hollow needles or tubes are loaded with iridium-192 sources and a second session is frequently given after removal of the radioisotope. A drawback to this type of interstitial hyperthermia is the discomfort and possible misalignment of rigid metallic needles which must remain in place for several days. More flexible, teflon catheters (16 gauge angiocaths) are used for microwave interstitial heating. Coaxial microwave antennas are inserted inside each catheter for subsequent heating. The catheters are evenly spaced 10-12 mm apart. Afterloading iridium-192 ribbons are positioned inside each catheter after the patient has returned to the hospital room. The radioisotope is temporarily removed for the hyperthermia sessions, which are spaced 72-96 hours apart. Separate catheters are placed into the tumor volume for thermometry pur-

poses. Disadvantages include restriction to 4-5 cm heating volume and poor heating at the terminal portion of each antenna.

Clinical trials utilizing low dose rate interstitial radiation with interstitial hyperthermia have reported encouraging results (ARISTIZABAL and OLESON 1984; EMAMI et al. 1984; COSSET et al. 1985; PUTHAWALA et al. 1986; GOFFINET et al. submitted 1988). Complete response rates of 70-80% have been obtained in patients who have previously failed high dose definitive or preoperative irradiation. Follow-up evaluation has been short, often three to six months. Since similar response rates have been observed in closely matched patients who received interstitial radiation therapy alone, additional investigations regarding the efficacy of interstitial thermoradiotherapy is needed.

References

Aristizabal SA, Oleson JR (1984) Combined interstitial irradiation and localized current field hyperthermia: Results and conclusions from clinical studies. Cancer Res 44: 4457s-4760s

Ash CL (1961) Oral cancer: A twenty-five year study (Janeway Lecture) Am J Roentgenol 87: 417-430

Ashley FL, McConnell OV, Machida R, Sterling HE, Galloway D, Grazer F (1965) Carcinoma of the lip. A comparison of five year results after irradiation and surgical therapy. Am J Surg 110: 549-551

Atkinson CH, Harwood AR, Cummings BJ (1984) Ameloblastoma of the jaw. A reappraisal of the role of megavoltage irradiation. Cancer 53: 869-873

Aygun C, Salazar DM, Sewchand W, Amornmarn R, Prempree T (1984) Carcinoma of the floor of mouth: A 20-year experience. Int J Radiat Oncol Biol Phys 10: 619–626

Baker SR, Krause CJ (1950) Carcinoma of the lip. Laryngoscope 90: 1–9

Barker JL, Fletcher GH (1977) Time, dose and tumor volume relationships in megavoltage irradiation of squamous cell carcinoma of the retromolar trigone and anterior tonsillar pillar. Int J Radiat Oncol Biol Phys 2: 407–414

Beumer J, Harrison R, Sanders B, Kurrasch M (1983) Post radiation dental extractions: A review of the literature and a report of 72 episodes. Head Neck Surg 198: 581–586

Bloom ND, Spiro RH (1980) Carcinoma of the cheek mucosa. A retrospective analysis. Am J Surg 140: 556–559

Bradfield JS, Scruggs RP (1983) Carcinoma of the mobile tongue: Incidence of cervical metastases in early lesions related to method of primary treatment. Laryngoscope 93: 1332–1336

Brown RG, Poole MD, Calamel PM, Bakamjian VY (1976) Advanced and recurrent squamous carcinoma of the lower lip. Am J Surg 132: 492–497

Burns HP, van Nostrand P, Palmer JA (1980) Verrucous carcinoma of the oral cavity: Management by radiotherapy and surgery. Can J Surg 23: 19–25

Byers RM, O'Brien J, Waxler J (1978) The therapeutic and prognostic implications of nerve invasion in cancer of the lower lip. Int J Radiat Oncol Biol Phys 4: 215–217

Byers RM, Anderson B, Schwarz EA, Fields RS, Meoz R (1984) Treatment of squamous carcinoma of the retromolar trigone. Am J Clin Oncol 7: 647–652

Byers RM, Newman R, Russell N, Yue A (1981) Results of treatment for squamous cell carcinoma of the lower gum. Cancer 47: 2236–2238

Callery CD, Spiro RH, Strong EW (1984) Changing trends in the management of squamous carcinoma of the tongue. Am J Surg 148: 449–454

Campos Jl, Lampe I, Fayos JV (1977) Radiotherapy of carcinoma of the floor of mouth. Radiology 99: 677–682

Carter I, Barr LC, O'Brien CJ, Soo KC, Shaw HJ (1985) Transcapular spread of metastatic squamous cell carcinoma from cervical lymph nodes. Amer J Surg 150: 495–499

Chu A, Fletcher GH (1973) Incidence and causes of failures to control by irradiation the primary lesion in squamous cell carcinomas of the anterior two-thirds of the tongue and floor of mouth. Am J Roentgen 3: 502–508

Conley J, Sadoyama JA (1973) Squamous cell carcinoma of the buccal mucosa. A review of 90 cases. Arch Otolaryngol 97: 330–333

Cossett JM, Dutreix J, Haie C, Gerbaulet A, Janoray P, Dewar JA (1985) Interstitial thermoradiotherapy: a technical and clinical study of 29 implantations performed at the Institut Gustave-Roussy. Int J Hyperthermia 1: 3–13

Crissman JD, Gluckman J, Whitely J, Quenelle D (1980) Squamous cell carcinoma of the floor of mouth. Head Neck Surg 3: 2–7

Davis JC, Dunn JM, Gates GA, Heimbach RD (1979) Hyperbaric oxygen. A new adjunct in the management of radiation necrosis. Arch Otolaryngol 105: 58–61

Decroix Y, Ghossein NA (1981a) Experience of the Curie Institute in treatment of cancer of the mobile tongue I. Treatment policies and result. Cancer 47: 496–502

Decroix Y, Ghossein NA (1981b) Experience of the Curie Institute in treatment of carcinoma of the mobile tongue II. Management of the neck nodes. Cancer 47: 503–508

Dreizen, Daley T, Drane J (1977) Prevention of xerostomia-related dental caries in irradiated cancer patients. J Dental Res 56: 99–103

Emami B, Marks JE, Perez CA, Nussbaum GH, Leybovich L, Von Gerichten D (1984) Interstitial thermoradiotherapy in the treatment of recurrent/residual malignant tumors. Am J Clin Oncol 7: 699–704

Fayos FV (1972) Management of squamous cell carcinoma of the floor of mouth. Am J Surg 123: 706–711

Fayos JV (1973) Carcinoma of the mandible. Result of radiation therapy. Acta Radiol [Ther] (Stock) 12: 376–386

Fayos JV, Lampe I (1967) Radiotherapy of squamous cell carcinoma of the oral portion of the tongue. Arch Surg 94: 316–321

Fayos JV, Lampe I (1972) The therapeutic problem of metastatis neck adenopathy. Am J Roentgen 114: 65–75

Fazekas JT, Sommer C, Kramer S (1983) Tumor regression and other prognosticators in advanced head and neck cancers: A sequel to the RTOG methotrexate study. Int J Radiat Oncol Biol Phys 9: 957–964

Fee WE, Goffinet DG, Paryani S, Goode RL, Levine PA, Hopp ML (1983) Intraoperative iodine 125 implants: Their use in large tumors in the neck attached to the carotid artery. Arch Otolaryngol 109: 727–730

Flamant R, Hayem M, Lazar P, Denoix P (1964) Cancer of the tongue. A study of 904 cases. Cancer 17: 377–385

Fletcher GH (1972) Elective irradiation of subclinical disease in cancer of the head and neck. Cancer 29: 1450–1454

Flynn MB, Mullins FX, Moore C (1973) Selection of treatment in squamous carcinoma of the floor of mouth. Am J Surg 126: 477–481

Frazell EL (1971) The James Ewing Lecture. A review of the treatment of cancer of the mobile portion of the tongue. Cancer 28: 1178–1181

Frazell EI, Lucas JC (1962) Cancer of the tongue. Report of the management of 1554 patients. Cancer 15: 1085–1099

Frierson HF, Cooper PH (1986) Prognostic factors in squamous cell carcinoma of the lower lip. Human Pathology 17: 346–354

Fu KK, Lichter A, Galante M (1976a) Carcinoma of the floor of mouth: An analysis of treatment results and the sites and causes of failures. Int J Radiat Oncol Biol Phys 1: 829–837

Fu KK, Ray JW, Chan EK, Phillips TL (1976b) External and interstitial radiation therapy of carcinoma of the oral tongue. A review of 32 years' experience. Am J Roentgen 126: 107–115

Gilbert EH, Goffinet DR, Bagshaw MA (1975) Carcinoma of the oral tongue and floor of mouth: 15 years experience with linear accelerator therapy. Cancer 35: 1517–1524

Gladstone WD, Kerr HD (1958) Epidermoid carcinoma of the lower lip. Results of radiation therapy of the local lesion. Am J Roentgen 79: 101–113

Goffinet DR, Gilbert EH, Weller SA, Bagshaw MA (1975) Irradiation of clinically uninvolved cervical lymph nodes. Cancer J Otolaryngol 4: 927–933

Goffinet DR, Martinez A, Pooler D, Palos B, Cox R (1981) (Book Chapter) Brachytheray Renaissance Frontiers of Radiation Therapy and Oncology. Karger, Basel 15: 43–57

Goffinet DR, Martinez A, Fee WA (1985) 125/I vicryl suture implants as a marginal adjuvant in cancer of the head and neck. Int J Radiat Oncol Biol Phys 11: 399–402

Goffinet DR, Prionas SD, Kapp DS, Fessenden P, Hahan CM, Lohrbach AW, Mariscal JM, Bagshaw MA (submitted May 1988) Interstitial ^{192}Ir flexible catheter radiofrequency hyperthermia treatments of head and neck and recurrent pelvic carcinomas

Griffin TW, Gerdes AJ, Simko TG, Parker RG (1977) Peroral irradiation for limited carcinoma of the oral cavity. Int J Radiat Oncol Biol Phys 2: 333–335

Guillamondegui OM, Oliver B, Hayden R (1980) Cancer of the anterior floor of mouth. Am J Surg 140: 560–562

Hardingham M, Dalley VM, Shaw HJ (1977) Cancer of the floor of mouth: Clinical features and results of treatment. Clinical Oncol 3: 227–246

Harrold CC (1971) Management of cancer of the floor of mouth. Am J Surg 122: 487–493

Heller KS, Shah JP (1979) Carcinoma of the lip. Am J Surg 138: 600–603

Hendricks JL, Mendelson BC, Woods JE (1977) Invasive carcinoma of the lower lip. Surg Clin North Am 57: 837–844

Hong WK, Endicott J, Itri LM, Doos W (1986) 13-is-retinoic acid in the treatment of oral leukoplakia. NEJM 315: 1501–1505

Horiuchi J, Okuyama T, Shibuya H, Takeda M (1982) Results of brachytherapy for cancer of the tongue with special emphasis on local prognosis. Int J Radiat Oncol Biol Phys 8: 829–835

Hornback NB, Shidnia H (1978) Carcinoma of the lower lip. Treatment results at Indiana University Hospitals. Cancer 41: 352–357

Ildstad ST, Bigelow ME, Remensynder JP (1983a) Intraoral cancer at the Massachusetts General Hospital. Squamous cell carcinoma of the floor of mouth. Ann Surg 197: 34–41

Ildstad ST, Bigelow ME, Remensnyder JP (1983b) Squamous cell carcinoma of the mobile tongue. Clinical behavior and results of current therapeutic modalities. Am J Surg 145: 443–449

Jesse RH (1977) The philosophy of treatment of neck nodes. Ear Nose Throat J 56: 58–63

Jesse RH, Barkley HT, Lindberg RD, Fletcher GH (1970) Cancer of the oral cavity. Is elective neck dissection beneficial? An J Surg 120: 505–508

Jorgensen K, Elbrond D, Anderson AP (1973) Carcinoma of the lip. A series of 869 cases. Acta Radiol 12: 177–190

Kalnins IK, Leonard AG, Sako K (1977) Correlation between prognosis and degree of lymph node involvement in carcinoma of the oral cavity. Am J Surg 134: 450–454

Konrad HR, Canalis RF, Calaterra TC (1978) Epidermoid carcinoma of the palate. Arch Otolaryng 104: 208–212

Kraus FT, Perez-Mesa C (1966) Verrucous carcinoma. Clinical and pathologic study of 105 cases involving oral cavity, larynx and genitalia. Cancer 19: 26–38

Landa SJF, Zarem HA (1973) Cancer of the floor of mouth and the gingiva. Surg Clin N Am 53: 135–145

Lee JG, Litton WB (1972) Symposium on malignancy II. Occult regional metastasis: carcinoma of the oral tongue. Laryngoscope 1273–1281

Lee ES, Wilson JSP (1973) Carcinoma involving the lower alveolus. An appraisal of past results and an account of current management. Brit J Surg 60: 85–107

Leipzig B, Hokanson JA (1982) Treatment of cervical lymph nodes in carcinoma of the tongue. Head Neck Surg 5: 3–9

Leipzig B, Cummings CW, Johnson JT, Chung CT, Sagerman RH (1982) Carcinoma of the anterior tongue. Ann Otol Rhinog Laryngol 91: 94–97

Lindberg R (1972) Distribution of cervical lymph node metastases for squamous cell carcinoma of the upper respiratory and digestive tract. Cancer 6: 1446–1449

Looser KG, Kuehn PG (1976) Primary tumors of the mandible. A study of 49 cases. Am J Surg 132: 608–614

Love R, Stewart IF, Coy P (1977) Upper alveolar carcinoma – a 30 year survey. J Otolaryngol 6: 393–398

MacComb WS (1967) Cancer of the head and neck. Baltimore, Williams & Wilkin pp 89–151

MacKay EN, Seller AH (1964) A statistical review of carcinoma of the lip. Can Med Assoc J 90: 670–672

Mahoney LG (1969) Resection of cervical lymph nodes in carcinoma of the lip. Results in 12 patients. Can J Surg 12: 40–43

Marchetta FC, Sako K (1975) Preoperative irradiation for squamous cell carcinoma of the head and neck. Does it improve five year survival or control figures? Am J Surg 130: 487–488

Marcus RB, Million RR, Mitchell TP (1980) A preloaded, custom-designed implantation device for stage T_1–T_2 carcinoma of the floor of mouth. Int J Radiat Oncol Biol Phys 6: 111–113

Marks JE, Lee F, Freeman RB, Zivnuska FR, Ogura JH (1981) Carcinoma of the oral tongue: A study of patient selection and treatment results. Laryngoscope 91: 1548–1559

Marks JE, Lee F, Smith PG, Ogura JH (1983) Floor of mouth cancer: Patient selection and treatment results. Laryngoscope 93: 475–480

Mashberg A, Meyers H (1976) Anatomical site and size of 222 early asymptomatic oral squamous cell carcinomas. A continuing prospective study of oral cancer. Cancer 37: 2149–2157

McDonald JS, Crissman JD, Gluckman JL (1982) Verrucous carcinoma of the oral cavity. Head Neck Surg 5: 22–28

McQuarrie DG (1986) Carcinoma of the tongue - selecting appropriate therapy. Curr Probl Surg 23: 562–653

Medina JE, Dichtel W, Lunda MA (1984) Verrucous-squamous carcinomas of the oral cavity. A clinicopathologic study of 104 cases. Arch Otolaryngol 110: 437–440

Memula N, Ridenhour G, Doss Ll (1980) Radiotherapeutic management of oral cavity verrucous carcinoma (abstr). Int J Radiat Oncol Biol Phys 6: 1404

Mendelson BC, Woods JE, Beahrs OH (1976) Neck dissection in the treatment of carcinoma of the anterior two-thirds of the tongue. Surg Gyn & Obstet 143: 75–80

Mendenhall WM, Million RR, Cassisi NJ (1980) Elective neck irradiation in squamous cell carcinoma of the head and neck. Head Neck Surg 3: 15–20

Mendenhall WM, Van Cise WS, Bova FJ, Million RR (1981) Analysis of time-dose factors in squamous cell carcinoma of the oral tongue and floor of mouth treated with radiation therapy alone. Int J Radiat Oncol Biol Phys 7: 1005–1011

Meoz RT, Fletcher GH, Lindberg RD (1982) Anatomical coverage in elective irradiation of the neck for squamous cell carcinoma of the oral tongue. Int J Radiat Oncol Biol Phys 8: 1881–1885

Million RR (1974) Elective neck irradiation for TxN0 squamous carcinoma of the oral tongue and floor of mouth. Cancer 34: 149–155

Mohit-Tabutabai MA, Sobel HT, Rush BF, Mashberg A (1986) Relation of thickness of floor of mouth stage I and II cancers to regional metastasis. Am J Surg 152: 351–353

Molnar L, Ronay P, Tapolosanyi L (1974) Carcinoma of the lip. Analysis of the material of 25 years. Oncology 29: 101–121

Monaco AP, Buckley M, Raker JW (1962) Carcinoma of the oral cavity I. Carcinoma of the anterior two thirds of the tongue: Results of surgical treatment. N Engl J Med 266: 575–579

Mustard RA, Rosen B (1963) Cervical lymph node involvement in oral cancer. Am J Roent 90: 978–989

Nakissa N, Hornback NB, Shidnia H, Sayoc E (1978) Carcinoma of the floor of the mouth Cancer 42: 2914-2919

Neblett DL, Syed AMN, Puthawala AA, Harrop R (1985) An interstitial implant technique evaluated by contiguous volume analysis. Endo/Hyperth/Oncol 1: 213-222

Northrop M, Fletcher GH, Jesse RH, Lindberg RD (1972) Evolution of neck disease in patients with primary squamous cell carcinoma of the oral tongue, floor of mouth, and palatine arch, and clinically positive neck nodes neither fixed nor bilateral. Cancer 29: 23-30

O'Brien CJ, Lahr CJ, Soong S, Gandour MJ, Jones JM, Urist MM, Maddox WA (1986) Surgical treatment of early-stage carcinoma of the oral tongue - Would adjuvant treatment be beneficial? Head and Neck Surg 8: 401-408

Palos BB, Pooler D, Goffinet DR, Martinez A (1980) A method for inserting ^{124}I seeds into absorbable sutures for permanent implantation in tissue. Int J Radiat Oncol Biol Phys 6: 381-385

Panje WR, Smith B, McCabe BF (1980) Epidermoid carcinoma of the floor of mouth: Surgical therapy vs combined therapy vs radiation therapy. Otolaryngol Head Neck Surg 88: 714-720

Perez CA, Kraus FT, Evan JC, Powers WE (1966) Anaplastic transformation in verrucous carcinoma of the oral cavity after radiation therapy. Radiology 86: 108-115

Petrovich Z, Kuisk H, Tobochnik N, Hittle RE, Barton R, Jose L (1979) Carcinoma of the lip. Arch Otolaryngol 105: 187-191

Petrovich Z, Parker RG, Luxton G, Kuisk H, Jepson J (1987) Carcinoma of the lip and selected sites of head and neck skin. A clinical study of 896 patients. Radiotherapy and Oncology 8: 11-17

Pierquin B, Chassagne D, Baillet F, Castro JR (1971) The place of implantation in tongue and floor of mouth cancer. JAMA 215: 961-963

Pigneux J, Richard PM, Lagarde C (1979) The place of interstitial therapy using ^{192}Iridium in the management of carcinoma of the lip. Cancer 43: 1073-1077

Puthawala AA, Syed AMN, Neblett D, McNamara C (1981) The role of afterloading iridium (IR^{192} implant in the management of carcinoma of the tongue. Int J Radiat Oncol Biol Phys 7: 407-412

Puthawala AA, Syed AMN, Sheikh KMA, Seyed R (1986) Thermoendocurietherapy for recurrent and/or persistent head and neck cancers (abstr). Int J Radiat Oncol Biol Phys 12 *suppl 1) 110

Ratzer ER, Schweitzer RJ, Frazell El (1970) Epidermoid carcinoma of the palate. Am J Surg 119: 294-297

Sandor J, Palos B, Goffinet DR, Martinez A, Fessenden P (1979) Dose calculation for planar arrays of 192 Ir and 125 I seeds for brachytherapy. Appl Radiol 8: 41-44

Schleuning AJ, Summers GW (1972) Carcinoma of the tongue: Review of 220 cases. Laryngoscope 82: 1446-1454

Schneider JJ, Fletcher GH, Barkley HT (1975) Control of irradiation alone of non-fixed clinically positive lymph node from squamous cell carcinoma of the oral cavity, oropharynx, supraglottic larynx and hypopharynx. Am J Roentgen 123: 42-48

Schwade JG, Wara WM, Dedo GH, Phillips TL (1976) Radiotherapy for verrucous carcinoma. Radiology 120: 677-679

Silverberg E, Lubera J (1988) Cancer statistics, 1988. Ca-a Cancer J for Clinicans 38: 5-15

Simpson JR, Thawley SE, Matsuba HM (1984) Adenoid cystic salivary gland carcinoma: treatment with irradiation and surgery. Radiology 151: 509-512

Simpson JR, Matsuba HM, Thawley SE, Mauney M (1986) Improved treatment of salivary adenocarcinomas: planned combined surgery and irradiation. Laryngoscope 96: 904-907

Son YH, Kapp DS (1985) Oral cavity and oropharyngeal cancer in a younger population. Review of literature and experience at Yale Cancer 55: 441-444

Southwick HW (1973) Cancer of the tongue. Surg Clin No Amer 53: 147-148

Spiro RH (1985) Squamous cancer of the tongue. CA-a Can J Clinicians 35: 252-256

Spiro RH, Strong EW (1971) Epidermoid carcinoma of the mobile tongue. Treatment by partial glossectomy alone. Am J Surg 122: 707-710

Spiro RH, Strong EW (1974) Surgical treatment of cancer of the tongue. Surg Clin No America 54: 759-765

Spiro RH, Koss LG, Hajdu SI, Strong EW (1973) Tumors of minor salivary origin. A clinicopathologic study of 492 cases. Cancer 31: 117-129

Spiro RH, Huvos AG, Wong GY, Spiro J, Gnecco CA, Strong EW (1986) Predictive value of tumor thickness in squamous carcinoma confined to the tongue and floor of the mouth. Am J Surg 152: 345-350

Strong EW (1969) Preoperative radiation and radical neck dissection. Surg Clin No America 49: 271-276

Strong EW (1979) Carcinoma of the tongue. Otolaryngol Clin No America 12: 107-114

Swearingen AG, McGraw JP, Palumbo VD (1966) Roentgenographic pathologic correlation of carcinoma of the gingiva involving the mandible. Am J Roentgen 96: 15-18

Syed AMN, Feder BH, George FW (1977) Persistent carcinoma of the oropharynx and oral cavity re-treated by after loading interstitial 192 Ir implant. Cancer 39: 2443-2450

Teichgraeber JF, Clairmont AA (1984) The incidence of occult metastases for cancer of the oral tongue and floor of the mouth: treatment rationale. Head Neck Surg 7: 15-21

Vandenbrouck C, Sancho-Garnier H, Chassagne D (1980) Elective versus therapeutic radical neck dissection in epidermoid carcinoma of the oral cavity. Results of a randomized clinical trial. Cancer 46: 386-390

Vegers JWM, Snow GB, van der Waal I (1979) Squamous cell carcinoma of the buccal mucosa. A review of 85 cases. Arch Otolaryngol 105: 192-195

Vermund H, Brennhovd IO, Kaalhus O, Poppe E (1984a) Squamous-cell carcinoma of the tongue: preoperative interstitial radium and external irradiation. Part I: Local and regional control. Radiology 154: 499-503

Vermund H, Brennhovd I, Kaalhus O, Poppe E (1984b) Incidence and control of occult neck node metastases from squamous cell carcinoma of the anterior two-thirds of the tongue. Int J Radiat Oncol Biol Phys 10: 2025-2036

Vikram B, Hilaris BS, Anderson L, Strong EW (1983) Permanent iodine 125 implants in head and neck cancer. Cancer 51: 1310-1314

Vikram B, Strong EW, Shah JP, Spiro R (1984) Failure at distant sites following multimodality treatment for advanced head and neck cancer. Head Neck Surg 6: 731-733

Wallner PE, Hanks GE, Kramer S, McLean CJ (1986) Patterns of care study. Analysis of outcome survey data - anterior two thirds of tongue and floor of mouth. Am J Clin Oncol 9: 50-57

Wang CC (1983) Radiation therapy for head and neck neoplasms. Indications, techniques, and results. Littleton, Wright-PSG Inc pp 73-134

Wang CC, Doppke KP, Biggs PJ (1983) Intra-oral cone radiation therapy for selected carcinomas of the oral cavity. Int J Radiat Oncol Biol Phys 9: 1185–1189

Ward GE, Hendrick JW (1950) Results of treatment of cancer of the lip. Surgery 27 (3): 321–342

White D, Byers RM (1980) What is the preferred initial method of treatment for squamous carcinoma of the tongue? Amer J Surg 140: 553–555

Whitehouse GH (1976) Radiological bone changes produced by intraoral squamous carcinomata involving the lower alveolus. Clin Otolaryng 1: 45–52

Whitehurst JO, Droulias CA (1977) Surgical treatment of squamous cell carcinoma of the oral tongue. Arch Otolaryngol 103: 212–215

Willin R, Nathanson A, Moberger G, Anneroth G (1975) Squamous cell carcinoma of the gingiva. Histological classification and grading of malignancy. Acta Otolaryngol 79: 146–154

Yco MS, Cruizkshauk JC (1986) Treatment of stage I carcinoma of the anterior of the floor of the mouth. Arch Otolaryngol Head Neck Surg 112: 1085–1089

7 Oropharynx

WILL WISBECK and GEORGE E. LARAMORE

CONTENTS

7.1 Introduction

Oropharyngeal carcinomas are being diagnosed with increasing frequency in the United States. Classically, these tumors occurred in 60 to 70 year old males. Now they are being found with increasing frequency in patients who are in the fourth and fifth decades of life, and the male to female ratio is declining.

Tumors of the oropharynx are best managed by a multidisciplinary team including a radiation oncologist, an otolaryngologist, and often a medical oncologist. Proper management decisions require knowledge of the etiology, anatomy, histopatholo-gy, and clinical behavior of these lesions, as well as familiarity with the various methods of treatment and their expected outcomes. The multidisciplinary team must help the patient choose the most appropriate therapy.

Even when an oropharynx cancer has been controlled, careful follow-up examinations are required. Malignancies of the oropharynx have the highest associated incidence with second primary malignancies of any head and neck tumor site. JESSE and SUGARBAKER (1976) reported a 37% incidence of second primary tumors of the upper aerodigestive tract in patients who survived more than five years following treatment of an oropharynx tumor. Half of these new cancers developed in patients with stage I or II disease – those who had the best chance of being "cured" of their first malignancy and hence, of living long enough to develop a second primary tumor.

7.2 Anatomy

The oropharynx is continuous anteriorly with the oral cavity, superiorly with the nasopharynx and inferiorly with the supraglottic larynx and hypopharynx. Four anatomic regions comprise the oropharynx; the base of tongue, soft palate, tonsillar region, and pharyngeal walls (Fig. 7-1).

The base of the tongue is anatomically divided from the anterior two-thirds of the tongue that lies in the oral cavity by the terminal sulcus and the foramen cecum (Fig. 7-2). Just anterior to the V-shaped terminal sulcus lie the circumvilate papillae. At the apex of the "V" is the foramen cecum with marks the site of the thyroglossal duct outpouching from the floor of the pharynx during the embryological development of the thyroid gland. The terminal sulcus also marks a division in innervation of the tongue. The anterior portion of the tongue receives somatic innervation and the posterior portion receives visceral. The inferior border of the tongue is at the level of the epiglottis. Here lie the

WILL WISBECK, M.D., GEORGE E. LARAMORE, Ph.D., M.D., Department of Radiation Oncology, RC-08, University of Washington, 1959 N.E. Pacific Street, Seattle, Washington 98195, U.S.A.

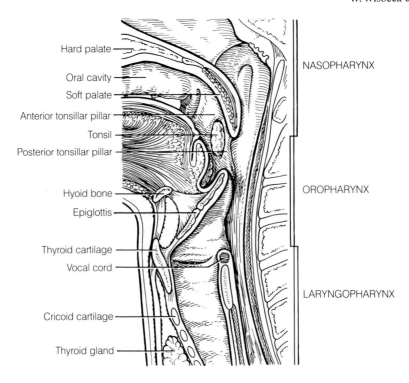

Hard palate

Oral cavity

Soft palate

Anterior tonsillar pillar

Tonsil

Posterior tonsillar pillar

Hyoid bone

Epiglottis

Thyroid cartilage

Vocal cord

Cricoid cartilage

Thyroid gland

NASOPHARYNX

OROPHARYNX

LARYNGOPHARYNX

Fig. 7-1. Sagittal section through the head and neck

lingual valleculae, bounded by the median glosso-epiglottic fold (between the base of tongue and the apex of the epiglottis) and the lateral glossoepiglottic folds (extending from the lateral surface of the

Fig. 7-2. Transverse section through the neck

tongue to the lateral and inferior margins of the epiglottis). The lateral border of the tongue base is the glossopharyngeal sulcus.

The soft palate separates the nasopharynx from the oral cavity and oropharynx and serves to seal the nasopharynx during swallowing. It is also important in speech. Structurally, it is a complex of five muscles; the tensor veli palatini, levator veli palatini, palatoglossus, palatopharyngeus, and uvular muscles. The soft palate is covered by squamous

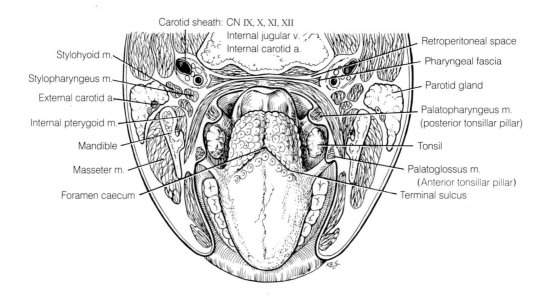

Carotid sheath: CN IX, X, XI, XII

Internal jugular v.
Internal carotid a.

Stylohyoid m.

Stylopharyngeus m.

External carotid a.

Internal pterygoid m.

Mandible

Masseter m.

Foramen caecum

Retroperitoneal space

Pharyngeal fascia

Parotid gland

Palatopharyngeus m.
(posterior tonsillar pillar)

Tonsil

Palatoglossus m.
(Anterior tonsillar pillar)

Terminal sulcus

mucosa on the side of the oropharynx and by respiratory mucosa on the side of the nasopharynx. The soft palate contains the uvula in the midline and is continuous laterally with the tonsillar pillars. Innervation of the soft palate is through branches of the pharyngeal plexus derived from cranial nerves IX, X and XI. Cranial nerve XI plays a minor role innervating only the stylopharyngeus muscle.

The tonsillar region makes up the lateral wall of the oropharynx. This is a triangular area bounded anteriorly by the anterior tonsillar pillar (palatoglossus muscle), posteriorly by the posterior tonsillar pillar (palatopharyngeal muscle), and inferiorly by the glossopharyngeal sulcus and the pharyngoepiglottic fold. The palatine tonsil lies within the triangle. Lateral to the tonsillar region lie the pharyngeal constrictor muscle, the internal pterygoid muscle, the mandible, and the lateral pharyngeal space. Tumor invasion through the tonsillar region to the internal pterygoid muscle produces trismus. Just behind the posterior tonsillar pillar lies the carotid sheath containing the internal carotid artery, internal jugular vein, and cranial nerves X, XI, and XII. If tumor penetrates the carotid sheath, it may invade the nerves and vessels or extend perineurally to the periphery or to the base of skull.

The posterior wall of the oropharynx begins at the lower border of the nasopharynx and extends to the pharyngoepiglottic fold. The wall of the oropharynx is composed of squamous mucosa, submucosa, the pharyngobasilar fascia, the superior constrictor muscle, and the buccopharyngeal fascia. The buccopharyngeal fascia is separated from the paravertebral fascia by a potential space and a layer of loose areolar tissue. The buccopharyngeal fascia is a potent barrier to tumor penetration. Often tumors of the oropharyngeal wall extend into the superior constrictor muscle and are arrested in the buccopharyngeal fascia. Once tumor extends through the paravertebral fascia, it is usually unresectable.

7.3 Histology

Lesions of the oropharynx may be broadly categorized as either inflammatory or neoplastic processes. Benign neoplasms occur more commonly in the oral cavity than in the oropharynx. Benign tumors of the oropharynx include fibromas, granular cell tumors, hemangiomas, leiomyomas, lipomas, lymphangiomas, schwannomas, neurofibromas, papillomas, and a few others. Pre-malignant lesions are similarly more common in the oral cavity than the oropharynx. These include leukoplakia secondary to hyperkeratosis (with or without atypia), erythroplasia, lichen planus, and nicotine mucositis. In the oropharynx the majority of pre-malignant lesions are found on the soft palate.

Leukoplakia is a vague descriptive term applied to many white mucosal plaques. On microscopic examination, biopsy of a leukoplakic plaque may reveal hyperkeratosis with or without atypia, or early invasive carcinoma. Leukoplakic lesions are more common in smokers.

Erythroplasic lesions are red, flat or slightly elevated plaques and tend to be well-circumscribed. Underlying tumors are more likely to be associated with erythroplasic than leukoplakic lesions. Lichen planis appears as a white, lacy lesion on the soft palate. Heavy smoking may lead to nicotine mucositis-a constellation of changes ranging from leukoplakic, hyperkeratotic areas to flat, erythematous plaques or small raised lesions. Distinguishing benign lesions from early malignancy may be difficult.

Ninety to ninety-five percent of malignant tumors of the oropharynx are squamous cell carcinomas. Verrucous carcinomas rarely occur. The lymphoid tissues of the palatine and lingual tonsils give rise to occasional lymphomas which account for about 5% of tonsillar malignancies and 1–2% of base of tongue malignancies. Unusual tumors of the oropharynx include minor salivary gland malignancies, plasmacytomas, and others.

7.4 Etiology

Alcohol and tobacco have been implicated as etiologic agents of nearly all squamous cell head and neck cancers. The use of either substance alone increases a patient's risk of developing a tumor and together alcohol and tobacco act synergistically. ROTHMAN and KELLER (1972) studied risk factors for squamous cell carcinoma of the oral cavity. Consumption of more than 1.5 ounces of alcohol per day was associated with a relative risk for carcinoma of the oral cavity of 2.33. Smoking more than 40 cigarettes per day had a relative risk of 2.43. Patients who both drank more than 1.5 ounces of alcohol per day and smoked more than 40 cigarettes per day had a relative risk of 15.5.

7.5 Staging

Ideally a cancer staging system provides information than can be useful in planning treatment and predicting prognosis. It should provide a basis for the reporting of results and the comparison of treatment outcomes between series. The TNM classification schemes are based on anatomic extent of disease as determined clinically, radiographically, and if possible, histopathologically.

Tumors of the oropharynx are commonly staged according to the American Joint Commission's

Table 7-1. TNM staging system for cancer of the oropharynx following the recommendations of the American Joint Committee for Cancer Staging and End Result Reporting

T-Staging

Tis	Carcinoma in sutu
T_1	Tumor 2 cm or less in greatest diameter
T_2	Tumor more than 2 cm but not more than 4 cm in greatest diameter
T_3	Tumor more than 4 cm in greatest diameter
T_4	Massive tumor more than 4 cm in diameter with invasion of bone, soft tissues of neck, or root (deep musculature) of tongue

N-Staging

N_X	Nodes cannot be assessed
N_0	Clinically negative nodes
N_1	One clinically positive homolateral node 3 cm or less in diameter
N_2	A single clinically positive homolateral node more than 3 cm but less than 6 cm in diameter or multiple clinically positive homolateral nodes, none of which are more than 6 cm in diameter
	N_{2a} Single homolateral node between 3 and 6 cm in diameter
	N_{2b} Multiple homolateral nodes, none of which are more than 6 cm in diameter
N_3	Massive homolateral node(s), bilateral nodes or contralateral node(s)
	N_{3a} One clinically positive homolateral node greater than 6 cm in diameter
	N_{3b} Bilateral clinically positive nodes. Each side of neck should be separately staged
	N_{3c} Clinically positive contralateral node(s)

M-Staging

M_X	Metastatic disease not assessed
M_0	No known distant metastases
M_1	Distant metastases present

Stage grouping

Stage I	$T_1 N_0 M_0$
Stage II	$T_2 N_0 M_0$
Stage III	$T_3 N_0 M_0$
	T_1, T_2, or $T_3 N_1 M_0$
Stage IV	$T_4 N_0 M_0$
	Any *T*-stage, N_2 or $N_3 M_0$
	Any *T*-stage, any *N*-stage, M_1

TNM classification outlined in Table 7-1 which also shows the stage groupings within the AJC System. Staging of oropharyngeal tumors can be quite difficult. It may be impossible to determine the site of origin of a large tumor. Generally, smaller lesions of th soft palate can be accurately classified. Tonsillar region tumors, however, may extend to the retromolar trigome, palate and pharyngeal wall and can be confused with extensive primary tumors arising in these locations. Base of tongue lesions may involve the lingual valleculae and epiglottis. Distinguishing these from primary tumors of the supraglottic larynx may be impossible.

Classifying a tumor as T_3 vs. T_4 is frequently difficult in the oropharynx. A large lymph node may be mistaken for soft tissue extension of the primary tumor. Bimanual palpation and CT or MR scanning may be helpful in determining the extent of the primary tumor. On physical examination, fixation of the tongue implies invasion of the deep tongue musculature. Similarly, tonsillar lesions that produce trismus or cranial nerve signs should be classified as stage T_4.

The T-stage for oropharyngeal tumors increases with increasing maximum tumor dimension, but often it is not the tumor's greatest dimension that is the best predictor of prognosis. For example, a superficial, plaque-like tumor arising from the anterior tonsillar pillar and extending over the retromolar trigome for a distance of 4 cm would be staged T_3 but a spherical tumor in the tonsillar fossa measuring 3.5 cm in diameter would be staged T_2. The spherical T_2 tumor might contain a greater volume of cells (and possible hypoxic cells) and be potentially less radiocurable than the plaque-like T_3 tumor.

7.6 Patient Evaluation

Unfortunately, tumors of the oropharynx are often not discovered until they are relatively advanced. Sore throat is perhaps the most common presenting symptom. Referred otalgia, mediated through cranial nerves IX or X is another common presenting complaint (Fig. 7-3). In some patients, cervical adenopathy is the first sign of disease.

Evaluation of the patient with cancer of the oropharynx begins with a complete history and physical exam. The patient's alcohol and tobacco use history should be determined. Heavy alcohol and tobacco users are at risk for multiple or subsequent primary head and neck tumors. The patient's past

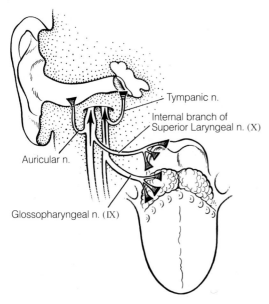

Tympanic n.

Internal branch of
Superior Laryngeal n. (X)

Auricular n.

Glossopharyngeal n. (IX)

Fig. 7-3. Pathways for referred otalgia from head and neck tumors

medical history and review of systems may be helpful in determining his fitness to undergo surgery or radiation therapy.

A general physical examination is in order for all patients. Following this, attention is turned to the head and neck. The object of the examination is to determine the location and extent of the primary tumor and to be sure there are no other suspicious lesions present. In the clinic an indirect examination is made using laryngeal and nasopharyngeal mirrors. The condition of the patient's dental work is noted. Next, the floor of mouth and base of tongue are palpated bimanually. Following this, the neck and supraclavicular fossae are carefully examined and the location, size, and consistency of any suspicious nodes is recorded. It is important to note whether nodes are mobile or fixed.

The neck examination is then repeated under general anesthesia. Some smaller nodes may now be palpable with the muscles relaxed. Panendoscopy is then performed including nasopharyngoscopy, laryngoscopy, esophagoscopy, and bronchoscopy. Again, the intent is to characterize the primary lesion and be sure there are no other tumors present. Biopsies of the primary tumor and any suspicious lesions are taken.

Computed tomography (CT) can help delineate the extent of oropharyngeal tumors. CT scans are also useful in radiation treatment planning. Magnetic resonance imaging (MRI) is being used with increasing frequency to study head and neck tu-

mors. Bone artifact, which limits the utility of CT in some regions, is not a problem with MRI. Additionally, MRI can provide sagittal and coronal images with good spatial resolution.

All patients should have a chest x-ray and liver function tests to rule out metastatic disease. Because of the high prevalence of alcohol abuse and alcohol-associated liver disease in head and neck tumor patients, the significance of elevated liver enzymes may be uncertain. When enzymes are elevated and there is a moderate to high likelihood of liver metastases, imaging tests should be ordered. A baseline complete blood count and general chemistry panel (with creatinine) should be done. A bone scan may be indicated in selected cases.

7.7 General Principles of Radiation Therapy

Early-stage oropharyngeal tumors have a reasonable probability of cure with definitive radiation therapy. Patients can be spared the functional and cosmetic losses associated with surgical resection. Unfortunately, many tumors of the oropharynx are discovered at advanced stages when the chance of cure with radiation, surgery, or combined therapy is dramatically reduced.

Radiation treatments for tumors of the oropharynx are delivered through fields designed to encompass the primary lesion, areas of possible tumor extension, and nodal areas at risk for metastatic spread. Generally treatments are given through opposed lateral fields encompassing the primary tumor with at least a 2 cm margin, as well as any possible extension anteriorly into the oral cavity, superiorly into the nasopharynx, and inferiorly into the hypopharynx and larynx. The cervical lymph nodes at risk for metastatic spread are also generally included within the lateral fields.

When clinically uninvolved cervical nodes are considered at risk, they are carried to a dose of 5000 cGy in 5 to 5½ weeks. The treatment of clinically-positive nodes is more variable. For nodes larger than 3 cm, elective neck dissection may be recommended. If extracapsular extent of tumor is seen, postoperative irradiation to 6000 cGy in 6 to 6½ weeks is indicated. When neck dissection is not done, small clinically positive nodes are carried to 6500 cGy and larger nodes receive doses comparable to those prescribed for similar-sized, primary tumors.

The posterior neck field is blocked to protect the spinal cord at 4500 cGy. The blocked field is then boosted with electrons to achieve the desired nodal dose.

7.8 Base of Tongue

7.8.1 Presentation and Patterns of Spread

The American Cancer society estimated that 5700 new cases of tongue carcinoma were discovered in 1987 (SILBERBERG and LUBERA 1987). Since tumors of the oral tongue outnumber base of tongue lesions by about four to one, this means that roughly 1150 patients were discovered to have carcinoma of the base of tongue. Carcinoma of the tongue is more common in males but the incidence in females is increasing. For 1987 the male to female ratio is expected to fall to 1.85:1.

Squamous cell carcinoma of the base of tongue tends to early, silent, deep infiltration. Sore throat or referred otalgia may be the first symptoms. Patients may complain of the sensation of a lump in the throat or report a palpable mass. Dysphagia is common. Infiltration of the deep tongue musculature may lead to pain that increases with swallowing or movement of the tongue. A characteristic "hot potato in mouth" speech may result. Advanced tumors may involve the pterygoid muscles producing trismus. They may extend superiorly to the tonsillar region and inferiorly to the vallecula, epiglottis, and pharyngeal walls. Deep penetration of tumor into the glossotonsillar sulcus allows the tumor to escape into the neck since there is no effective muscular barrier in this region.

The base of tongue is richly supplied with lymphatics. It is a midline structure and the incidence of bilateral lymph node metastases is high. The first echelon subdigastric nodes are most often involved by tumor. Jugular chain nodal metastases are also common. Posterior cervical nodes are involved less frequently but should be included in neck radiation ports (LINDBERG 1972). In Lindberg's series, 78% of patients with carcinoma of the base of tongue had clinically positive neck nodes on admission and 29% had bilateral adenopathy. The incidence of occult disease in clinically negative necks is reported to be 22% (OGURA et al. 1971); however this estimate may be low considering that smaller lesions were selected for operation and some patients in the series received preoperative irradiation (MILLION and CASSISI 1984 p 301).

7.8.2 Selection of Treatment

Excellent local control rates have been reported for early stage base of tongue carcinomas with either surgery or radiation alone. Definitive radiation therapy is the treatment of choice for most early (T_1 and T_2) base of tongue carcinomas and for extensive lesions that would require total glossectomy, laryngectomy, and bilateral neck dissection. Surgery is usually combined with postoperative radiation for resectable T_3 and T_4 lesions.

Definitive surgical management of a T_1 or T_2 lesion generally involves a mandibular osteotomy and ipsilateral neck dissection. Patients with close margins or more than pathologic N_1 neck disease are generally referred for postoperative radiation therapy. More extensive tumors require a composite resection, neck dissection, flap reconstruction, and usually postoperative radiation.

Base of tongue carcinomas that involve the vallecula are a difficult surgical problem. Elderly patients and those with poor pulmonary function require total laryngectomy, rather than a more conservative procedure, to prevent subsequent aspiration. Well-lateralized, vallecular lesions may be managed with a voice-sparing supraglottic laryngectomy if the following conditions are met: (1) There must be no gross involvement of the pharyngoepiglottic fold; (2) Preservation of one lingual artery must be possible; (3) Resection must entail the removal of less than 80% of the base of tongue; (4) Pulmonary function must be adequate for supraglottic laryngectomy, and (5) Medical condition must be suitable for a major operation. Lesions that cross the midline are generally unresectable because a procedure to excise such a tumor would involve sacrifice of both lingual arteries.

7.8.3 Radiation Treatment Technique

7.8.3.1 External Beam Irradiation

Carcinoma originating in the base of tongue is treated through opposed lateral fields which encompass the base of tongue, valleculae, suprahyoid epiglottis, superior portion of the pre-epiglottic space, pharyngeal walls, and varying amounts of the oral tongue depending on the anterior extent of the tumor. The base of tongue is a midline structure and there is a relatively high incidence of bilateral nodal metastases. Accordingly, the lateral radiation portals should encompass the ipsilateral and contralateral cervical nodes at risk. These include the first echolon subdigastric nodes, and the jugular chain, junctional, and spinal accessory nodes. When there is known or likely cervical lymphadenopathy, an anteroposterior-only field is added to cover the supraclavicular nodes.

Adequate nodal coverage with the initial lateral portals is ensured by careful attention to field borders (Fig. 7-4). The superior border is placed at a line connecting the zygomatic arch with a point about 3 cm superior to the mastoid tip. This ensures

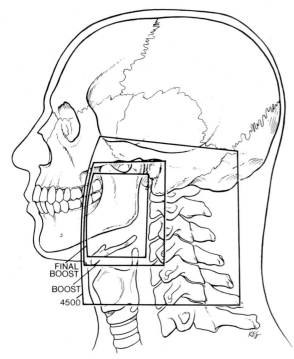

Fig. 7-4. General field arrangement for squamous cell carcinomas of the base of tongue. Parallel opposed fields are used to deliver 4500 cGy to a wide field encompassing the base of tongue, valleculae, epiglottis, pharyngeal walls, and a portion of the oral tongue. When there are clinically positive neck nodes or when the risk of nodal metastases is high the subdigastric, jugular, junctional, and spinal accessory nodes are included. The superior border is at a line connecting the zygomatic arch with a point about 3 cm above the mastoid tip. The inferior border is at or below the thyroid notch. Often an anteroposterior-only, supraclavicular fossa field is matched to the lateral fields. The spinal cord is blocked out of the lateral fields after 4500 cGy. Following this, the posterior neck is boosted with electrons. After the desired nodal dose has been delivered, the field size may be reduced to boost the primary tumor region. Of course, any clinically positive nodes must also be boosted. When neck nodes appear uninvolved and there is only a limited risk of nodal metastases, the lateral fields are sometimes modified to spare the larynx. In this case, the bottom border of the lateral fields is placed at the top of the thyroid cartilage. An anteroposterior only field with a full midline block covering the lower neck and supraclavicular nodes is matched to the lateral neck field

adequate coverage at the base of skull. The lower neck is always treated. The inferior border is matched to the superior border of the supraclavicular field. The posterior border is designed to spare a strip or skin on the posterior neck but cover the spinal accessory nodes. The spinal cord is blocked after 4500 cGy and the posterior neck is boosted with electrons. The anterior border is placed just ahead of the anterior tonsillar pillars unless the tumor extends toward the oral tongue. A ^{60}Co source or a 4 MeV or 6 MeV accelerator is used to deliver the initial 5000 cGy to midplane through these fields.

Following the initial course of wide field irradiation, the region of the primary tumor in the base of tongue receives an additional boosting dose. The amount of radiation prescribed and the manner in which it is delivered is influenced by characteristics of the tumor, the patient's condition, and the resources and skill of the radiation oncologist. Smaller lesions confined to the base of tongue may be suitable for an interstitial implant boost. Alternatively, the primary tumor region may be boosted through reduced-size, lateral external beam fields or through a single submental port as described by MILLION and CASSISI (1984 p 307).

7.8.3.2 Interstitial Implantation

Interstitial implantation is an attractive means in which to deliver a boosting dose of radiation to tumors in the base of tongue. Using an implant, a high local dose of radiation can be delivered to the tumor while the surrounding normal tissues receive a substantially lower dose.

While interstitial implantation may offer some improvement in local tumor control, there are several disadvantages to this method of boost delivery. First, general anesthesia is required for the placement and safe removal of the implant, and hospitalization is necessary while the radioactive sources are in place. The base of tongue is technically more difficult to implant than the oral tongue. Vital structures such as the carotid arteries are just adjacent to the implant site and great care must be taken to avoid serious injury. Tumors of the base of tongue are more difficult to localize by palpation for implant planning than are those of the oral tongue. An improperly constructed implant will underdose areas of the tumor.

Patients must be carefully selected for implantation boost. The location and extent of the tumor must be precisely known. Patients should be examined after two weeks of radiation therapy. A tu-

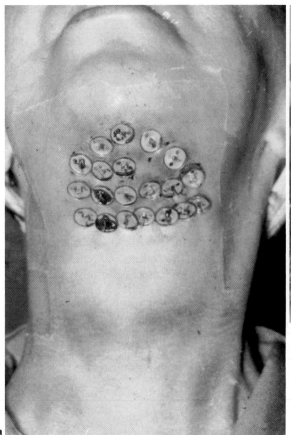

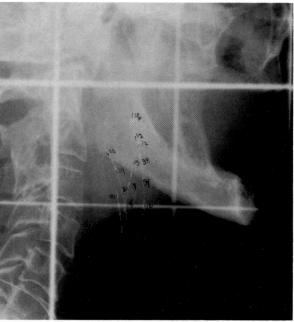

Fig. 7-5 a, b. An interstitial implant in the base of tongue. A number of implant techniques are possible. Commonly, wide bore stainless steel needles are passed through the neck and base of tongue. Plastic tubing is then passed through one needle and looped out through another as the needles are withdrawn. At the mucosal surface, the segments of tubing are kinked to prevent ^{192}Ir sources loaded into one segment of tubing from slipping into the other. The tubing is then secured at the skin surface with plastic "buttons" (**a**). When the patient recovers from anesthesia, dummy sources are loaded into the implant tubes and films are taken for dosimetry (**b**). The photograph shows only a portion of the tubes being loaded to facilitate seed identification on orthogonal films. Finally, the ^{192}Ir sources are loaded

mor that initially appeared small and confined may now appear larger and be seen to extend beyond the base of tongue. This is the so called "tumoritis" reaction. If the tumor does extend beyond the base of tongue, it may not be possible to achieve an adequate dose distribution with an interstitial implant and an external beam boost is indicated.

Implantation is only recommended for those patients able to safely undergo general anesthesia. A number of implantation techniques have been de-

scribed (Henschke et al. 1963; Levin and Wasserman 1978; Vikram and Hilaris 1981). Today, radium needles are seldom used. Instead most implants are constructed with plastic tubing and afterloaded with iridium-192 seeds (Fig. 7-5). Computer dosimetry is essential in planning the implant.

While the implant is in place patients are maintained on antibiotics to reduce the chance of infection and on dexamethasone to reduce swelling in the tongue. It is important that the initial dose of dexamethasone be administered at the beginning of the implant procedure (usually 10 mg IV) in order to prevent severe tongue swelling which may make the procedure difficult to complete. If significant swelling in the tongue occurs after the procedure, the implant geometry can be distorted and areas may be under or over dosed. When the desired dose has been delivered the iridium-192 sources are removed in the patient's room and the tubes are removed in the operating room under general anesthesia. Usually, tubing removal is simple and uncomplicated, however the risk of hemorrhage is significant and without general anesthesia, it may be difficult to control.

7.8.4 Treatment Results

Generally speaking, definitive radiation therapy is relatively successful in controlling early stage base of tongue tumors, but the results with advanced lesions are disappointing. Control rates for T_1 ant T_2 lesions treated with definitive radiation therapy compare favorably with control rates in surgical series. Unfortunately, the excellent control rates for early lesions treated surgically are often obtained at the cost of significant functional loss.

Local control rates by T-stage for patients treated with definitive radiation therapy are shown in Table 7-2. The series reported by GARDNER et al. (1987) includes patients treated by conventional and split course radiation. Some of the patients reported by GARDNER et al. (1987) and all of the patients treated by PUTHAWALA et al. (1985) received an interstitial implant. In general, better local control is achieved when a portion of the definitive radiation therapy is delivered through an interstitial implant (PUTHAWALA et al. 1985; BLUMBERG et al. 1979; HOUSSET et al. 1987). This, of course, implies selection of appropriate patients for implantation. The University of Florida data, by contrast, show rates of local recurrence and complications that were higher in patients who received an implant boost (GARDNER et al. 1987; PARSONS et al. 1982). Split course radiation was found to yield a similar rate of late complications and poorer local control than conventional course radiation (GARDNER et al. 1987).

Table 7-2. Local control of base of tongue tumors with definitive radiation therapy

T-Stage	GARDNER et al. 1987		BLUMBERG et al. 1979	
T_1	7/ 9	78%	5/ 5	100%
T_2	15/23	65%	8/10	80%
T_3	22/29	76%	6/13	46%
T_4	5/29	17%	1/ 4	25%

Patients had two years minimum follow-up. Here control rates are reported according to T-stage of the primary tumor. Nodal status is not considered.

Table 7-3. Carcinoma of the base of tongue: absolute 5-year survival by nodal stage for all T-stages (PARSONS et al. 1982)

N_0	6/ 9	66%
N_1	5/10	50%
N_{2A}	1/ 8	13%
N_{2B}	3/10	30%
N_{3A}	3/ 7	43%
N_{3B}	3/21	14%

Table 7-4. Local control of T_1 and T_2 base of tongue tumors by treatment technique[a] (HOUSSET et al. 1987)

	Control rate
External beam irradiation alone	31/54 (57%)
Surgery and postoperative external beam irradiation	22/27 (81%)
External beam irradiation and interstitial implant boost	23/29 (79%)

[a] Minimum follow up 4 years

Reporting of local control by T-stage allows one to roughly compare the efficacy of different treatment modalities in eradicating disease in the base of tongue, but the status of the neck nodes an the presence or absence of distant metastases must also be determined before definitive treatment plans are made. Tumor control is better in lower "overall" stage disease. For a given T-stage the probability of tumor control declines with increasing N-stage (Table 7-3). Overall five year survival is related to the stage of disease at presentation.

A number of investigators have searched for tumor and patient characteristics that carried prognostic significance. RILEY et al. (1983) found that well-differentiated histology, low T-stage, and the absence of clinically detectable neck disease were statistically significant predictors of improved survival. ROLLO et al. (1981) similarly found that poorly differentiated histology and the presence of more than three lymph nodes involved by tumor in the neck dissection specimen were indicators of poor prognosis. Furthermore, they report that the absence of histologic response of tumor to preoperative radiation therapy was associated with a four times higher recurrence risk than that seen in patients who did respond.

Surgery has been combined with postoperative radiation therapy in an attempt to improve tumor control. In a retrospective study reported by HOUSSET et al. (1987) examining the treatment of T_1 and T_2 base of tongue lesions, patients treated with surgery and postoperative external radiation fared no better than those treated by external beam radiation followed by an interstitial implant boost. External irradiation alone, however, yielded inferior control rates (Table 7-4). In general, early stage lesions are highly curable with either surgery or carefully planned definitive radiation. For early lesions definitive radiation therapy should be employed when surgery would leave a moderate to severe functional or cosmetic defect. Surgery should be reserved for salvage of radiation failures. The doses of radiation required to control early stage lesions are lower than those employed with more advanced lesions and are thus associated with fewer complications. For more advanced lesions the disappointing results with either radiation or surgery alone make combined approaches more attractive.

7.8.5 Time-Dose Relationships

Time-dose relationships for definitive radiation therapy of squamous cell carcinoma of the base of tongue have been reported. SPANOS et al. (1976) studied 174 patients treated with megavoltage external beam irradiation using conventional treatment times. More than 90% of T_1 lesions were locally controlled with between 6000 cGy in 6 weeks and 6500 cGy in 6½ weeks and no recognizable pattern for failure could be discerned from examination of a time-dose scattergram. A dose response curve was elicited for T_2 and T_3 tumors. There were few failures in patients receiving more than 2000 ret (approximately 7500 cGy in 7½ weeks). Interestingly, for tumors of the glossopalatine sulcus there were no failures above 2000 ret. Few T_4 lesions were controlled and thus a dose response curve could not be constructed.

GARDNER et al. (1987) analyzed treatment outcomes in 114 patients with squamous cell carcinoma of the base of tongue who underwent definitive megavoltage external beam radiation therapy at the University of Florida between 1964 and 1981. As in the M. D. Anderson series discussed above, (SPANOS et al. 1976) no time-dose relationship was found for T_1 and T_4 tumors. A time-dose relationship was found for T_2 and T_3 lesions. Local control was achieved in 17/18 (94%) of patients receiving greater than 6500 cGy in 6½ to 7 weeks and in only 11/18 (61%) of patients whose time-dose schedules fell outside this range.

7.8.6 Complications

Radiation portals for most tumors of the oropharynx are similar in that they encompass a significant portion of the major salivary glands, oral mucosa, and taste buds. Varying degrees of xerostomia, mucositis, and diminished taste sensation are thus expected during the course of radiation. The mucositis generally resolves within a few weeks of completion of radiation. Taste sensation is slower to return and may be permanently altered. Whether or not salivary function returns depends on the absorbed dose in the salivary glands.

MARKS et al. (1981) examined the relationship between absorbed dose in the parotid gland and parotid function. Parotid salivary flow was measured in 44 patients who received varying doses of radiation. Measurements were recorded at 5 to 47 months (mean 23.7 months) post irradiation. A progressive reduction in salivary flow with increasing doses of radiation was seen. Only 20% of parotids receiving between 4000 and 6000 cGy had measurable salivary flow and no parotid that received more than 6000 cGy showed measurable salivary flow.

Necrosis of soft tissues and bone is a potentially more serious complication than xerostomia. In most reports soft tissue necrosis is more common than bone necrosis. These side effects are more commonly seen when a portion of the radiation is delivered with an interstitial implant (PARSONS et al. 1982; HOUSSET et al. 1987). In PARSON'S (1982) series of 89 patients treated with definite radiation therapy, no severe soft tissue or bone necrosis was observed. The overall incidence of necrosis was 13% in soft tissue and 7% in bone. Necrosis was observed in 7/64 (11%) patients treated exclusively with the external beam and in 11/25 (44%) patients who received an interstitial implant. Unfortunately, the doses each group received were not specified. Two patients in the series developed hypoglossal nerve palsies secondary to entrapment of the nerve in the lateral pharyngeal space.

Preoperative and postoperative radiation therapy increase the risk of fistula and delayed wound healing. Soft tissue and bone necrosis are uncommon with doses of 6000 cGy or less.

7.9 Tonsillar Region

7.9.1 Presentation and Patterns of Spread

The tonsillar region is the most common site of malignancy in the oropharynx and the second most common site of malignancy in the head and neck, superseded only by the larynx. Tonsillar region malignancies account for about 0.5% of all malignant tumors in men in the United States according to the Surveillance, Epidemiology, and End Results Report (SEER) of the National Cancer Institute.

Roughly 95% of tonsillar region malignancies are squamous cell carcinomas and lymphomas account for approximately the other 5%. The discussion in this section will focus on squamous cell carcinomas. These tumors are more common in males with series reporting male to female ratios of 4:1 to 5:1. The incidence of tonsillar carcinoma increases with age, being most frequently diagnosed in the sixth and seventh decades of life. Small tumors of the tonsillar region are often asymptomatic and may be detected during the course of a routine dental or medical exam. Ipsilateral sore throat and otalgia, often worse with food or drink, are the most common symptoms of tonsillar region tumors. Lesions extending out of the tonsillar fossa or up the anterior pillar to the hard palate or gum may cause dentures to fit poorly. Extensive lesions extending through the tonsillar fossa to the pterygoid muscles may produce trismus.

The tonsillar region, unlike the base of tongue, is easily visualized. Early lesions on the anterior tonsillar pillar may appear as areas of leukoplakia. As these lesions enlarge, they may spread superficially or become infiltrative and develop central ulceration. Spread may occur anteriorly to the retromolar trigone or laterally to the buccal mucosa. Once tumor has involved the buccal mucosa, occult spread to the buccal fat pad may take place. Tumor may extend from the tonsillar pillar or tonsillar fossa superiorly to involve the soft and hard palate, or laterally to involve the base of the tongue. PEREZ et al. (1982) reported that of 218 patients presenting with squamous cell carcinoma of the tonsillar region, 60% had involvement of the soft palate and 55% had extension to the base of tongue. Tumor is rarely confined to the posterior pillar.

The location and extent of the primary tumor is important in predicting which lymph node groups may harbor metastatic disease. LINDBERG (1972) reported that clinically positive cervical adenopathy was present in 76% of patients with tonsillar fossa tumors. The subdigastric group was most commonly involved and the submaxillary, junctional, and spinal accessory nodes were also common sites of metastatic disease. Contralateral nodes were detected in only 11% of patients (LINDBERG 1972). The incidence of occult disease after preoperative irradiation was found in one series to be 22% (ROLANDER et al. 1971). The actual risk of occult nodal disease at presentation (all T-stages) is estimated to be 50% to 60% (MILLION and CASSISI 1984).

The pattern of lymph node metastases from lesions of the anterior tonsillar pillar/retromolar trigone differs somewhat from the pattern seen with tonsillar fossa lesions. LINDBERG (1972) reported an overall 45% incidence of clinically positive cervical adenopathy with anterior tonsillar pillar/retromolar trigone lesions. The subdigastric, submaxillary and jugular lymph nodes were most commonly involved

but the junctional and spinal accessory nodes often were spared. The incidence of contralateral cervical adenopathy was only 5% (LINDBERG 1972). Approximately 10% to 15% of clinically negative necks were found to contain nodal metastases at elective neck dissection (SOUTHWICK 1971).

7.9.2 Radiation Treatment Technique

Small (T_1 and T_2) carcinomas of the tonsillar region are generally treated with definitive radiation therapy. Small, very well-localized lesions may be suitable for conservative excision but for larger lesions, adequate surgical excision may require resection of the mandible, tonsillar region including the anterior and posterior pillars, a portion of the soft palate, and sometimes a portion of the tongue. Such a procedure may be necessary for "salvage" in a patient who has had prior radiation therapy, but generally the functional and cosmetic deficits that results from such a surgical procedure make radiation the treatment of choice in a *de novo* presentation.

When planning a course of treatment, it is important to consider the known prognostic factors. Survival and local control are clearly related to T and N stage, but treatment results can not be completely explained on the basis of initial stage (OREGGIA et al. 1983). Most investigators agree that extension of tonsillar carcinoma to the base of tongue indicates poor prognosis. All T_3 cases in Tong's series that failed at the primary site had base of tongue involvement (TONG et al. 1982). WANG (1972) reported a 55% disease free survival in tonsillar carcinomas without base of tongue involvement and a 25% disease free survival with involvement. Infiltrative or ulcerative tumors were found to have a significantly worse prognosis than exophytic lesions on the anterior tonsillar pillar and retromolar trigome in a review by Lo et al. (1987).

Radiation portals for tonsillar tumors are tailored to each patient's situation. Patients with small, well-lateralized lesions and no associated adenopathy may receive radiation only to the primary site and ipsilateral neck in an attempt to spare the contralateral parotid and prevent xerostomia. MURTHY and HENDRICKSON (1980) reported on 20 patients with T_1-T_4 N_0-N_1 disease who received radiation to the primary site and ipsilateral neck only. There were no isolated failures in the contralateral neck. TONG et al. (1982) reported that in 13 similarly treated patients with T_1-$T_2 N_0$ disease, there were no failures in the contralateral neck. It thus seems reasonable to avoid irradiation of the contralateral neck in patients with $T_1 N_0$ or $T_2 N_0$ disease where the tumor does not extend to the soft palate or tongue base.

A number of treatment techniques may be employed to spare the contralateral parotid. Very selected, small, well-demarcated lesions on the anterior tonsillar pillar may be treated partially or entirely by intraoral cone therapy using orthovoltage x-rays or electrons. When intraoral cone therapy is used, a generous margin on the tumor should be planned initially. The patient is carefully examined after 1000 to 2000 cGy has been delivered. The "tumoritis" reaction that occurs may suggest that the tumor is actually larger than it initially appeared. If intraoral cone therapy appears still possible, the tumor boundaries should be marked with sutures or India ink tattoos. Occasionally, a tumor will respond completely to the radiation before the prescribed dose has been delivered. In such cases, if there are no boundary markers, it can be difficult to reproducibly set up the field and regions of the target may be underdosed.

Today, few centers regularly use intraoral cone radiation therapy in the treatment of tonsillar region carcinomas and most patients are treated with external beam radiation. Tumors that do not extend toward midline may be treated through a single lateral external beam portal with a mixture of high energy x-rays and electrons. For patients with T_1–$T_2 N_0$ lesions of the anterior tonsillar pillar, FLETCHER (1980 p. 320) suggests it may be necessary to treat only the ipsilateral subdigastric nodes. Patients with less well differentiated or more extensive lesions should receive radiation to at least the entire ipsilateral neck. Clinically negative nodal regions receive 5000 cGy. Following this, a reduced size external beam field or an interstitial implant may be used to deliver the boost dose.

When tumor extends beyond the tonsillar region toward the midline, the contralateral neck is a risk. Opposed lateral fields (60 Co, 4 MeV or 6 MeV x-rays) are used to treat the neck and primary tumor region (Fig. 7-6). Generally the spinal accessory and lower jugular nodes are included in the neck fields. An anteroposterior supraclavicular fossa field is matched to the lateral neck fields. A number of techniques may be used to ensure that the spinal cord is not overdosed at the field junction. When there is no lower cervical adenopathy, a midline block may be included in the supraclavicular fossa field to protect the cord.

Often when bilateral nodal regions are treated, the fields are weighted 2:1 or 3:2 to the side of the primary tumor. If such weighting is considered, the

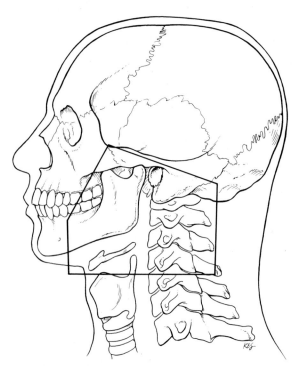

Fig. 7-6. Field arrangement for tonsillar carcinomas extending toward the midline with a risk of nodal metastases. Parallel opposed fields are designed to encompass the tonsillar region and any anterior tumor extension. The subdigastric, jugular and spinal accessory nodes are included within the lateral fields. The superior border is placed at a line connecting the zygomatic arch and the mastoid tip. The inferior border is placed at or below the level of the thyroid notch. An anteroposterior only supraclavicular fossa field with a midline spinal cord block is matched to the lateral fields. When the desired nodal dose has been delivered, the region of the primary tumor is boosted. Some possible boost techniques include mixed unilateral electrons and photons, a wedged pair of photon fields, and interstitial implants

radiation oncologist must pay careful attention to the dose distribution to be sure no region is underdosed. It is important in such situations to consider not just the total dose to given areas, but also the effective dose per fraction. Consider, for example a situation in which a dose of 6400 cGy is delivered to a tumor volume in 32 fractions (Fig. 7-7). The treatment plan is normalized to a point in the tumor and the tumor volume receives the prescribed dose of 6400 cGy at 200 cGy per fraction. Contralateral lymph nodes receive approximately 6000 cGy in 32 fractions, equivalent to treating this side of the neck at about 190 cGy per day.

The precise field arrangements for an individual patient are planned after careful clinical and radiographic examination. Generally the superior field border is placed at a line connecting the zygomatic

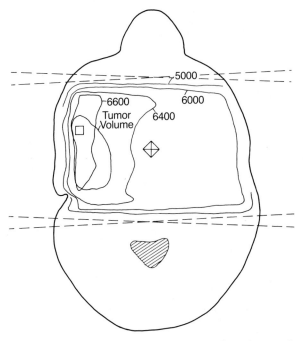

Fig.7-7. Isodose distribution for treatment of carcinoma of the tonsillar region with a risk for bilateral nodal metastases. Parallel opposed 6 MeV photon fields are employed. The normalization point is in the center of the tumor (square). Fields are weighted 2:1 to the side of the tumor

T_3 and T_4 lesions are treated with definitive radiation therapy the primary tumor should receive 7000–7500 cGy. If an implant boost is used, the final tumor dose is usually in the range of 8000 cGy.

7.9.3 Results

Definitive radiation therapy alone yields excellent control rates for T_1 and T_2 lesions but the control rates for larger tumors are disappointing. Even radiation doses in excess of 7500 cGy are inadequate to control many T_3 and most T_4 tumors. Often radiation is combined with surgery in an attempt to improve local control of large lesions.

Table 7-5 shows local control rates by T-stage for patients treated by definitive radiation therapy. All analyses were retrospective and thus may show selection bias. The results presented in the table are merely intended to show that good local control of T_1 and T_2 lesions is possible with definitive radiation therapy, and reasonable control rates can also be achieved with T_3 lesions.

The control rates shown in Table 7-5 for T_3 lesions are better than those reported in most other series. This may reflect the selection of appropriate T_3 lesions for radiation therapy. In the series reported by REMMLER et al. (1985) local control was achieved in 8/9 (89%) $T_3 N_0$ patients and only 7/12 (58%) T_3 – node positive patients. When the T_3 tumor invaded the base of tongue, local control was achieved in 5/8 (63%) with nodes negative and only 3/10 (30%) with nodes positive.

7.9.4 Time-Dose Relationship

Time, dose and treatment volume relationship to control of tonsillar region squamous cell carcinoma have been reported by a number of investigators. SHUKOVSKY and FLETCHER (1973) analyzed treatment results for 129 patients who underwent definitive megavoltage radiation therapy at M. D. Anderson Hospital between 1954 and 1968. All T_1 lesions were controlled and thus a dose response curve

arch and a point just above the mastoid tip. The anterior border is designed to allow a 2 cm margin beyond the tumor. The inferior border is at the level of the thyroid notch if only upper cervical nodes are to be included. When lower cervical nodes are to be irradiated as well, the inferior field border is placed as low as the shoulders will permit and an anterior-only, supraclavicular fossa field is matched to this border. The placement of the posterior border similarly varies depending on which nodal groups are to be irradiated. When the spinal accessory nodes are included, the cord must be blocked after 4500 cGy. The posterior neck is boosted with electrons.

Several studies have demonstrated that good control is possible with 6000 to 6500 cGy for T_1 lesions and 6500 to 7000 cGy for T_2 lesions (SHUKOVSKY and FLETCHER et al. 1973; PEREZ et al. 1976). When

Table 7-5. Local control of tonsillar lesions treated by radiation therapy alone

	AMORNMARN et al. 1984		GARRETT et al. 1985		REMMLER et al. 1985		TONG et al. 1982		PEREZ et al. 1976	
T_1	16/17	94%	41/ 47	87%	14/14	100%	14/16	88%	11/12	92%
T_2	32/40	80%	109/161	68%	31/35	89%	22/33	67%	20/28	72%
T_3	38/74	51%	82/164	50%	34/50	68%	19/39	49%	20/35	57%
T_4	5/26	19%	–		4/17	24%	1/16	6%	9/30	30%

could not be constructed. Dose response relationships were found for T_2 and T_3 lesions (Table 7-6). Baset on these results, the authors recommend 6500 cGy over 6½ weeks (1850 rets) for T_1 lesions, 7000 cGy over 7 weeks (1950 rets) for T_2 lesions and 7500 cGy over 8 weeks for T_3 and T_4 lesions.

PEREZ et al. (1976) followed 105 patients treated at the Malinkrodt Institute between 1955 and 1973. Control rates by T-stage are shown in Table 7-5. Dose response curves were contructed and failures were analyzed with respect to tumor dose and treatment volume. Only one of twelve T_1 lesions recurred locally. This patient received 4750 cGy while the others received 5000 to 7000 cGy. In the T_2 group, 8 of 28 patients failed locally; five of these received less than 6000 cGy and the other three received 6000 to 6500 cGy. One of the patients treated to between 6000 and 6500 cGy failed as the result of a geographical miss. Most T_3 tumors that recurred locally received less than 6000 cGy. Five of seven T_3 tumors treated to between 6500 and 7000 cGy were controlled. Local recurrences with T_4 lesions occurred predominantly in patients treated with less than 6500 cGy. Five of six T_4 lesions were locally controlled with doses of 6500 to 7000 cGy. On the basis of these findings, the authors recommend 6000 cGy for T_1 lesions, 6500 cGy for T_2, 7000 cGy for T_3 and 7500 cGy for T_4 lesions.

More recently, a review of 372 patients with squamous cell carcinoma of the tonsillar region treated between 1970 and 1979 at the Princes Margaret Hospital was reported by GARRETT et al. (1985). Control rates by T-stage are shown in Table 7-5. Time, dose, and volume relationships were sought to explain recurrences. No statistically significant improvement in local control could be demonstrated for any stage disease when the dose was increased from 5000 to 6500 cGy, although there was a trend toward improved control of T_1 and T_2 lesions when the dose was increased in this range. Interestingly, a statistically significant improvement in local control of T_1 and T_2 lesions was seen when field sizes of 80 cm^2 or more were employed. This underscores the importance of allow-

Table 7-6. Local control of tonsillar fossa carcinoma according to NSD and stage (SHUKOVSKY and FLETCHER 1973)

NSD (rets)	T_1	T_2	T_3 and T_4
< 1900	8/8 (100%)	9/12 (75%)	8/16 (50%)
1900–2000	3/3 (100%)	8/10 (80%)	8/13 (62%)
≥ 2000	1/1 (100%)	6/ 6 (100%)	12/13 (92%)

Table 7-7. Local control of T_3 carcinomas of the tonsillar region according to dose (MILLION and CASSISI 1984)

Dose cGy	Control rate
5500–5900	0/ 2
6000–6900	2/ 5 (40%)
7000–7900	6/10 (60%)
≥ 8000	7/ 8 (88%)

ing adequate radiation field margins to cover possible gross and microscope extensions of tumor. These investigators advocate a policy of moderate dose definite radiation therapy for tonsillar carcinomas.

MILLION and CASSISI (1984, p 311) reported local control rates for T_3 tonsillar region carcinomas according to dose (Table 7-7). Both higher local control and complication rates were achieved with higher doses of radiation.

7.9.5 Complications

Acute reactions to radiation therapy for tonsillar carcinomas are similar to those that occur with radiation for base of tongue lesions. Varying degrees of xerostomia, mucositis and diminished taste sensation occur. Likewise, soft tissue and bone necrosis are the most common serious late complications. The incidence and severity of late complications is influenced by patient and tumor characteristics, the total dose of radiation, the dose per fraction, and the field arrangements used.

SHUKOVSKY and FLETCHER (1973) analyzed complication rates for 129 patients who underwent definitive radiation therapy for squamous cell carcinomas of the tonsillar fossa. The incidence of late complications in patients surviving an minimum of 18 months was analyzed with respect to field size and nominal standard dose (NSD). They found that the incidence of mandibular osteonecrosis requiring surgery was 5% or less for doses up to 2100 rets delivered to a field 100 cm^2 or less in area. The overall incidence of osteonecrosis requiring surgery in the series was 9%.

More recently improved dental care and refinements in treatment planning have helped lower the incidence of bone and soft tissue necrosis. REMMLER et al. (1985) reported a 6% incidence of osteonecrosis of the mandible requiring surgery in 143 patients treated with definitive radiation therapy at M. D. Anderson between 1968 and 1979. In a Princess Margaret Hospital series GARRETT et al.

(1985) reported a 3% incidence of osteonecrosis for patients treated between 1970 and 1979.

The incidence of mandibular osteonecrosis is in part related to field arrangement. Equal-ret doses delivered through different portal arrangements may well result in different complication rates (SHUKOVSKY and FLETCHER 1973). When a single homolateral field or wedged pair fields are used to treat a tonsillar region tumor, careful attention to dosimetry is required. The mandible and overlying soft tissues may receive a higher dose with these fields than would be delivered through opposed lateral ports.

The complication rate for definitive radiation therapy of tonsillar region tumors, similar to that for base of tongue lesions, is higher when an interstitial implant boost is used. MILLION and CASSISI (1984, p. 312) observed roughly twice the incidence of soft tissue and bone necrosis when an implant was employed.

7.10 Soft Palate

7.10.1 Presentation and Patterns of Spread

Primary tumors arising on the soft palate are relatively rare. Small tumors can easily be classified as to site of origin but the true origin of large tumors involving the soft palate can be difficult to determine. Carcinomas arising in the tonsillar region may extend to the soft palate and in some cases may be indistinguishable from a primary soft palate carcinoma that has extended to the tonsillar region.

Tumors originating in the soft palate occur almost exclusively on the anterior surface. Only advanced tumors involve the posterior surface. It is unusual for even large nasopharyngeal tumors to invade the soft palate. Small white lesions on the soft palate may represent leukoplakia, carcinoma-in-situ or invasive carcinoma; differentiation among these may require biopsy. Heavy smokers may have areas of leukoplakia and injection. Distinguishing which lesions are significant is difficult. When biopsy of a small lesion on the soft palate does prove squamous cell carcinoma, it may be difficult to delineate the borders of the lesion. Following the first week of radiation therapy, adjacent mucosa that initially appeared normal may become injected suggesting the tumor is more extensive than initially appreciated. This again, is the so called "tumoritis" reaction.

Most tumors of the soft palate are discovered early. Undetected lesions spread first laterally down the tonsillar pillars and anteriorly to the hard palate. Larger lesions may lead to ulceration of the hard palate. Laterally, the tumor may extend to involve the pharyngeal walls where extension through the superior constrictor muscles to the pterygoid muscles may produce trismus.

The subdigastric nodes are the most common site of nodal spread from tumors of the soft palate. The spinal accessory and submandibular nodes are less often involved. In Lindberg's series 44% of patients with soft palate primaries had clinically-positive cervical adenopathy with bilateral neck disease being found in 16% (LINDBERG 1972).

7.10.2 Radiation Treatment Technique

A few patients with very small tumors of the soft palate may be suitable candidates for a definitive surgical procedure. However, for larger tumors adequate surgical resection can only be achieved at the expense of significant functional loss. Generally, lesions larger than 5 mm are treated with definitive radiation therapy.

Squamous cell carcinomas of the soft palate may be treated by intraoral cone, interstitial implant and external beam irradiation. The major portion of a patient's therapy is usually delivered through external beam portals since the soft palate is a midline structure and there is significant risk for bilateral nodal metastases. The upper jugular chain and subdigastric nodes are most commonly involved and should be included in the initial lateral portals. Equally-weighted parallel opposed fields are designed to encompass the soft palate, tonsillar region, and nodes at risk (Fig. 7-8). The patient with a clinically negative neck receives 5000 cGy in 5-5½ weeks. Following this a boosting dose of radiation is delivered through a smaller field.

The radiation boost is planned to suit the individual patient's situation. Well localized tumors confined to the soft palate may be suitable for an intraoral cone boost. Intraoral cone boosts are often given prior to the external beam therapy when the lesion is clearly visible and oral mucositis has not developed. If the intraoral cone boost is to be delivered following external beam therapy, care must be taken in order to avoid a geographic miss. The tumor boundaries as seen following 1-2 weeks of external beam therapy should be marked by sutures or tattoos. Allowing the patient to receive a modest dose of radiation before outlining the boost volume

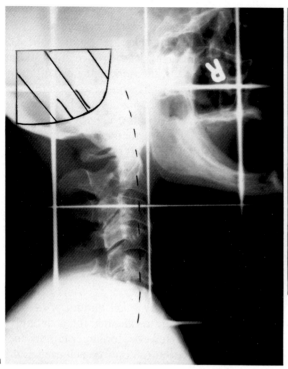

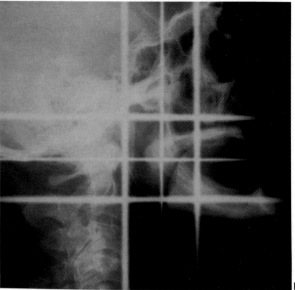

a

b

Fig. 7-8 a, b. A 66 year old man received radiation therapy following resection of a T_2N_0 squamous cell carcinoma of the uvula. The tumor measured 2.5 cm in situ and was excised with clear margins. Initially, opposed lateral fields (**a**) and a matched supraclavicular fossa field were treated to 5040 cGy in 28 fractions. Following this, the soft palate region was boosted through reduced-sized portals (**b**). Similar fields could be employed for definitive radiation therapy of such a lesion. The final boost dose would be between 6500 and 7000 cGy

allows visualization of any tumoritis reaction that may occur.

Alternatively, the boost may be delivered by way of an interstitial implant. A number of implant techniques have been described using radioactive wires and seeds (SEALY et al. 1984; GOFFINET et al. 1977). The principal advantage to boosting with either an implant or the intraoral cone is that a high local dose can be delivered while keeping the dose to surrounding normal tissues down. When reduced size external beam fields are used to boost the soft palate region the parotids are invariably included in the field. Even with a high energy accelerator, significant dose is absorbed in the parotid and xerostomia results.

7.10.3 Treatment Results

The literature regarding treatment of soft palate carcinomas is sparse. No good prospective controlled trials have been reported. The few papers that are available report on small numbers of cases or on cases that were accrued over several decades. In one of the more recent reports FEE et al. (1979) conducted a retrospective analysis of 106 patients with squamous cell carcinomas of the soft palate treated between 1956 and 1977. Not surprisingly, they found statistically significant improved survival for patients with clinically negative necks and for patients with well and moderately differentiated tumors. Interestingly, they report that patients that received less than 6300 cGy had statistically significant improved survival relative to patients that received more than 6300 cGy. They suggest that squamous cell carcinoma of the soft palate may be more radiosensitive than other squamous cell carcinomas of the oropharynx. This suggestion warrants closer inspection of their data. The two treatment groups did not differ significantly with respect to patient age, sex, or tumor stage but the lower dose group contained more poorly differentiated carcinomas (10% vs. 23%). Perhaps in part because of this fact, the low dose group also contained more patients who underwent radiation combined with

al Cancer Institute, SEER Program (1984) Cancer incidence and mortality in the United States 1973–1981. Bethesda, MD

Vikram B, Strong EW, Shah JP, Spiro R (1984) Failure at the
primary site following multimodality treatment in advanced head and neck cancer. Head & Neck Surgery 6:
720–723

Vikram B, Hilaris BS (1981) A non-looping afterloading technique for interstitial implants of the base of tongue. Int J
Rad Onc Biol Phys 7: 419–422

Wang CC (1972) Management and prognosis of squamous
cell carcinoma of the tonsillar region. Radiology 104:
667–671

8 Nasopharynx

MELVIN L. GRIEM and DAVID TZE-CHUN CHIANG

CONTENTS

8.1 Perspective

Cancer of the nasopharynx is a disease which is managed by radiation therapy as the major method of treatment. The disease location and its propensity for spread to the lymph nodes of the neck limits the surgical approach to the treatment of this disease. As the cancer has a tendency to be localized

MELVIN L. GRIEM, M.D., Department of Therapeutic Radiology, University of Chicago, Box 442, 5841 South Maryland Avenue, Chicago, IL 60637, USA

DAVID TZE-CHUN CHIANG, M.D., Illinois Masonic Hospital, Chicago, IL 60637, USA

in the head and neck region in its clinical course and is reasonably sensitive to radiation, the role of adjuvent chemotherapy for this disease has yet to be established. In addition, the tumor burden and histology, an epithelial malignancy, limits the use of chemotherapy. As the disease becomes more advanced, the tumor invades the base of the brain with destruction of the sphenoid bone. Distant metastases may develop in the liver, lungs and bones. In the treatment of this tumor, local control can be achieved both in the primary lesion and in the lymph nodes with proper treatment. The dose limiting tissues include the brain, spinal cord, and mandible and in some clinical situations, the orbital contents may also become a dose limiting tissue. Retreatment of the primary lesion has also been accomplished following failure in some situations.

8.2 Epidemiology

Nasopharyngeal cancer is found among the Chinese people living in the Southeast Provinces of China, the Provinces of Fukein, Kwangsi, Kwangtung (Canton) and Taiwan. (CHIANG and GRIEM 1973). The disease is also very prevalent in Hong Kong, which geographically can be considered part of the Kwangtung Province. Biopsy data from these Provinces mentioned indicate that nasopharyngeal carcinoma is the most frequent cancer in the male and in the female it ranks third behind carcinoma of the uterine cervix and breast. The highest incidence which has been reported comes from the Kwangtung Province, where nasopharyngeal constitutes 17.4% of the 4026 malignancies biopsied in women, and 56.9% of the tumors in 3010 men who have been biopsied for tumor. The incidence declines steadily in people living in the interior and the North of China. In Peking, nasopharyngeal carcinoma was found in 4% of 5037 tumors biopsied in males. Since Chinese from the Southeast Provinces of China have immigrated to Indo-China, India, Taiwan, the Philippine Islands and to the

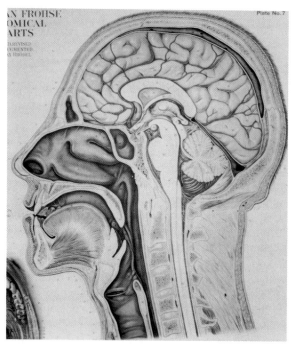

Fig. 8-1. Sagittal section of head and neck demonstrating nasopharynx in relation to base of skull, brain and pharynx

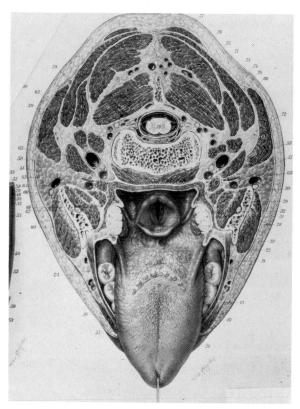

Fig. 8-2. Transverse section below nasopharynx demonstrating pharyngeal anatomy, salivary gland location and lymph nodes

United States, there is a relatively high incidence of this tumor found in these Chinese immigrants and their offspring (YEH and COWDRY 1954; MUIR and SHANMUGARATNAM 1967). In Korea and Japan this tumor is an uncommon malignancy. An interesting incidence of this tumor has been reported by Lederman occurring on the Island of Malta, and the disease may be seen in certain areas of Africa (LEDERMAN 1961). Steiner feels that this tumor has a strong genetic factor related to race, rather than an environmental cause (STEINER 1954). In both Caucasians and Chinese, nasopharyngeal cancer is more common in men than in women, with a ratio of about 2.5 to 1. Both Lederman and Chiang indicate that the peak incidence of this tumor in both males and females is seen at a mean age of approximately 40 to 50 years, whereas it is seen about 10 years later in the English and in the Maltese series (LEDERMAN 1961).

8.3 Etiology

Dobson considers the accumulation of smoke in poorly ventilated Chinese houses as a causative factor. However, Chinese living in New York and in Honolulu have a high incidence of this tumor. This

suggests that there may be a genetic trait, which make these people more susceptible for this disease (ZIPPIN 1962). No chromosomal aberration has yet been identified, and no genetic pattern among families or relatives has yet been described. In the Chinese who have immigrated to other countries, the locally born younger Chinese have a lower incidence of this tumor, than their parents who were born in China and immigrated. Whether the way of living, dietary habits such as frequent drinking of tea, use of alcohol, or cigarettes or whether environmental factors such as ventilation are contributing factors has yet to be worked out.

The possible role of a virus has been studied in the past. Of the Chinese patients with nasopharyngeal cancer, there was a higher incidence of infection with adeno-virus titer (types 7 and 12) in the serum of patients with tumors, when compared with a control group, (HENLE 1970; LAING 1969). In a study done in Hong Kong, the serologic data was correlated with the disease distribution and stage classification and the incidence of high titer was shown to be 45% in patients with early disease. This

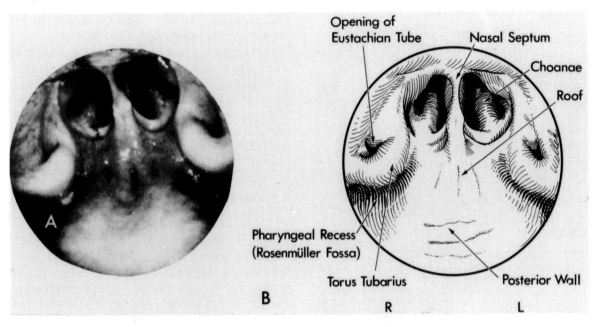

Fig. 8-3. Nasopharyngeal camera view with regional anatomy identified

incidence approached 100% in patients with advanced disease.

8.4 Anatomy of the Nasopharynx

The choana of the nasal cavity represents the anterior limit of the nasopharynx. The roof of the nasopharynx is attached to the base of the skull, and slopes backward and downward in a gradual arc to become continuous with the posterior wall of the nasopharynx which becomes continuous with the posterior oropharyngeal wall. Laterally, the nasopharyngeal walls are perforated by the orifice of the Eustachian tube surrounded by the elevated ridge superiorly and posteriorly called the Torus Tubarius. At the junction of the posterior wall and the lateral wall, there is an elongated depression called the pharyngeal recess of Rosenmuller's fossa. An imaginary plane separates the nasopharynx from the oropharynx and represents the floor of the nasopharynx, which is situated at the level of the soft palate and uvula. Figure 8-1 shows the nasopharynx demonstrating the anatomy. Figure 8-2 is a cross sectional drawing of the region showing the relationship with the brain stem and structures of the head and neck.

Using a nasopharyngeal camera with a wide angle lens, the nasopharyngeal anatomy is demonstrated in Figure 8-3. This camera which is commercially available, is an invaluable tool in the examination of the nasopharynx and provides a means of identifying early disease by observation of the mucosal changes and provides a means of recording the anatomy and pathology as well as providing a means of observing the response of the tumor to treatment. These nasopharyngeal camera devices are available in both rigid and flexible fiberoptic designs with various illuminating devices attached.

The regional anatomy is very important in understanding the pathophysicological changes and manifestations this tumor presents. Because of the unique anatomical site, the clinical findings can be readily explained.

Above the nasopharynx is situated the sella turcica and slightly laterally, the foramen rotundum, foramen ovale and foramen lacerum of the base of the skull which commonly become involved with extension of this tumor superiorly. Posteriorly, there is a strong impervious pre-vertebral fascia anterior to the vertebral bodies preventing extension of the tumor posteriorly into the clivus and cervical vertebra. Laterally, the internal acoustic meatus and the Eustachian tube connect the nasopharynx to the middle ear and the tumor commonly obstructs the Eustachian tube.

There is a rich network of lymphatics, which includes the lymph node of Rouviere, situated behind the fossa of Rosenmuller and anterior to the pre-

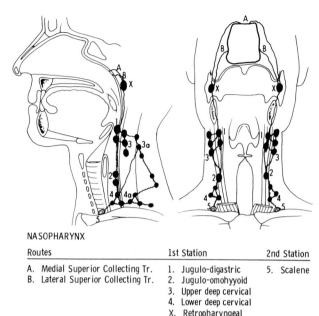

NASOPHARYNX

Routes	1st Station	2nd Station
A. Medial Superior Collecting Tr. B. Lateral Superior Collecting Tr.	1. Jugulo-digastric 2. Jugulo-omohyyoid 3. Upper deep cervical 4. Lower deep cervical X. Retropharyngeal	5. Scalene

Fig. 8-4. Diagram of lymphatic drainage

vertebral fascia. In addition, the lymphatic drainage extends into the posterior, middle and anterior neck nodes as shown in Figure 8-4. In the para-pharyngeal space one finds the parotid salivary gland and the mandible adjacent to the fossa of Rosenmuller. Figure 8-4 shows a cross section slightly below the plane separating the nasopharynx from the oropharynx, and shows the above anatomical considerations as would be seen in a CT scan. Slightly posterior and lateral to the retro-pharyngeal region the internal carotid artery, internal jugular vein and cranial nerves 9 to 12 are situated along with the cervical sympathetic nerve trunk. This close association of the nasopharynx and the rich lymphatic network together with the cranial nerves results in combinations of nerve palsies which will be described.

Superior to the sphenoid bone within the middle cranial fossa and lateral to the pituitary and sella turcica is the cavernous sinus, the circle of Willis and the cranial nerves II to VI innervating the eye, the extra-ocular muscles and providing sensory reception for the face and motor function to the muscles of mastication. The seventh and eighth cranial nerves exit the skill through the internal acoustic foramen and are protected in the temporal bone through a lengthy intracranial course before reaching the middle ear. These nerves, because of the protected anatomical course, are rarely involved by tumor extension. When the tumor extends into the nasal cavity anteriorly, involvement of the cribiform

plate is possible, and loss of the function of the first cranial nerve is occasionally seen.

The lining epithelium of the nasopharynx is covered by a mucosal membrane made up of ciliated epithelium and cylindrical epithelium along with goblet cells. In addition, lymphoid tissue making up Waldeyer's ring is situated posteriorly and laterally adjacent to the opening of the Eustachian tube and posteriorly as the adenoids.

8.5 Pathology

The gross appearance of the nasopharyngeal carcinoma may take a variety of configurations as demonstrated in Figures 8-5 and 8-6. These photographs made by one of the authors are representative of the pathology seen in 179 consecutive patients analyzed using the nasopharyngeal camera. The tumor presentation may range in size from a small swelling less than 5 mm in size with cervical adenopathy to lobulated tumors involving several anatomic regions. When the tumor is situated on the posterior wall, the border may become less well-defined. Infiltrating lesions and ulcerating lesions are infrequently seen.

In analyzing the histology of 350 patients seen in a period of September, 1961 to March, 1970, more than 90% of the tumors seen were epithelial in origin – Table 8-1 (CHIANG and GRIEM 1973). In a recent analysis the presence of keratinizing squamous cell carcinoma indicated a poorer prognosis (HSU et al. 1987). Hodgkin's disease and non-Hodgkin's lymphomas may present in the nasopharynx and must be considered in the differential diagnosis of a non-ulcerating lobulated mass in this region. Unusual tumors may also present as a mass in the nasopharynx. These tumors will be discussed in the differential diagnosis.

Table 8-1. Histology of Veterans General Hospital, Taiwan series (CHIANG and GRIEM 1973)

Types	No. of patients	% of 350 patients
Epidermoid carcinoma	151	43.1
Transitional cell carcinoma	133	38.0
Anaplastic carcinoma	37	10.6
Lymphoepithelioma	9	2.6
Angiosarcoma	1	0.3
Unclassified	19	5.4
Total	350	100.0

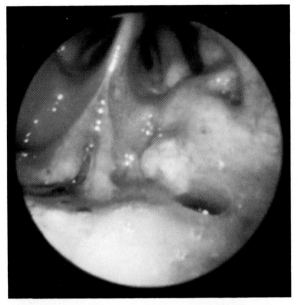

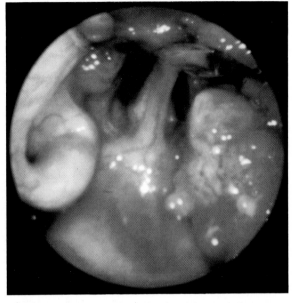

Fig. 8-5. Early 3 mm lesion in nasopharynx. Patient had neck adenopathy

Fig. 8-6. Exophytic lobular lesion involving several areas

There is some controversy among pathologists on the interpretation and classification of the epithelial tumors of the nasopharynx. Reverchon and Coutard in France, and Schmincke in Germany, simultaneously reported on the tumor described as a lymphoepithelioma, which has been considered to be the classic histologic type of nasopharyngeal tumor. This is probably and epithelial tumor with a lymphoid response to the malignancy. This incidence of this tumor varies from series to series (HSU et al. 1987).

8.6 Clinical Manifestations

8.6.1 General Comments

In the series of 350 patients seen at the Veterans' General Hospital in Taiwan, the signs and symptoms can be divided into several groups (CHIANG and GRIEM 1973). The patient may present with signs and symptoms related to the primary tumor itself, where as other patients may present with lymphadenopathy as the intial manifestation of this disease. Other patients present with symptoms related to the extension of the tumor to encompass cranial nerves inside the skull or outside the skull at the level of the retro-pharyngeal nodes. As the disease progresses, one may see distant metastases in the lung, liver or bone.

8.6.2 Local Tumor Manifestations

Table 8-2 presents the common local symptoms of nasopharyngeal cancer (CHIANG and GRIEM 1973). The percentage is greater than 100 since some patients present with several symptoms simultaneously. Nasal bleeding, obstruction of the airway and headache are common findings. Symptoms related to hearing, including impaired hearing and ringing of the ears are also common findings. When the tumor involves the Eustachian tube, symptoms

Table 8-2. Common presenting symptoms in Veterans General Hospital Series (CHIANG and GRIEM 1973)

Common symptoms	No. of patients	% of 350 patients
Nasal bleeding	155	44.2
Nasal obstruction	106	30.3
Headache	144	40.2
Stuffiness, impaired hearing	79	22.6
Tinnitus	73	20.8
Diplopia, visual disturbance	70	20.0
Numbness of face	42	12.0
Sore throat	30	8.6
Hoarseness, voice change	18	5.3
Swallowing, disturbance	15	4.3

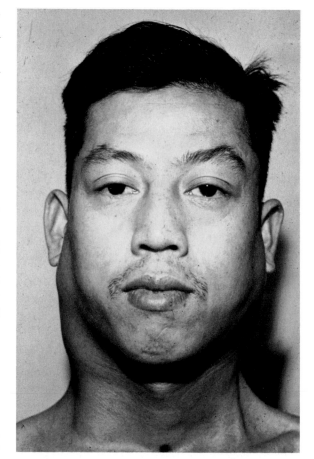

Fig. 8-7. Bilateral lymph node involvement demonstrated

of otitis media, tinnitus, and impaired hearing and stuffiness of the nose may be elicited. When the tumor involves the nasal cavity, bleeding may be seen and nasal obstruction, change in voice and difficulty breathing may be observed with breathing through the mouth as a late symptom.

8.6.3 Regional Manifestations

8.6.3.1 Lymphatic Structures

Regional disease manifests principally as metastases to the cervical lymph nodes. In the Veterans' General Hospital series, Table 8-3 demonstrates the high frequency of cervical lymph node metastases seen in nasopharyngeal carcinoma (CHIANG and GRIEM 1973). Similar observations have been made at the MD Anderson Hospital, (LINDBERG 1972). Lymph node involvement may be bilateral as shown by the patient in Figure 8-7 and involvement of the posterior cervical nodes is common as shown by the patient in Figure 8-8. The most common node involved is at the anterior margin of the ster-

noclidodomastoid muscle just below the ear lobe and posterior to the angle of the mandible. The jugulo-diagatric node is the next most common node involved with spread to the spinal accessory chain, mid-jugular chain and with spread to the retropharyngeal nodes (Fig. 8-9).

8.6.3.2 Non-lymphatic Structures

With the tumor spreading laterally and superiorly to the base of the skull, one finds invasion of the base of the skull and bone destruction. Cranial nerves inside the skull posteriorly through the jugular foramen are commonly involved. On CT scan or MRI, involvement of the cranial nerves may be seen inside the skull or at the base of the skull in the region of the retropharyngeal nodes. In an analysis of 350 patients, 25.4% had cranial nerve involvement and all cranial nerves can be involved to a varying degree (Fig. 8-10), (CHIANG and GRIEM 1973). The most common cranial nerve involved is

Table 8-3. Cervical lymph node metastases in Veterans General Hospital Series (CHIANG and GRIEM 1973)

Clinically positive	No. of patients	% of 350 patients
Unilateral	149	42.5
Single node	90	25.7
Multiple nodes	59	16.8
Bilateral	138	39.5
Single node	16	4.5
Multiple nodes	122	35.0
Total	287	82.0

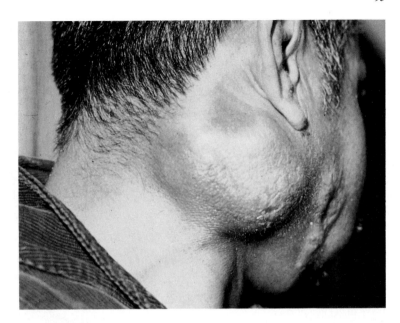

Fig. 8-8. Posterior node involvement demonstrated

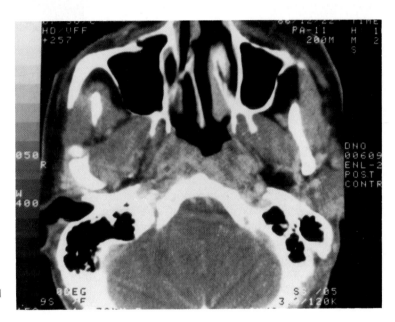

Fig. 8-9. CT scan showing retropharyngeal node involvement

the 6th cranial nerve in the frequency distribution shown in that series. Figure 8-11 demonstrates a patient with a squint due to involvement of the *6th* cranial nerve. The patient also has trismus suggesting that the tumor has extended into the pterygoid region. A Horner's syndrome can be seen as the retropharyngeal node involvement impinges on the cervical sympathic trunk. These nerve palsies have been subclassified and identified as to the first author who described the finding in an excellent review in Lederman's book (LEDERMAN 1961). Two

principal palsies can be identified; one called the retroparotidian syndrome, usually involving the 9th, 10th, 11th and 12th cranial nerves; the other syndrome called the petro-sphenoidal syndrome involving the 3rd, 4th, 5th, and 6th cranial nerves commonly, (and occasionally the 2nd nerve caused by extension superiorly through the foramen lacerum into the middle cranial fossa lateral to the sella). Figure 8-11 demonstrates a patient with 6th nerve involvement. The 1st cranial nerve lies quite anteriorly and is rarely involved and the 7th and 8th cra-

Cranial Nerve Involvement in Nasopharyngeal
Carcinoma

Total Number of Patients With Cranial Nerve Involvement	Percent of 350 Patients
89	25.4

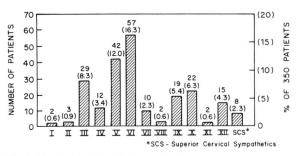

Fig. 8-10. Graph of cranial nerve involvement

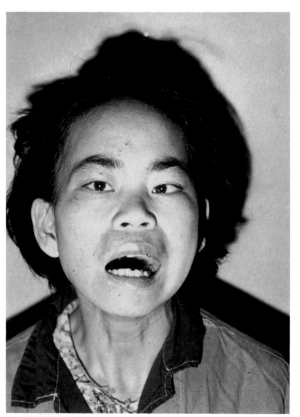

Fig. 8-11. Patient with squint due to cranial nerve involvement

nial nerves are not commonly involved because of the protected course of these nerves as they traverse the skull in the internal acoustic foramen.

8.6.4 Other Manifestations

Table 8-4 demonstrates the incidence of local invasion of contiguous structures. This tumor may invade the pterygoid plate and when the retropharyngeal tissue and pharyngeal constrictor muscles are invaded, the patient may complain of sore throat and difficulty swallowing. With invasion anteriorly, the pterygoid muscle involvement may produce trismus. The tumor may grow into the nasal cavity, extend into the antrum, ethmoid and orbit. A large mass extending into the oropharynx may be an interesting late finding.

Table 8-4. Local invasion of contiguous structures in Veterans General Hospital Series (CHIANG and GRIEM 1973)

Structures	No. of patients	% of 350 patients
Base of skull (including sphenoid sinus)	60	17.2
Oropharynx	28	8.0
Pterygoid fossa	15	4.3
Paranasal sinuses (excluding sphenoid)	7	2.0
Whole nasal fossa	5	1.4
Orbit	3	0.9

8.7 Detection and Diagnosis

8.7.1 General Comments

Patients of Chinese background deserve frequent screening exams of the nasopharyngeal area and query into symptoms related to the nasal cavity and nasopharynx. Patients with unexplained cervical adenopathy should be evaluated by examination of the nasopharynx. Needle aspiration and biopsy of the lymph nodes may help in establishing the diagnosis.

8.7.2 Mirror Examination

The nasopharynx can be examined by a skilled examiner without difficulty using a small angled mirror heated to body temperature. For patients who gag easily, topical anesthetics may be sprayed into the oropharynx. Some patients who are extremely nervous may require premedication. In examining some patients with a very thick tongue, a small nasopharyngeal cavity, or a short neck, retraction of the uvula using a special retractor and topical anesthesia of the uvula and pharynx becomes part of the procedure.

8.7.3 Nasopharyngeal Camera

The nasopharyngeal camera provides an excellent means of examining the nasopharynx. These units, either flexible or rigid, have a special lens (wide angle – fish eye type) and camera which allows visualization, special illumination and photography. The device inserted through the mouth can visualize the whole nasopharynx. Topical anaesthesia is applied to the oropharynx and a uvular retractor is used in combination with the optical system. This camera and optical unit is very useful in demonstrating small lesions and provides a permanent record of the extent of disease, and important in providing a serial documentation of the lesion as it responds to radiation therapy.

8.7.4 X-ray Examination and Other Imaging Procedures

The nasopharyngeal cavity can be opacified using a nasopharyngeogram and has been advocated in the past as a method of pretreatment evaluation. X-ray examination of the base of the skull is useful in determining the extent of bony involvement, however, with modern CT scanning, the extend of disease in the nasopharynx is carefully documented using high resolution CT procedures. Figure 8-12 demonstrates the lateral pharyngeal involvement. Lymph node metastases especially the lymph node groups in the retropharyngeal region are well demonstrated with high resolution CT scans. In treatment planning the CT scans are very important to help in determining beam direction and can be used as basic data for the treatment planning computer for electron density corrections (KESSLER et al. 1987). The role of magnetic resonance imaging (MRI) in the detection, diagnosis and management of this cancer appears to play a very important role in detecting edema and early extension to the regional structures including the sphenoid sinus. One may expect to see MRI become an important procedure (KESSLER et al. 1987). Nuclear magnetic resonance procedures on blood samples may also play a role in detection. As yet, ultrasound and isotope scanning have not been useful imaging procedures in detection or management of this epithelial cancer. Galli-

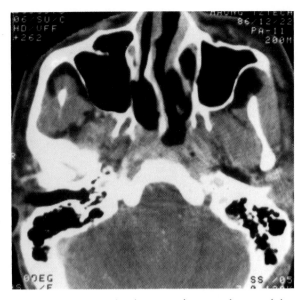

Fig. 8-12. CT scan showing extensive nasopharyngeal involvement

um tumor scanning will image lymphomas which may, on occasion, present in the nasopharynx. Whether radioactive monoclonal antibodies can be made to target this disease is a future prospect for both diagnosis and ultimate therapy.

8.7.5 Diagnosis

With all of the details presented above, the diagnosis of this tumor is based on the recognition of the symptoms of nasal bleeding, nasal obstruction and the detection of lymphadenopathy particularly of the posterior cervical nodes and the recognition of the multiple cranial nerve syndromes which may point to a tumor in the nasopharynx. The final diagnosis is based on histological tissue taken by biopsy from the nasopharynx. In some instances, the tumor is so small that the initial examination dose not view the primary lesion. A diagnosis of cancer of the nasopharynx based on the histology found in neck node sampling is not an ideal method of establishing the diagnosis, however, occasionally the primary lesion disappears leaving only the neck node disease.

8.7.6 Differential Diagnosis

A number of disease may produce a mass in the nasopharynx. A list of these possibilities is given in Table 8-5.

Table 8-5. Differential diagnosis of nasopharyngeal mass

Mass in nasopharynx
 1 Malignant tumors
　(a) Carcinoma (squamous cell, adeno, unclassified)
　(b) Sarcoma (rhabdo, fibro, chondro, unclassified)
　(c) Lymphoma
　(d) Mixed salivary type tumor
　(e) Plasmacytoma
　(f) Malignant melanoma
　(g) Metastasis
 2 Benign tumors
　(a) Juvenile angiofibroma
　(b) Chordoma
　(c) Odontoma
　(d) Chondroma
　(e) Neurofibroma
　(f) Angioma
 3 Hypertrophy of adenoids
 4 Granulomatous disease
 5 Sarcoidosis
 6 Nasal polyp
 7 Tumors of sphenoid
 8 Thornwall cyst
 9 Parotid gland tumor
10 Meningioma of base of skull
11 Wegener's

8.8 Treatment

8.8.1 General Comments

The treatment of choice for cancer of the naso-pharynx has been radiation therapy. The primary tumor is rather sensitive and the lymph node metastases respond dramatically to ionizing radiation. The site of the primary tumor limits any curative attempt by surgery. (Surgical removal of the base of the skull is possible, however, a functional patient with a good outcome is not readily achievable with current surgical techniques.) Likewise, chemotherapy has made great strides in the management of certain tumors highly sensitive to combination chemotherapy, however, in this epithelial malignancy the role of chemotherapy has yet to be defined (VILLAR et al. 1987), (TANNOCK et al. 1986). The risks of injury of normal tissue by radiation therapy are well-defined for this region. The tolerance of the nervous system is well known particularly for late injury (GRIEM 1987; GLASS et al. 1984; MARKS et al. 1981; WARA et al. 1975; ABBATUCCI et al. 1978; SHUKOVSKY and FLETCHER 1972). Data concerning the nervous system and certain cancer chemotherapeutic drugs suggest an interaction between some drugs and radiation (VAN DER KOGEL and SISSINGH 1985; DANOFF 1983). Drug concentra-

tions in the blood vary widely from patient to patient adding another confounding factor which may decrease the tolerance of normal tissue to ionizing radiation particularly the central nervous system. At this point adjuvant chemotherapy coupled with radiation therapy is experimental. There may be some evidence that pretreatment with chemotherapy changes the tumor doubling time to a short time interval making radiation therapy more difficult. If chemotherapy is used, the patient should be on some experimental protocol and the patient should understand the risks involved and give informed consent to such experiments. At the present time treatment by radiation therapy alone should be used at a dose optimum for its maximum benefit (METZ et al. 1982; ANDREWS 1985).

8.8.2 Techniques of Radiation Therapy

Most centers, using megavoltage photon radiation therapy or Cobalt-60 radiation in the treatment of this tumor have improved the 5-year survival when compared with the kilovoltage era (LEDERMAN 1972). The ability to deliver photon radiation to the site of the tumor and the lymph node metastases yet sparing the skin and avoiding sensitive structures has made a significant change in outcome (HUANG 1980). High energy electron therapy coupled with photon therapy has allowed the therapist to irradiate the superficial lymph node regions of the neck without injuring the deep structures such as the cervical spinal cord (GRIEM et al. 1979).

Prior to initiating treatment, it is essential to obtain a dental consultation to evaluate the condition of the teeth. After approximately 1000 cGy there is frank dryness of the mouth with a major reduction in the production of saliva (MOSSMAN et al. 1979). Serous cell function is curtailed above 1000 cGy while mucus gland function continues until somewhat higher does are reached. Although submaxillary salivary glands may be excluded from the field of radiation, the parotid salivary glands which are in the field of radiation represent the major contribution to saliva production in the mouth. With dryness of the mouth, serious oral problems ensue including changes in the teeth as cavities occur around the neck of the tooth and the level of the junction of the enamel and dentin. These problems can be minimized by applying high concentration of fluoride to the teeth using fluoride compounds as a past or solution in custom fabricated dental carriers for this application. This procedure hardens the surface of the teeth and prevents cavities. The diet should be changed to reduce the sugar in the diet. Any diseased teeth should be fixed if possible or removed prior to treatment (BEDWINEK et al. 1976; CHENG and WANG 1974).

CT scans of the nasopharynx and of the regional nodes of the neck as well as information of the position of critical structures of the brain, base of the brain, cervical spinal cord and eye may be used in the detailed treatment planning procedure. Information about the extend of disease in the nasopharynx base of the skull, nasal cavity, and pterygoid regions can provide important information for the treatment planning procedure, so as to minimize the dose in the normal tissues and maximize the dose in the disease and the regional metastatic sites. Figure 8-13 a and Figure 8-13 b show the immobilization procedure used prior to simulation for the laterally directed beams and show the anterior low neck field as well. Figure 8-14 shows the simulator

film with the fields to be used. Figure 8-15 demonstrates the custom blocks for the initial lateral fields. The verification films for these initial fields are shown in Figure 8-16. A reduced field directed at the primary lesion when cervical spinal cord tolerance is approached and is demonstrated in Figure 8-17. The posterior nodes are treated simultaneously with electron fields. The isodose curves for such a plan are shown in Figure 8-18.

8.8.3 Dose Strategy

The primary lesion which has a histological diagnosis of squamous cell carcinoma or lymphoepithelioma will require a dose of 6500 to 7200 cGy depending upon tumor size and upon the decision making process in which the probability of tumor control is considered as a principal factor in the treatment

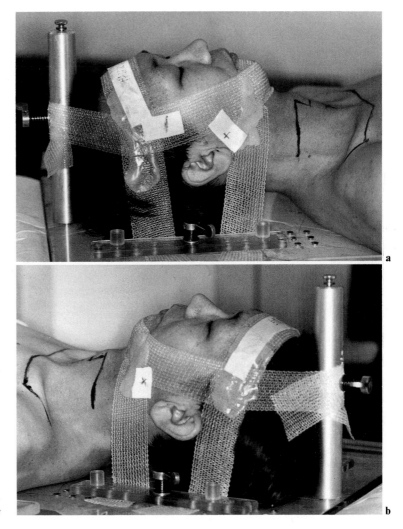

Fig. 8-13. a Patient immobilization for lateral field placement. **b** Opposite side view

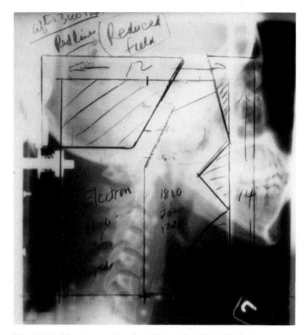

Fig. 8-14. Simulator planning film with initial field placement

equation. With standard fractionation of 180–200 cGy per day it is essential to attempt to complete the treatment without a break or interruption. In an analysis of related head and neck epithelial tumors made by Withers, lengthening the treatment time decreased the probability of tumor control (WITHERS 1986).

Several authors have been treating epithelial tumors of this region with accelerated fractionation or with hyperfractionation. The Massachusetts General Hospital experience with twice a day treatment (BID) has shown some excellent results where the separation between treatments has been 4 to 6 hours. In this series, the formula for success is as follows: 160 cGy per fraction is given BID, 5 days a week until a dose of 3840 cGy has been given to the tumor; a rest period of 10 days to 14 days is inserted and the treatment resumed using like 160 cGy fractions BID until a total tissue dose of 6400 cGy is given to the tumor. There are 12 treatment days in the first part, a 10 to 14 day break and 8 treatment days in the second part. In the second part of the treatment, the cervical spinal cord is NOT treated (WANG 1986).

In the M.D. Anderson fractionation technique, there is no break and the dose per fraction is 120 cGy given BID with a 6 hour interval between the two fractions. A tissue dose of 6800 to 7200 cGy is planned in this technique.

In addition to the external radiation it is possible to add additional radiation locally with a brachytherapy technique described by C.C. Wang (WANG et al. 1975). This is a afterloading technique which can add 1000 to 2000 cGy to the local area without giving a significant dose to the brain or spinal cord. The technique can be done on an outpatient basis and is not of great discomfort to the patient. His overall local control rate with the BID accelerated fractionation and the intracavitary boost is 85% (WANG 1986).

8.8.4 Therapy of Cervical Lymph Nodes

Since approximately 90% of the patients have cervical lymphadenopathy containing tumor, treatment of the lymph nodes of the neck should be routine. Both sides of the neck are at risk and both necks should be treated in the initial treatment plan (Figure 8-13a and Figure 8-13b). The posterior lymph nodes are commonly involved. There is no real role for surgical treatment as an alternative because of

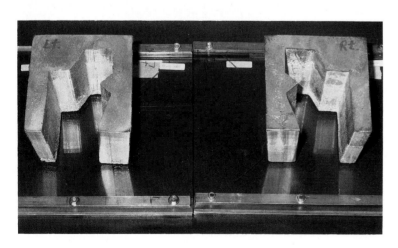

Fig. 8-15. Custom blocks for initial field

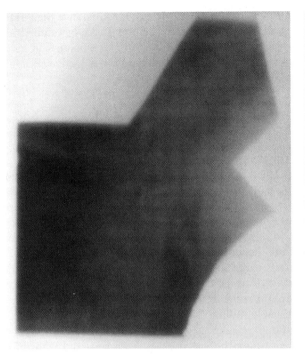

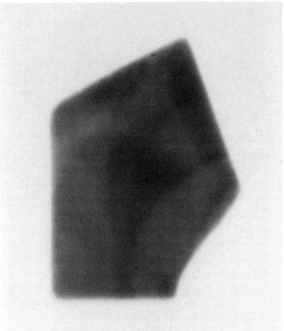

Fig. 8-16. Verification films. Note extension of field posteriorly. Field will be reduced as cord tolerance is approached

Fig. 8-17. Reduced field shown on verification film to avoid exceeding tolerance of cervical spinal cord. Lateral fields treated with electrons at this point

the retropharyngeal node involvement found in this disease. There is no combined surgery and radiation therapy series showing any superiority of the adjuvant surgery with or without chemotherapy. The details of the treatment plan should be designed to cover the neck nodes while avoiding a high dose to the cervical spinal cord. Matching anterior photon and posterior electron beam fields can be used (GRIEM et al. 1979), Figure 8-18. An anterior supraclavicular field can be added to treat microscopic disease extension in the lower neck (Figure 8-13). Half block techniques may be used for field matching so as to provide a uniform dose at the junction of two fields. For these techniques, a cast or customized patient positioning devise should be used to insure the day-to-day reproducability of the treatment plan (Figure 8-15). Some therapists use a bite block in the immobilization process; however, the rigid custom cast technique provides greater accuracy of setup (MILLION and BOVA 1987).

Custom made blocks should be used to protect normal tissue and to make the patient better tolerate the radiation therapy. Following the completion of 5000 cGy (if 180 to 200 cGy daily fractionation is used) with large lateral fields including the whole primary lesion and all of the regional lymphatics,

additional radiation therapy is given to modified fields (Figure 8-17). As the primary tumor requires 7000 cGy with the above daily fractionation, the port of radiation for the primary should be shrunk to avoid normal tissue, the pons, brain stem, and cervical cord and orbital contents but adequate to include the nasopharyngeal cavity and its walls including the imaginary wall of anterior nasopharynx (Figure 8-13). Additional radiation to the lymph nodes may be necessary and should be customized depending on the distribution and extent of involvement. This treatment of the lymphatics should be given so as to avoid the cervical spinal cord. Matched lateral electron beam fields adjusted for the penetration of the particular energy of the accelerator being used is an important part of the planning process at this point. An additional 1000 to 2000 cGy may be needed for the adenopathy depending on the initial degree of involvement and response of the nodes. The low neck nodes are infrequently involved and the anterior low neck field is not an essential part of the treatment. As treatment of the primary lesion and neck nodes progresses, careful observation of the primary lesion should be done and is easily accomplished and documented with the nasopharyngeal camera. Tumor regression and normal tissue reactions should be recorded.

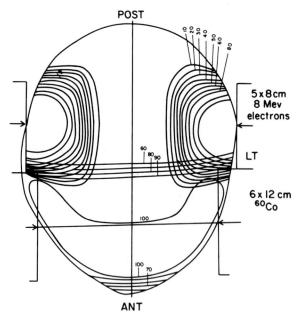

Fig. 8-18. Composite isodose curves showing laterally directed anterior photon and posterior electron beams, as would be used in Figure 8-17

Several weeks after the external beam therapy is complete, intracavitary brachytherapy can be considered.

8.8.5 Special Problems and Unusual Diseases

8.8.5.1 Nasopharyngeal Angiofibroma

This is a benign disease usually found in males as they enter puberty. The tumor may be highly vascular and produce nasal obstruction, epistaxis with difficulty in breathing and phonation. The extend of tumor can be seen on CT scan and vascular studies may show the relation of the lesion to the vascular structures at the base of the skull. The first approach to this disease is surgical and may involve embolization; however, in a number of patients, repeated surgical procedures have not controlled this benign lesion. In some patients, the disease may extend into the orbit and floor of the middle cranial fossa making removal difficult (KADIN et al. 1974). This lesion responds very favorably to radiation therapy (FITZPATRICK and RIDER 1973). Radiation directed to the lesion giving 3500 cGy in 16 fractions in 3 weeks to does a high as 6000 cGy are cited in an excellent review of the subject found in the Federal Food and Drug publication on benign diseases (KOPICKY and ORDER 1977). In selecting radi-

ation for a benign lesion, one must balance the risks of treatment against the minimal risk of tumor induction. A review of radiation carcinogensis in humans has placed this problem in perspective (BOICE and FRAUMANI 1984).

8.8.5.2 Nasopharyngeal Lymphoma

The nasopharynx has a rich lymphatic network, particularly situated in the posterior nasopharynx, a part of Waldeyer's ring. Primary presentation of a lymphoma can occur at this site and it is essential to examine a patient with early lymphoma of the neck for tumor in the nasopharynx. Hodgkin's disease and the non-Hodgkin's lymphomas may be seen. The result of treatment of early disease either stage I or early stage II may be very favorable. Treatment with regional radiation therapy including elective radiation of the neck should be carried out after thorough staging (MARKS et al. 1974). Excellent long term survival has been reported with diffuse histiocytic lymphoma (VOKES et al. 1985; WANG 1969).

8.8.5.3 Plasmacytoma

A solitary plasma cell tumor may occur in the nasopharynx. This tumor if localized may be treated and controlled with a dose of 6000 cGy in five weeks as with other presentations in the head and neck region (KOTNER and WANG 1972).

8.8.5.4 Minor Salivary Gland Tumors

A tumor with a histological diagnosis of a salivary gland may be seen in the nasopharynx. It should be managed by radiation therapy as discussed in the chapter on salivary gland tumors.

8.8.5.5 Miscellaneous Tumors

Various tumor presentations may be seen in the nasopharynx. These may include a chordoma, a variety of sarcomas, and melanoma. Benign tumors such as neurofibroma may also present in the nasopharynx. Because of the unique location and disease distribution, radiation therapy may play a major role in the management of this unique treatment situation.

8.8.5.6 Mid-line Granuloma

This lesion presents an enigma. A review by Eichel suggests that this might be subclassified into two diseases; Wegener's granulomatosis and midline malignant reticulosis (EICHEL 1968; KASSEL et al. 1969). Eichel also points out that other lymphomas, including mycosis fungoides, and a variety of inflammatory conditions can simulate these two lesions.

The differentiation between these two ulcerating lesions seems to be the angitis found in Wegener's type and the fact that this condition may also be found as necrotizing lesions in the upper and lower respirator tract, focal glomerulitis and generalized focal necrotizing vasculitis (ALDO et al. 1970). Wegener's granulomatosis responds to immunosuppressive agents particularly the alkylating agents (ALDO et al. 1970; HOLLANDER and MANNING 1967; NOVAK and PEARSON 1971). The lesion may be found in the nasopharynx frequently and may even involve the heart (CARRINGTON and LIEBOW 1956). Wolff also discusses this disease in depth (FAUCI and WOLFF 1973; WOLFF 1974).

Midline malignant reticulosis appears to be a malignant neoplasm of lymphoreticular cells with an admixture of inflammatory cells (FECHNER and LAMPPIN 1972). Vasculitis is not a major feature of this histology. In that review, several patients with localized disease were without disease after being treated with radiation of doses between 3500 and 6000 cGy. Although the series is small, patients receiving lower doses than 3500 cGy did not do well.

8.9 Follow-up

Important in the overall support and follow-up program is the care of the post-radiation oral mucosa and the mucosa of the nasopharynx, and oropharynx. The secretions of the salivary glands and the mucus and serous glands of the mucosa are decreased. The epithelium is less able to respond to stress. Humidification of the patient's environment will help symptomatically. Irritation of the mucosa should be avoided. Such irritants as smoking, alcohol, hot and spicy food should be avoided. The diet should consist of soft foods which will not abrade the heavily irradiated mucosa. The patient will always complain of a dry mouth. It is essential that the patient return to the dentist for frequent follow-up care and management of any small dental carries that may occur.

Follow-up may be conducted at monthly intervals for the first several months. If the patient is recovering satisfactorily, the follow-up sequence can then be extended to visits every three months for the first two years. Twice a year follow-up is then suggested through the five year point, with yearly follow-up thereafter. Inspection of the nasopharynx, oropharynx, mouth and laryngopharynx should be done as well as an evaluation of the status of the neck. A chest x-ray is suggested to search for pulmonary metastases in the early follow-up period. A general physical exam with palpation of the abdominal viscera, particularly the liver, should be done since this is a common site for metastases.

8.10 Retreatment

Wang has reported on the retreatment of patients who have failed the first course of treatment (WANG and SCHULZ 1966). He has retreated the same region with some success without seeing unacceptable side effects in those patients referred to him for such treatment where the first course of radiation was not given with an optimum technique or an effective dose.

8.11 Outcome Analysis

The results of treatment have improved significantly over the past two decades. With the use of higher doses of radiation and the addition of hyperfractionation and intracavitary therapy, local control of 85% has been reported. Shukovsky and his collaborators at the M.D. Anderson Hospital have reported a dose response curve for epithelial tumors in this region (SHUKOVSKY 1970; MESIC et al. 1981). Others have reported on the radiosensitivity of this tumor (BOHORQUEZ 1976; HOPPE et al. 1976). The University of California group has analyzed the response of T_1 tumors in terms of percent local control (MOENCH and PHILLIPS 1972). Marks and his associates confirmed the existence of such a dose response curve for similar tumors in the pharynx (MARKS et al. 1982). Tokars and his colleagues have analyzed the dose response curve for epithelial tumors of the nasopharynx separating the T_1 and T_2 tumors from the advanced T_3 and T_4 disease patients and found a dose response curve for these two groups of T stages and compared the outcome with complications in the nervous systems a result of irradiation of the cervical spinal cord (TOKARS et al. 1979). High dose photon therapy of the cervical spinal cord has also been evaluated recently by Kim and Fayos (KIM 1978). Metz has taken Tokars data to provide a decision making analysis curve for cancer of the nasopharynx (METZ 1982). Andrews recently has reviewed this decision making process for radiation therapy sighting head and neck malignancies as a place where these concepts can be applied. The outcome depends on the dose delivered and the time in which the treatment is given (ANDREWS 1985). Cure rates of over 60% can be achieved in the modern era (WANG 1986).

8.12 Summary

The results of treatment of the epithelial malignancy are very good. Radiation therapy is the treatment of choice following recognition and diagnosis. High risk groups have been identified and should be screened regularly for this tumor. Megavoltage radiation therapy with modern methods of treatment planning with CT scanning coupled with proper preparation of the patient, particularly dental care, have resulted in an excellent outcome.

References

Abbatucci JS, Delozier T, Quint R, et al. (1978) Radiation myelopathy of the cervical spinal cord: Time, dose and volume factors. Int J Radiat Oncol Biol Phys 4: 239–248

Aldo MA, Benson MD, Comerford MB, Cohen AS (1970) Treatment of Wegener's granulomatosis with immunosuppressive agents. Arch Intern Med 126: 298–305

Andrews JR (1985) Benefit, risk and optimization by ROC analysis in cancer radiotherapy. Int J Radiat Oncol Biol Phys 11: 1557–1562

Boice J, Fraumani R (1984) Radiation Carcinogenesis. Raven Press, New York (eds)

Bedwinek JM, Shukovsky LJ, Fletcher GH, et al. (1976) Osteonecrosis in patients with treated with definitive radiation therapy for squamous cell carcinoma of the oral cavity naso- and oropharynx. Radiology 119: 665–667

Bohne BA, Marks JE, Glasgow GP (1985) Delayed effects of ionizing radiation on the ear. Laryngoscope 95: 818–828

Bohorquez J (1976) Factors that modify the radio-response of cancer of the nasopharynx. Am J Roentgenol 126: 863–876

Cai WM, Zhang HX, Hu YH, Gu XZ (1983) Influence of biopsy on nasopharyngeal carcinoma – a critical study of biopsy from the nasopharynx and cervical lymph node of 649 patients. Int J Rad Onc Biol Phys 9: 1439–1444

Carrington CB, Liebow AA (1956) Limited forms of angiitis and granulomatosis of Wegener's type. Am J Med 41: 497–527

Chen KL, Fletcher GH (1971) Malignant tumors of the nasopharynx. Radiology 99: 165–171

Cheng VST, Wang CC (1974) Osteoradionecrosis of the mandible resulting from external megavoltage radiation therapy. Radiology 112: 685–689

Chiang TC, Jung PF (1977) Nasopharyngoscope and camera examination of primary carcinoma of the nasopharynx. Cancer 40: 2353–2364

Chiang TC, Griem ML (1973) Nasopharyngeal cancer. Surg C1 N Am 53: 121–133

Danoff BF (1983) Complications and late effects of irradiation of brain tumors. In: Syllabus: Therapy of CNS Tumors. Marks JE, Griem ML. (eds) RSNA Chicago

Eichel BS, Mabery TE (1968) The enigma of lethal midline granuloma. Laryngoscope 78: 1367–1386

Fauci AS, Wolff SM (1973) Wegener's granulomatosis; studies in eighteen patients and a review of the literature. Medicine 52: 535–561

Fechner RE, Lamppin DW (1972) Midline malignant Reticulosis. Arch Otolaryng 95: 467–476

Fitzpatrick GM, Rider WD (1973) The radiotherapy of nasopharyngeal angiofibroma. Radiology 109: 171–178

Glass JP, Hwang T-L, Leavens ME, Libshitz HI (1984) Cerebral radiation necrosis following treatment of extracranial malignancies. Cancer 54: 1966–1972

Griem ML, Kuchnir FT, Lanzl LH, Skaggs LS, Sutton HG, Tokars R (1979) Experience with high energy electron beam therapy at the University of Chicago. In: Chu FCH, Laughlin JS (Eds) Proceedings of the Symposium on Electron Beam Therapy - Memorial Sloan Kettering Cancer Center. Pages 99–104 Aubrion Press, New York

Griem ML (1987) Radiation therapy treatment planning for tumors of the central nervous system. In: Veath JM and Meyer J. (Eds) Treatment Planning in Radiation Therapy of Cancer. Krager, Basel, Schweiz

Hendrickson FR (1977) Management guidelines for carcinoma of the nasopharynx. In: Management Guidelines for Head and Neck Cancer. USPHS, Bethesda, Maryland

Henle W, Henle G, Ho CH, et al. (1970) Antibodies to Epstein-Barr virus in nasopharyngeal carcinoma, other head and neck neoplasms and control groups. J Nat Cancer Inst 44: 225–231

Ho HC (1967) Nasopharyngeal carcinoma in Hong Kong. In: Muir CS and Shanmugaratnum K. (Eds) Cancer of the Nasopharynx-UICC Monograph Series 1: 58–63

Ho JHC (1978) An epidemiologic and clinical study of nasopharyngeal carcinoma. Int J Radiat Oncol Biol Phys 4: 183–198

Hollander D, Manning RT (1967) The use of alkylating agents in the treatment of Wegener's granulomatosis. Ann Int Med 67: 393–398

Hoppe RT, Goffinet DR, Bagshaw MA (1976) Carcinoma of the nasopharynx: Eighteen years' experience with megavoltage radiation therapy. Cancer 37: 2605–2612

Hoppe RT, Williams J, Warnke E, et al. (1978) Carcinoma of the nasopharynx; significance of histology. Int J Rad Oncol Biol Phys 4: 199–205

Hsu HC, Chen CL, Hsu MN, Lynn TC, Tu SM, Huang SC (1987) Pathology of nasopharyngeal carcinoma: Proposal of a new histologic classification correlated with prognosis. Cancer 59: 945–951

Huang SC (1980) Nasopharyngeal cancer: A review of 1605 patients treated radically with cobalt-60. Int J Rad Oncol Biol Phys 6: 401–407

Hwang HN (1983) Nasopharyngeal carcinoma in the People's Republic of China: incidence, treatment and survival. Radiology 149: 305–309

Kadin MR, Thompson RW, Benton JR, Ward PH, Calcetena

TC (1974) Angiographic evaluation of the regression of an extensive juvenile nasopharyngeal angiofibroma after radiation therapy - a case report with therapeutic implications. Br J Radiol 47: 902-905

Kassel SH, Echevarria RA, Guzzo FP (1969) Midline malignant reticulosis (so-called lethal midline granuloma). Cancer 23: 920-935

Kessler ML, Pithluck S, Chen GTY (1987) Techniques and applications of image correction in radiotherapy treatment planning. In: Veath JM and Meyer J (eds) Treatment Planning in the Radiation Therapy of Cancer. Kager, Basel, Schweiz

Kim YH, Fayos JV (1978) Radiation injury of the cervical cord. Int J Radiat Oncol Biol Phys 5: 105, Supp. 2

Kopicky J, Order SE (1977) Survey and analysis of radiation therapy of benign diseases. USPHS FDA, Rockville, Maryland

Kotner L, Wang CC (1972) Plasmacytoma of the upper air and food passages. Cancer 30: 414-418

Laing D (1969) Virus as a cause of rhinopharyngeal carcinoma. Acta Otolaryng 67: 190-199

Lederman M (1961) Cancer of the Nasopharynx - Its Natural History and Treatment. Charles C. Thomas Pub. Springfield, Illinois, USA

Lederman M (1972) Megavoltage advances vs the orthovoltage era. JAMA 220: 398-400

Lindberg RD (1972) Distribution of cervical lymph node metastases from, squerous cell carcinoma of upper respiratory and digestive tracts. Cancer 29: 1446-1449

Marks JE, Moran EM, Griem ML, Ultmann JE (1974) Extended mantle radiotherapy in Hodgkin's disease and malignant lymphoma. Am J Roentgenol 121: 772-788

Marks JE, Baglan RJ, Prasad SC, Bland WF (1981) Cerebral necrosis; Incidence and risk in relation to dose, time, fractionation and volume. Int J Radiat Oncol Biol Phys 7: 243-252

Marks JE, Bedwinek JM, Lee F, Purdy JE, Perez CA (1982) Dose response analysis for nasopharyngeal carcinoma. Cancer 50: 1042-1050

Metz CE, Tokars RP, Kronman HB, Griem ML (1982) Maximum likelihood estimation of doseresponse parameters for therapeutic operating characteristic (TOC) analysis of carcinoma of the nasopharynx. Int J Radiat Oncol Biol Phys 8: 1185-1192

Mesic JB, Fletcher GH, Goepfert H (1981) Megavoltage irradiation of epithelial tumors of the nasopharynx. Int J Radiat Oncol Biol Phys 7: 447-453

Million RR, Bova FJ (1987) General principles for treatment planning for squamous cell carcinoma of the head and neck. In: Vaeth JM and Meyer J (eds) Treatment Planning in the Radiation Therapy of Cancer. Karger, Basel

Moench HC, Phillips TL: Carcinoma of the nasopharynx (1972) Review of 146 patients with emphasis on radiation dose and time factors. Am J Surg 124: 515-518

Mossman K, Chencharik J, Henkin R (1979) Radiation-induced changes in saliva and taste acuity in cancer patients. 6th Int. Congress of Rad Res Abstract A-29-8, pp. 10, Tokyo, Japan

Muir CS, Shanmugaratnam K (1967) Cancer of the Nasopharynx. UICC Monograph series Vol. 1, Copenhagen, Muntersgard

Novak SN, Pearson CM (1971) Cyclophosphamide therapy in Wegener's granulomatosis. N Eng J Med 284: 938-942

Petrovich Z, Cox JD, Roswit B, et al. (1982) Advanced carcinoma of the nasopharynx. Radiology 144: 905-908

Scanlon PW, Rhodes RE, Jr, Wooner LB, et al. (1967) Cancer of the nasopharynx. Am J Roentgenol 99: 313-325

Shibuya H, Kamiyama RI, Watanabe I, Horiuchi JI, Suzuki S (1987) Stage I and Stage II Waldeyer's ring an oral-sinonasal non-Hodgkin's lymphoma. Cancer 59: 940-944

Shukovsky LJ (1970) Dose, time, volume relationship in squamous cell carcinoma of the supraglottic larynx. Am J Roentgenol 108: 27

Shukovsky LJ, Fletcher GH (1972) Retinal and optic nerve complications in a high dose irradiation technique of ethmoid sinus and nasal cavity. Radiology 104: 629-634

Steiner PE (1954) Cancer - Race and Geography. Williams and Wilkins; Baltimore, Maryland

Tannock I, Hewitt K, Payne D (1986) Chemotherapy given prior to radiation for nasopharyngeal cancer (NPC) produces a high response rate but does not improve survival. Proc of ASCO 5: 133

Tokars RP, Griem ML (1979) Carcinoma of the nasopharynx an optimization of radiotherapeutic management for tumor control and spinal cord injury. Int J Rad Onco Biol Phys 5: 1741-1748

Vaeth JM (1964) Nasopharyngeal malignant tumors: 82 consecutive patients treated in a period of 22 years. Radiology 77: 364-377

Van der Kogel AJ, Sissingh HA (1985) Effects of intrathecal methotrexate and cytosine arabinoside on the radiation tolerance of the rat spinal cord. Radiother Oncol 4: 239-251

Vikram B, Mishra UB, Strong EW, Manolotos S (1985) Patterns of failure in carcinoma of the nasopharynx I. Failure at the primary site. Int J Rad Onc Biol Phys 11: 1455-1459

Villar A, Pera J, Arellano A, Galiana R, Villa S, Farrus B, Hernandez M (1987) Induction chemotherapy with cisplatin, bleomycin and methotrexate in advance head and neck cancer - lack of therapeutic gain. Radioth and Oncol 10: 175-181

Vokes EE, Ultmann JE, Golomb HM, Gaynor ER, Ferguson DJ, Griem ML, Oleske D (1985) Long term survival of patients with localized diffuse histiocytic lymphoma. Am J Clin Oncol 3: 1309-1317

Wang CC (1983) Carcinoma of the nasopharynx. In: Radiation Therapy for Head and Neck Neoplasms. CC Wang, John Wright - PSG Inc. Littleton, Massachusetts, USA

Wang CC (1969) Malignant lymphoma of Waldeyer's ring. Radiology 92: 1335-1339

Wang CC, Schulz MD (1966) Management of locally recurrent carcinoma of the nasopharynx. Radiology 86: 900-903

Wang CC, Busse J, Gitterman M (1975) A simple afterloading applicator for intracavitary irradiation of carcinoma of the nasopharynx. Radiology 115: 737-738

Wang CC (1986) Personal communication

Wara W, Phillips TL, Sheline GE, Schwade JG (1975) Radiation tolerance of the spinal cord. Cancer 35: 1558-1562

Withers HR (1986) New approaches to dose fractionation. RSNA symposium RSNA Scientific Program 161 (P): 108

Wolff SM (1974) Wegener's granulomatosis. Ann Int Med 81: 513-525

Yeh S, Cowdry EV (1954) Incidence of malignant tumors in Chinese, especially in Formosa. Cancer 7: 425-436

Zippin C, Tekawa TS, Bragg KU, et al. (1962) Studies in heredity and environment on cancer of the nasopharynx. J Nat Cancer Inst 29: 283-290

9 Hypopharynx

Anantha K. Murthy, Dennis Galinsky, and Frank R. Hendrickson

CONTENTS

9.1 Introduction

9.1.1 Anatomy

The hypopharynx is that portion of the pharynx which envelops the larynx and lies lateral and posterior to the larynx. It extends from the level of the hyoid bone superiorly to the lower border of the cricoid cartilage inferiorly. (Fig. 9-1) It consists of the pyriform sinus, the posterior pharyngeal wall

---

Anantha K. Murthy, M.D., Director – Section of Radiation Oncology
Dennis Galinsky, M.D., Section of Radiation Oncology
Frank R. Hendrickson, M.D., Professor and Chairman
Department of Therapeutic Radiology, Rush Presbyterian St. Luke's Medical Center, 1653 West Congress Parkway, Chicago, IL 60612, USA

and the post-cricoid region. The posterior pharyngeal wall of the hypopharynx is contiguous with the oropharyngeal walls. Most authors analyze the oropharyngeal wall and the hypopharyngeal wall tumors together. Pyrifom sinus cancers form the majority of hypopharyngeal cancers. The incidence of post-cricoid tumors varies in different countries and is quite uncommon in the United States.

The hypopharynx extends from the level of the hyoid bone and the pharyngoepiglottic fold to the inferior border of the cricoid cartilage. It is widest at the cephalad portion and narrows caudally. The superior border of the hypopharynx corresponds to the 3rd cervical vertebra and the inferior border to the 6th cervical vertebra. The anterior wall of the hypopharynx is the laryngeal aperture superiorly, the arytenoids and the lamina of the cricoid inferiorly. The lateral and posterior walls of the hypopharynx are made up of inferior constrictor muscles. The anterior portion of the lateral wall is intimately related to the inner aspect of the thyroid cartilage and the thyro-hyoid membrane. (Fig. 9-2)

The hypopharynx is divided into 3 sections; the pyriform sinus, the posterior pharyngeal wall and the post-cricoid area. (Fig. 9-3) The pyriform sinuses are pear-shaped channels surrounding the larynx on both sides. They form part of the gastrointestinal tract and serve as passive passageways from the oropharynx to the cervical esophagus by transporting the bolus to either side of the larynx. The loose areolar tissue that is in contact with the mucosa of the pyriform sinus anteriorly allows the pyriform sinus to expand anteriorly to accommodate the food bolus. Superiorly bordered by the pharyngo-epiglottic fold it is wide in the cephalad portion and narrows to an apex as it extends caudally to the upper border of the cricoid cartilage. The medial wall of the pyriform sinus is formed by the aryepiglotic fold superiorly and the arytenoids inferiorly. The lateral wall of the pyriform sinus is continuous with the lateral oropharyngeal wall superiorly. The cephalad portion of the lateral wall of the pyriform sinus is related to the inner aspect of the thyro-hyoid membrane and is referred to as the

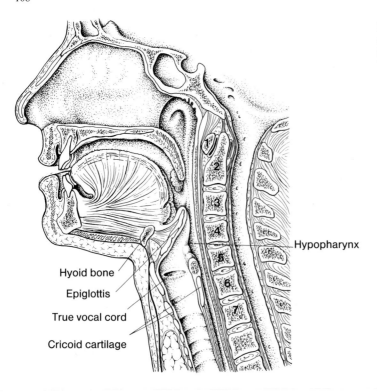

Fig. 9-1. Sagittal view of midplane of the neck showing the relationship of the hypopharynx to surrounding structures. (From CIBA/Netter Vol. 3, Pt. 1, § 1, Plate 16)

Hypopharynx

Hyoid bone
Epiglottis
True vocal cord
Cricoid cartilage

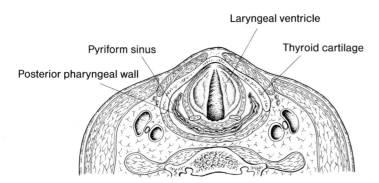

Laryngeal ventricle
Pyriform sinus
Thyroid cartilage
Posterior pharyngeal wall

Fig. 9-2. Cross-section of hypopharynx at the level of the laryngeal ventricle.

membranous portion of the pyriform sinus. More inferiorly, it lies against the inner aspect of the thyroid ala and is referred to as the cartilagenous portion. Posteriorly, the pyriform sinus is continuous with the pharyngeal cavity. The posterior pharyngeal wall is continuous with the oropharyngeal wall superiorly and the cervical esophagus inferiorly. Anteriorly, it is continuous with the lateral wall of the pyriform sinus in the cephalad portion and with the post-cricoid region in the caudal aspect.

The post-cricoid area covers the posterior surface of the larynx from the arytenoid cartilage to the inferior border of the cricoid. The lateral margin is the pyriform fossa superiorly and the post-pharyngeal wall inferiorly.

9.1.2 Lymphatics

The hypopharynx is drained by a rich network of lymphatics. The lymphatics exit through the thyrohyoid membrane and terminate in the retropharyngeal lymph nodes superiorly and the jugular chain laterally. The incidence of involvement of lymph nodes in carcinomas of the hypopharynx varies somewhat by the site of tumor involvement. Carcinomas arising in the pyriform sinus have the highest incidence of positive nodes at presentation. Compilation of selected literature for the incidence of positive nodes is shown in Table 9-1. Seventy-five percent of patients with pyriform sinus cancers have positive nodes on admission. Posterior pha-

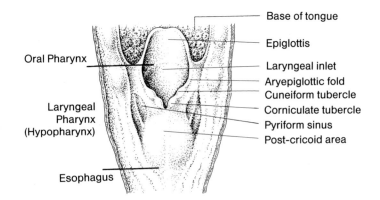

Fig. 9-3. Posterior view of the interior of the pharynx. (From CIBA/Netter Vol. 3, Pt. 1, § 1, Plate 17)

Table 9-1. Incidence of positive nodes by site

	No of Patients	%
Pyriform Sinus Cancers[a, b, c, d, e]	1112	75
Posterior Pharyngeal Wall Cancers[f, g, h, i]	381	56
Post-Cricoid Area[j, k]	200	37

[a] GOEPFETRT et al. (1981), [b] SHAH et al. (1976), [c] DRISCOLL et al. (1983), [d] MARTIN et al. (1980, [e] BATAINI et al. (1981), [f] MARKS et al. (1978 b), [g] TALTON et al. (1981), [h] MEOZ-MENDEZ et al. (1978), [i] PENE et al. (1978), [j] BRYCE (1967), [k] HIRANO et al. (1982).

Table 9-2. Contralateral neck failures

%	No of Patients
17[a]	35/203[a]
25[b]	5/19[b]
16[c]	13/82[c]
15[d]	20/137[d]

[d] EL BADAWI et al. (1982), [b] EISBACH and KRAUSE (1977), [c] CARPENTER et al. (1976), [d] MARKS et al. (1978 a, b)

ryngeal wall lesions have 50% positive nodes and approximately 35% of post-cricoid lesions have positive nodes.

The reported incidence of bilateral or contralateral nodal involvement is 3–10% (EL BADAWI et al. 1982; DRISCOLL et al. 1983; EISBACH and KRAUSE 1977; CARPENTER et al. 1976) in pyriform sinus cancers. Posterior pharyngeal wall lesions tend to spread bilaterally more frequently with the incidence varying quite widely (10–35%). (MEOZ-MENDEZ et al. 1978; WANG 1970)

Occult disease in clinically node negative patients is significant; SHAH et al. (1976) reported a 41% incidence of microscopic metastatic disease in patients with clinically negative neck nodes who underwent prophylactic node dissection. OGURA et al. (1980) reported an incidence of 38% sub-clinical disease in pyriform sinus and 66% in posterior pharyngeal wall lesions. When clinically negative neck nodes were left untreated, SHAH et al. (1976) reported a 25% incidence of failures in the neck.

Occult disease in the contralateral neck is also significant. Contralateral neck failures after surgery have been found to be 15–25% by various authors (EL BADAWI et al. (1982); EISBACH and KRAUSE 1977; CARPENTER et al. 1976; MARKS et al. 1978) (Table 9-2).

Jugulo-digastric lymph nodes are the most commonly involved group of nodes. Mid-jugular lymph nodes are the next most common. Like nasopharyngeal carcinomas, retropharyngeal lymph nodes are frequently involved. These lymph nodes are found posterior to the pharynx near the base of the skull and have been classified into medial and lateral groups. (Fig. 9-4) The lateral groups are intimately related to the internal carotid artery and the lymphatic chain. The medial group is more inferior and accessible by surgery. BALLENTYNE (1964) reported a 44% incidence of involvement of retropharyngeal nodes in pharyngeal wall tumors undergoing surgery.

9.1.3 Incidence and Epidemiology

Hypopharyngeal carcinomas are quite rare. Overall incidence was 1.0/100,000 population. That would mean approximately 2500 new cases per year. This constitutes 0.3% of all cancers and about 6% of all head and neck cancers. Laryngeal carcinoma is about 5 times as common as hypopharyngeal tumors. The male to female ratio is 4 to 1. The 1973–77 SEER (Surveillance, Epidemiology and End Results) program of the National Cancer Institute found the highest incidence rates among Hispanic males in Puerto-Rico (4.4/100,000) and Ha-

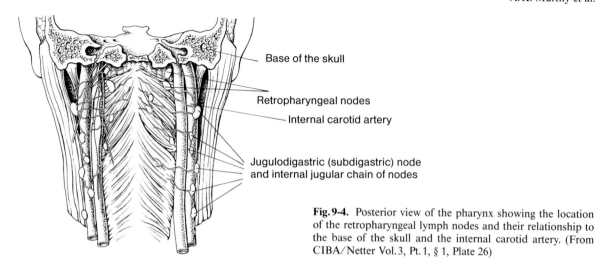

Base of the skull

Retropharyngeal nodes

Internal carotid artery

Jugulodigastric (subdigastric) node
and internal jugular chain of nodes

Fig. 9-4. Posterior view of the pharynx showing the location of the retropharyngeal lymph nodes and their relationship to the base of the skull and the internal carotid artery. (From CIBA/Netter Vol. 3, Pt. 1, § 1, Plate 26)

waiian males in Hawaii (3.5/100,000), followed by black males (2.8/100,000) and white males (1.6/100,000). Age specific incidence rates show increasing incidence from the 40–44 year old group (0.4/100.000) to 65–69 year old group (9.6/100,000) and then falling to 4.3/100,000 among the 85+ year old age group (white males) Among blacks, the incidence was seen to continue to increase with age and the highest incidence was quoted among the 85+ year old group with a rate of 15.8/100,000. Many series have shown a preponderance of women with post-cricoid carcinoma, CNAB-JONES (1961) showed that between one-third and two-thirds of patients with post-cricoid carcinoma have a history of the Patterson-Brown-Kelly syndrome. Carcinoma of the hypopharynx is usually associated with a history of heavy tobacco and alcohol abuse.

9.2 Pathology and Staging

Squamous cell carcinomas comprise more than 95% of carcinomas of the hypopharynx. In general, they are more poorly differentiated than endolaryngeal tumors. Minor salivary gland tumors have been reported in the hypopharynx (TOM et al. 1981; DAMIANI et al. 1981) as well as fibrosarcomas (BRADSHAW, VAN NOSTRAND 1971). The degree of differentiation has not been found to be of prognostic significance. (MARTIN et al. 1980; CARPENTER et al. 1976). Most of these tumors have infiltrating borders, but a small percentage (20%) (MARTIN et al. 1980) have pushing-type margins. However, the type of tumor-stromal interface has not been found to be of prognostic value in a multivariate

analysis by MARTIN et al. (1980). These tumors have a tendency towards submucosal spread and are usually found to have extension by 5–10 mm more than clinically suspected. (HARRISON et al. 1970).

The American Joint Committee staging for hypopharynx is used in literature originating from institutions in the United States. The International Union Against Cancer (U.I.C.C.) staging recommendations are more generally accepted throughout the rest of the world and are approved by the International Commission on Stage Grouping in Cancer and the Presentation of Results (ICPR) (with following in Australia, the United Kingdom and Western Europe), the Canadian National TNM Committee (CNC), and the Japanese Joint Committee (JJC). The "T" category descriptions are the same in both systems for hypopharyngeal primaries. However, the criteria for classification of nodal staging are quite different. Evaluation and comparison of literature using the two systems is difficult and should be borne in mind.

A.J.C. staging for T classification is shown in Table 9-3. Cervical node classification of both A.J.C. and U.I.C.C. is shown in Table 9-4. Stage grouping of TNM classification is similar to other head and neck cancers.

Table 9-3. Hypopharynx

T_{is}	Carcinoma in situ
T_1	Tumor confined to one site
T_2	Extension of tumor to adjacent region or site without fixation of hemilarynx
T_3	Extension of tumor to adjacent region or site with fixation of hemilarynx
T_4	Massive tumor invading bone or soft tissues of neck

Table 9-4. Cervical node classification (AJC and UICC)

Nodal Status	AJC	UICC
N$_0$	No regional node involvement	No regional node involvement
N$_1$	Single homolateral node 3 cm	Movable homolateral node(s)
N$_2$	a) Single homolateral node 3-6 cm b) Multiple homolateral nodes 6 cm	Movable contralateral or bilateral node(s)
N$_3$	a) Homolateral node(s) b) Bilateral nodes c) Contralateral node(s)	Fixed node(s)

"T" staging classification is satisfactory for lesions in the pyriform fossa. However, this staging system is quite inadequate for lesions of the posterior pharyngeal wall where tumors can grow to a large size and yet are limited to one or two sites.

9.3 Diagnostic Procedures

The initiation of staging work-up would consist of visualization of a tumor on indirect of direct laryngoscopy. Small lesions can often be difficult to identify. Lesions at the apex of the pyriform sinus or of the retrocricoid region are hard to visualize on indirect laryngoscopy. Unilateral arytenoid edema and pooling of secretions should alert one to underlying pathology. Biopsy requires examination under general anesthesia and direct visualization to get a positive biopsy. As in other cancers of the head and neck areas, a systematic evaluation of the entire upper aero-digestive mucosa with triple endoscopy is important. Significant incidence of second primary tumors have been found (McGUIRT et al. 1982; ATKINSON et al. 1982) on routine evaluation. A chest x-ray to detect distant disease should be part of the routine work-up. Lateral soft tissue radiographs and xerograms have been used to delineate posterior extension of pharyngeal wall tumors (Fig. 9-5). Anteroposterior conventional tomography with the Valsalva maneuver might be employed for better demonstration of the mouth of the esophagus and retrocricoid region.

Computerized tomographic scanning is replacing conventional radiographic procedures and taking an increasingly important role in evaluating head and neck cancers. Because of the fat content of the deep planes of the neck which serves as a good contrast medium, CT is an excellent procedure for delineating soft tissue neoplasms. In hypopharyngeal carcinomas with a significant incidence of submocosal spread, CT scanning is beneficial in evaluating the extent of the local disease (Fig. 9-6). CT scanning can also differentiate between pyriform sinus cancers and marginal tumors of the supraglottic area (LARSSON et al. 1981). The posterio-inferior spread of the tumor between the thyroid and arytenoid cartilages implies the spread of tumor within the pharyngeal space and usually signifies a primary site in the pyriform sinus. (SAGERMAN et al. 1979). Retropharyngeal adenopathy which is difficult to determine upon clinical examination can be defected (Fig. 9-7) (RUSSEL 1985). Extranodal extension of nodal disease as well as clinically unsuspected small contralateral nodal involvement can also be detected. Sometimes the soft tissue extension of primary disease into the neck can be confused with mid-jugular adenopathy. This can also be defined and differentiated by CT scanning. Coronal CT scans while phonating may show vocal cord mobility and laryngeal extension of pyriform sinus cancers; however, CT scans done immediately after a biopsy procedure might be misleading due to post-operative edema of traumatized tissues. This should be borne in mind in situations where carcinoma is highly suspected on clinical exam. In this case, CT scanning prior to a biopsy procedure is preferable (SILVERMAN et al. 1984). The normally irregular ossification of thyroid cartilage may lead to a false positive diagnosis of cartilagenous invasion (YEAGER et al. 1982; NATHAN et al. 1980).

CT has definitely proved useful in treatment planning by defining normal structures and determining anatomical relationship to tumor and its extension. This is certainly true in lesions of the hypopharynx which are deep to the neck and not readily visible or palpable. Definition of tumor extent can thus help to determine the ultimate course of therapy, whether it is primarily surgical or radiotherapeutic.

9.4 Pyriform Sinus

9.4.1 Presenting Symptoms, Signs, and Clinical Evolution

Pyriform sinus carcinomas make up the bulk of hypopharyngeal cancers. Compilation of distribution of hypopharyngeal tumors in various sites are

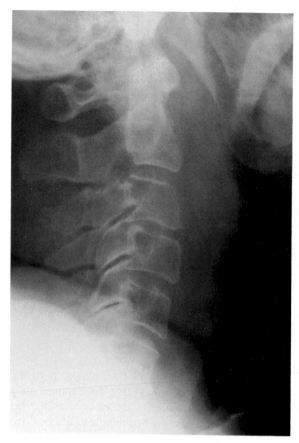

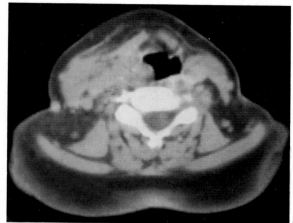

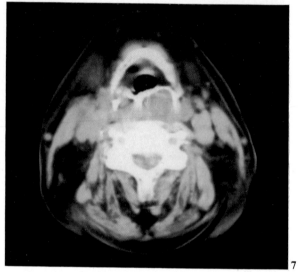

Fig. 9-5. Lateral soft tissue x-ray demonstrating a mass in the posterior pharyngeal wall

shown in Table 9-5. This varies somewhat among different authors mainly dependent on the frequency of post-cricoid lesions seen in their respective institutions and countries.

The most common presenting symptoms are odynophagia with later dysphagia and/or otalgia. These are the presenting symptoms in approximatly 50% of the patients (CARPENTER et al. 1976; KEANE 1982). The location of pain or swelling in the neck

Fig. 9-6. C. T. scan of the pyriform sinus showing the lesion in the left pyriform sinus

Fig. 9-7. C. T. scan showing clinically unrecognized retropharyngeal lymphadenopathy

is unusually unilateral and patients can direct the physicians attention to the site of disease. Persistent unilateral odynophagia associated with difficulty in visualization of the apex of the ipsilateral pyriform sinus should compel the physician to do a further workup. Otalgia is due to referred pain by way of the auricular branch (Nerve of Arnold) of the vagus nerve. (Fig. 9-8) This nerve is sensory to the back of the pinna and the posterior aspect of the external auditory canal. Patients usually report vague pain in the back of the ear. Dysphagia alone or a lump in the neck alone could be the sole presenting symptom. A neck mass without localizing symptoms occurs in approximately 20% of patients. (CARPENTER et al. 1976; HORWITZ et al. 1979). Hoarseness of

Table 9-5. Distribution of patient by site of lesion in hypopharyngeal cancers

	No	%
Pyriform Sinus	1571	76
Posterior Pharyn. Wall	347	17
Post-cricoid	148	7
Total	2069	

Pooled data from EL BADAWI et al. (1982), BATAINI et al. (1981), CARPENTER et al. (1976), SHAH et al. (1976), INOUI et al. (1983), LORD et al. (1973), KEANE (1982).

Fig. 9-8. Referral pathway for otalgia in carcinoma of the hypopharynx.

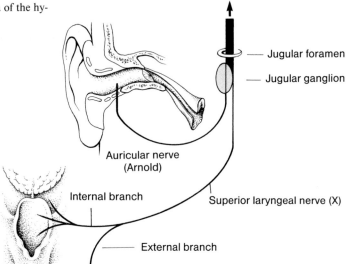

— Jugular foramen

— Jugular ganglion

Auricular nerve
(Arnold)

Internal branch

Superior laryngeal nerve (X)

External branch

voice (KEANE 1982; HORWITZ et al. 1979), hemoptysis, airway obstruction, and neck pain are often the presenting symptoms. Secondary infection of deep ulcerative lesions can give rise to malodorous breath. Duration of symptoms is fairly short. Median time is reported to be 2–3 months (KEANE et al. 1982; HORWITZ et al. 1979).

On examination of the hypopharyngeal region, early lesions can appear as a nodule or erythroplasia on either the medial or lateral wall of the pyriform sinus. Local exension of medial wall lesions is usually over the aryepiglottic fold or the arytenoids. Edema of these structures often obscures the lesion. (Fig. 9-9) Submucosal spread to the arytenoids or the false cord can appear as ipsilateral edema or swelling of the false cord. It is not uncommon to see secondary edema of the arytenoids without direct involvement. Extension could be more inferomedial to involve the post cricoid area and cross to the opposite pyriform sinus.

Tumors of the lateral wall can extend into the soft tissue of the neck, thyroid cartilage and thyroid gland. (Fig. 9-10) As the lesion advances tumor can invade the crycoarytenoid, the vocalis muscle to fix the vocal cord, the pre-epiglottic space, the parapharyngeal soft tissues and superiorly into the base of the tongue.

As noted previously, patients have a high incidence (75%) of palpable neck nodes at presentation. Approximately 10% will have bilateral nodal involvement. Because of dysphagia, along with malnutrition, it is not uncommon that patients present as cachectic and in poor general medical condition. Nineteen to twenty-seven percent of patients pre-

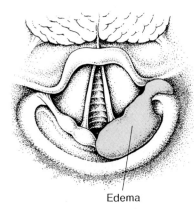

Edema

Fig. 9-9. Carcinoma of apex of pyriform sinus showing only edema of arytenoid obscuring the tumor

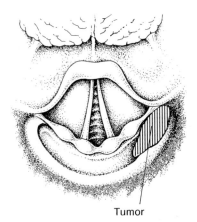

Tumor

Fig. 9-10. Carcinoma of lateral wall of pyriform sinus.

Table 9-6. Distribution and incidence of early stage pyriform sinus cancers

	T_1	T_2
N_0	21	37
	1047 (2%)	1047 (3.5%)
N_1	18	38
	1047 (1.7%)	1047 (3.6%)

Pooled data from EL BADAWI et al. (1982), AHMAD (1984), BATAINI et al. (1981), SAGERMAN et al. (1979), BYHARDT and COX (1980), PERSKY and DALY (1981).

Table 9-7. Distribution and incidence of advanced stage pyriform sinus cancers

	N_{0-1}	N_{2-3}
T_1	—	36 (3.4%)
		1047
T_2	—	80
		1047 (7.6%)
T_{3-4}	408 (39.9%)	408 (39.0%)
	1047	1047

Pooled data from EL BADAWI et al. (1982), AHMAD (1984), BATAINI et al. (1981), SAGERMAN et al. (1979), BYHARDT and COX (1980), PERSKY and DALY (1981)

sent in such condition, and therefore, are considered for palliative treatment only. (MARKS et al. 1978; KEANE et al. 1983; RAZACK et al. 1978)

Most pyriform sinus lesions will present in advanced stages. Table 9-6 shows the frequency of early stage presentation and ditribution within "T" and "N" classifications. Incidence of early stage presentations is 10% or less. Patients with early primaries have advanced nodal stages in approximately 10%. Eighty percent of the patients present with either advanced primaries or advanced nodal stages or both (Table 9-7).

9.4.2 Treatment Selection

9.4.2.1 General Remarks

For lesions limited to the cephalad portion of the pyriform sinus with or without early nodal disease, curative radiation therapy may be attempted with surgery reserved for salvage. Even among these patients, those with infiltrative lesions might have more disease than suspected. Exophytic lesions are felt to be the best type of lesions for radiation therapy. As can be seen in Table 9-6, less than 5% of the pat-

ients would be suitable for this therapy. For all other extensive lesions, combined surgery and radiation therapy is the treatment of choice. Even early lesions involving the apex of the pyriform sinus would be better of treated with combined treatment.

9.4.2.2 Surgery

Partial Laryngopharyngectomy (PLP). The partial laryngopharyngectomy would entail removal of the involved pyriform sinus and the supraglottic structures with preservation of the arytenoids and vocal cords. This procedure can be used in T_1 and T_2 lesions. Radical neck dissection is almost always combined with surgery for the primary. Early lesions involving the apex of the pyriform sinus are unsuitable for this type of surgery because of the proximity to the cricoid cartilage which cannot be removed. Voice conserving surgery has been reported in more advanced lesions as well with limited success. (GOEPFERT et al. 1981) However, FREEMAN et al. 1979 reported 8/85 patients treated with PLP for early pyriform sinus cancers lost their voice due to the need for complete laryngectomy or for tracheostomy. Most of the literature on combining radiation therapy with partial laryngeopharyngectomy has been administered as low dose pre-operative radiation therapy (MARKS et al. 1978; OGURA et al. 1980), although higher doses of post-operative radiation have been used with acceptable morbidity (GOEPFERT et al. 1981). Aspiration pneumonia is a major complication of voice conserving surgery and overall, fatal complications were found to be higher with partial laryngopharyngectomy than with total laryngopharyngectomy (FREEMAN et al. 1979).

Total Laryngopharyngectomy (TLP). In this surgical procedure, a total laryngectomy is combined with excision of the pharyngeal wall involved by tumor. As in PLP, a radical neck dissection is almost always combined with TLP. Primary closure of the pharyngeal wall is performed when only a portion of it is removed. In more advanced lesions when total pharyngectomy is necessitated, reconstruction by myocutaneous flap (LORE et al. 1982), or gastric transposition (SPIRO et al. 1983; LAM et al. 1981, HARRISON 1979) or jejunal replacement (ONG and WONG 1979) is done. Every attempt should be made to reduce the recovery period after extirpative surgery so as to enable the initiation of post-operative radiation within a 6 week period.

9.4.2.3 Combined Treatment

General Remarks. The rationale for a planned combination of surgery and radiation therapy is aimed to 1) reduce local recurrence at the primary site 2) to reduce local recurrence in the ipsilateral neck 3) to reduce the contralateral neck recurrence and 4) to convert unresectable lesions into resectable ones. The radiation can be delivered either pre-operatively or post-operatively.

Pre-operative Radiation. Radiation delivered pre-operatively has been the major way of combining radiation therapy and surgery in the past. Because of various factors to be discussed later in this chapter, post-operative radiation has become increasingly more popular. Still, there is a role for pre-operative radiation therapy. In selected exophytic lesions or early stages, a trial of irradiation can be started. At 4500–5000 cGy, the patient is re-evaluated. If the response is adequate, irradiation is continued to a definitive course. If not, surgery is performed and radiation therapy would be considered as preoperative. Another rationale for the use of pre-operative radiation is to convert unresectable neck nodal disease to resectable. Pre-operative radiation is used very little at our institutions.

Post-operative Radiation. Following surgery, radiation therapy is recommended in most situations. High risk factors for local recurrence include close or positive margins, multiple or large neck nodes, or extra-nodal extension. Even without high risk factors, we recommend post-operative radiation in pyriform sinus cancers, due to a significant risk of contralateral neck failures.

9.4.2.4 Radiation Therapy

Because of the tendency of carcinoma of the pyriform sinus to spread to the cervical lymph nodes at multiple levels, the entire neck, including the supraclavicular region needs to be treated. Even in patients with clinically negative neck nodes, there is a high probability of subclinical disease. Hence, treatment fields should include spinal accessary nodes, jugular and jugulodigastric nodes, retropharyngeal nodes as well as supraclavicular and lower jugular nodes. Because of subclinical mucosal spread, radiation fields for the primary region should be generous enough to include the oropharynx above and the cervical esophagus below. Treatment techniques used in clinical situations usually encountered are described below.

1) *Early T1 lesions with no nodes or a small node where curative radiation therapy is contemplated:* Parallel opposed lateral fields are used to include all of the primary and as much of the neck nodes as possible (Fig. 9-11) Superior borders should be at the base of the skull so as to include retropharyngeal lymph nodes which lie anterior to the C1 vertebrae. The posterior border should include the posterior cervical triangle. Anterior triangle lymph nodes, larynx and pre-epiglottic space should be included. Protection of a strip of anterior skin to facilitate lymphatic drainage by pulling skin out of the field by clothespins has been described. (MILLION and CASSISI 1984) We have not used this technique at this institution because of the proximity of the volume to be treated to the anterior skin. Inferiorly, the lower border should be as low in the neck as possible, with at least a 2 cm margin below the lower border of the cricoid. Occasionally, the inferior margin may not be adequate with ordinary lateral

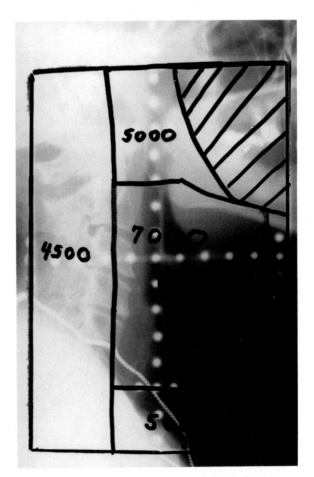

Fig. 9-11. Simulation film showing the outline of treatment fields and doses delivered with a shrinking field technique

fields because of the shoulders. In such instances, angulation of the couch in such a way as to direct the lateral fields inferiorly 5–10 degrees would help in obtaining adequate margins (ANDREW et al. 1984). An en face anterior field to treat these lower neck nodes is also added. A technique for matching these lateral fields and anterior fields will be discussed later in this chapter.

The supero-anterior portion of this field is shaped with blocks to protect the oral cavity and anterior portions of the oropharynx. A shrinking field technique is used and at 4500 cGy, the spinal cord is blocked. At 5000 cGy, the anterior field is terminated and the lateral fields are shrunk further. This then encompasses the primary tumor and nodal disease with safe margins. The total dose to the gross disease is 7000 cGy in 7 weeks at 200 cGy per fractions.

2) *More advanced lesions with large neck nodes:* Patients with more advanced primaries or nodal disease are generally treated with combined modality. However, due to the advanced age of the patient or general medical status, the patient might be considered medically inoperable. The treatment techniques used in such clinical situations is similar to that described above except when the nodal disease extends behind the plane of the spinal cord. After the lateral fields have been shrunk off the spinal cord, electron fields should be added to that area. However, if an electron beam is not available, a technique employing a combination of lateral pair

with postero-oblique fields with reversed wedge filters can be used to achieve optimum dose distribution to the tumor volume. (ELKON et al. 1978) (Fig. 9-12)

The major bulk of patients with carcinoma of the pyriform sinus are treated with a combination of surgery and irradiation. Pre-operative radiation is used infrequently. The pre-operative radiation dose is 4500 to 5000 cGy. Treatment techniques would be the same as described above. As radiation doses do not exceed spinal cord tolerance, a shrinking field technique is not necessary. Both the upper lateral fields and the lower anterior neck fields receive the same total dose.

Radiation is most often used post-operatively. Doses of 6000 cGy in 6 weeks are delivered to the pharyngeal walls, base of the tongue and upper and mid-jugular nodal areas. We normally deliver 6500 cGy when the margins are close or positive. The doses should be carried to 7000 cGy in such patients if the interval between surgery and the initiation of irradiation is prolonged. We also deliver 7000 cGy if there is suspicion of residual disease either in the primary site or the neck. The lower neck is treated to a total dose of 5000 cGy prescribed to a depth of 3 cm.

Because of the difficulty in radiating areas at risk in the upper neck as well as lower neck uniformly, no treatment technique is perfect. We use lateral opposed fields for the upper neck and an enface anterior field for the lower neck. The tracheostomy stoma is included in the lateral fields if possible.

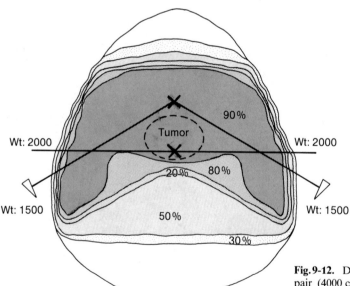

Fig. 9-12. Dose distribution combining a parallel opposing pair (4000 cGy, 10W × 12L, 80 SAD, Co^{60}) and 2 wedged beams at 120° (3000 cGy, 6W × 12L, 80 SAD, Co^{60})

Occasionally, angulation of the couch so as to direct the lateral fields inferiorly by 5° will allow inclusion of the stoma in these lateral fields. If the patient is unable to extend his neck far enough or cannot depress his shoulders sufficiently, the tracheostoma is included in the anterior field. If there is extensive subglottic extension, in order to prevent stomal recurrence (MANTRAVADI et al. 1981) the stoma is irradiated with a plastic tracheostomy tube in place. A donut-shaped applicator made of Play-Doh or other tissue-equivalent material (with a hole in the middle to facilitate breathing through it) will also suffice.

Unlike other head and neck cancers, in carcinoma of the hypopharynx abutment of lateral fields and anterior neck fields is complicated. The midline shield is generally used; however in hypopharyngeal cancers, the midline structures need to be treated for fear of microscopic extension of disease. Because of beam divergence of the anterior supraclavicular field, a portion of the spinal cord would be overdosed if included in both the lateral and anterior fields (DATTA et al. 1979; PARADELO et al. 1981). There have been several methods reported in the literature to avoid this problem. One involves using split beams both for lateral fields (DATTA et al. 1979; CHIANG et al. 1979) and anterior fields and another uses a small block to shield the spinal cord in the lateral fields at the junction of the lateral and anterior field (PARADELO et al. 1981; LEVITT 1984). A small partial transmission block at the junction in the midline of the anterior field can be used (FLETCHER 1973). Others have reported techniques such as anterior and posterior fields using a posterior spineblock with a 4:1 weighting for anterior fields with 10 MeV x-rays, (DOPPKE et al. 1980). Similarly, AP/PA fields with Cobalt 60 can be used to cord tolerance, followed by either lateral fields (PEZNER and FINDLAY 1981) or an anterior electron field (LEVITT 1984) for the rest of the desired dose. AP/PA techniques deliver radiation to the entire circumference of the neck which may result in more edema and may not address the retropharyngeal lymph nodes adequately. We use a 3-field technique with a shaped half-block for the anterior field, shaped to match the divergence of the lateral fields; thus avoiding the problem of cold spots or hot spots of an unshaped split beam (Fig. 9-13).

As in other head and neck cancers, it is important to use immobilization devices for daily reproducibility of the setup. Custom made blocks to protect the oral cavity and anterior portion of the oropharynx will minimize the volume of mucosa irradiated. Because of the extensiveness of the area irradi-

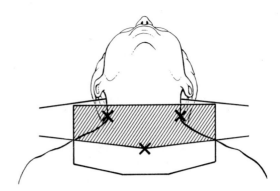

Fig. 9-13. Technique of making lateral neck fields to anterior low neck field with a half beam technique. Upper half of low neck field *(cross hatched area)* is blocked to make the divergent lower border of the lateral fields

ated, patients tolerate treatment poorly and strict attention should be given to proper nutrition, hydration and oral hygiene.

9.4.3 Treatment Results

9.4.3.1 General Remarks

The majority of pyriform cancers present in advanced stages. In a significant proportion of patients, high dose radiation therapy is delivered for palliative purposes. (MARKS et al. 1978; KEANE et al. 1982; RAZACK et al. 1978) Evaluation of treatment results reported in the literature is difficult because of the variation in selection factors for inclusion in analysis, variation in staging systems, types of surgery and doses of radiation. Some reports fail to subdivide results into specific primary sites and others include the aryepiglottic fold in their analysis. Reported overall survival rates vary widely in the literature and 3 year determinate survivals of 17% to 53% are reported (EEISBACH and KRAUSE 1977; CARPENTER et al. 1976; MARKS et al. 1978; YATES and CRUMLEY 1984) and 5 year rates of 12% to 41% (AHMAD 1984; CARPENTER et al. 1976; MARKS et al. 1978; RAZACK et al. 1978; BYHARDT 1980)

9.4.3.2 Radiation Therapy

Most reports show poor results with radiation therapy for pyriform sinus cancers. Three-year survival rates of 5–20% (DRISCOLL et al. 1983; EISBACH and KRAUSE 1977; SAGERMAN et al. 1979; KIRCHNER and OWEN (1977); INOUE et al. 1983) and 5 year rates of 0-26% (BADAWI et al. 1982; AHMAD 1984; BALLANTYNE 1964; EISBACH and KRAUSE 1977; RAZACK et al. 1978; PERSKY and DALY 1981; INOUE et al. 1983) are reported. All the reports are retrospective analyses and include reported results of various treatment modalities. Factors used for selection of different treatment are not always clear. Some authors have noted that radiation therapy was selected because of far advanced disease or poor general condition (RAZACK et al. 1978; CARPENTER et al. 1976). This negatively influences the treatment results obtainable by radiation therapy.

From the Institut Curie where radiotherapy has been the treatment of choice, BATAINI et al. (1982) reported 3 and 5 year determinate survivals of 47% and 41%. In that series, determinate survival rates for T_1 and T_2 lesions were 55% and 50% at 3 and 5 years, respectively. AHMAD (1984) reported at 100% and 56.5% actuarial 5 year survival for Stage II and III lesions.

EL BADAWI et al. (1982) reported a 48% 2 year NED survival on 48 patients treated with the Co^{60} machine in spite of the fact that 44% of their patients had T_3 and T_4 lesions and 65% had N_2 and N_3 disease.

MILLION (1984) reported a 41% 5 year determinate survival among patients treated with radiation therapy with or without node dissection. The rates were 83% for Stage I and II, 37.5% for Stage III and IV, respectively.

Loco-regional control is the major problem when radiation therapy is used as the sole treatment modality. Loco-regional control rates of 40% to 77% (BADAWI et al. 1982; AHMAD 1984; DRISCOLL et al. 1983; BATAINI et al. 1982; EISBACH and KRAUSE 1977) have been reported. MILLION (1984) reported 70% and 40% primary control rates in T_1 and T_2 and 47% for T_3 and T_4. Control of neck nodes was 100% for N_0 and N_1 and 63% for N_2 and N_3 without node dissection.

9.4.3.3 Surgery

Surgery alone as the treatment of choice has been reported by various authors. In all these reports, a fraction of the patients received additional radiation therapy either pre-operatively or post-operatively. Selection of patients for surgery or combination therapy is not always clear though a few authors note that more extensive disease was treated with combination therapy than surgery alone. Three year determinate survival rates of 24% to 65% are reported (DRISCOLL et al. 1983; EISBACH

and KRAUSE 1977; KIRCHNER and OWEN 1977; YATES and CRUMLEY 1984). Determinate survivals at 5 years were 24-56% (EL BADAWI et al. 1982; EISBACH et al. 1977; RAZACK et al. 1978; YATES et al. 1984). Primary recurrences range between 5-33% (DRISCOLL et al. 1983; EISBACH et al. 1977; RAZACK et al. 1978; YATES and CRUMLEY 1984). Contralateral nodal recurrences were noted in 15-25% of the patients (EL BADAWI et al. 1982; EISBACH and KRAUSE 1977; CARPENTER et al. 1976; MARKS et al. 1978).

9.4.3.4 Combined Treatment

Three year determinate survival ranges of 25-50% (DRISCOLL et al. 1983; EISBACH and KRAUSE 1977; SAGERMAN et al. 1979; KIRCHNER et al. 1977; YATES et al. 1984) and 5 year rates of 11-36% (EISBACH et al. 1977; MARKS et al. 1978; BYHARDT et al. 1980; PERSKY et al. 1981; YATES et al. 1984) have been noted. Primary failure rates of 5-28% (DRISCOLL et al. 1983; EISBACH and KRAUSE 1977; MARKS et al. 1978) and nodal failures of 13-27% (DRISCOLL et al. 1983; EISBACH and KRAUSE 1977; MARKS et al. 1978) have been reported. EL BADAWI et al. (1982) reported an 11% failure above the clavicle among 125 patients treated with planned post-operative radiation as compared to a 39% failure rate above the clavicle in 203 patients treated with surgery alone. The failure rate was 29% among 17 patients treated with pre-operative radiation.

Contralateral neck failure was very low (0-2%) with high dose radiation therapy (EL BADAWI et al. 1982; EISBACH and KRAUSE 1977). With 3000 cGy of post operative radiation, contralateral neck recurrence was 15% (MARKS et al. 1978).

Controversy exists in the literature regarding the added benefit adjuvant radiation offers over surgery alone. Several papers note no improvement in survival or loco-regional control in combined treatment groups as opposed to surgery only groups (EISBACH and KRAUSE 1977; CARPENTER et al. 1976; KIRCHNER et al. 1977; YATES and CRUMLEY 1984) whereas others do (EL BADAWI et al. 1982; DRISCOLL et al. 1983; INOUE et al. 1983). TERZ and LAWRENCE 1983) reviewed 34 papers for the purpose of comparing preoperative irradiation to surgery alone in head and neck cancers. These authors conclude from their review that there is no benefit to the combined approach. However, they did find that in the two randomized studies they reviewed, there was some improvement in survival for combination treated patients compared to surgery alone

(41% vs. 34%), though not statistically significant. Most benefit was seen in Stage III pharynx cancer (42% vs. 25%). Comparison of data from retrospective and randomized studies showed that patients treated with surgery alone in retrospective studies did significantly better than in randomized studies (51% vs. 34%). This implies that surgery alone treated patients in retrospective studies were a better group of patients due to the selection bias of treating physicians; whereas in randomized studies, this bias was eliminated.

9.4.4 Complications

Complications of treatment of pyriform sinus lesions could be due to surgery or radiation therapy or both. A review of the literature regarding complications by BYHARDT et al. (1980) revealed a major complication rate of 35% for surgery alone vs. 38% for the pre-operative radiation group. However, the fatal complication rate was 4% for surgery alone and 8% for the pre-operative group. Complications noted were pharyngo-cutaneous fistulae, carotid rupture and delays in would healing. BATAINI et al. (1982) reported a 2.5% fatal complication rate with radiation therapy alone; 11% had non-fatal major complications. Hemorrhage, cachexia, and aspiration pneumonia, were fatal complications. Laryngeal edema requiring tracheostomies, esophageal strictures and soft tissue necrosis were the non-fatal complications.

9.5 Posterior Pharyngeal Wall

9.5.1 Presenting Signs, Symptoms and Clinical Evolution

Posterior pharyngeal wall carcinomas make up 15-20% of all hypopharyngeal carcinomas. This varies in different series with a range of 7-35% (BADAWI et al. 1982; BATAINI et al. 1982; CARPENTER et al. 1976; SHAH et al. 1976; INOUE et al. 1973; LORD et al. 1973; KEANE et al. 1983). Evaluation of the literature on posterior wall tumors is difficult because these lesions are analyzed with other hypopharyngeal lesions or with oropharyngeal wall lesions. There are only a few reports addressing carcinoma of the posterior pharyngeal wall of the hypopharynx (TALTON et al. 1981; WANG 1970; RAINE et al. 1982). In females, there is a higher predilection for posterior pharyngeal wall tumors than pyriform fossa carcinomas. Male/female ratios reported are 2-3:1 rather than 4-5:1 for pyriform fossa cancers.

The common presenting symptoms are dysphagia and sore throat occurring in 50-90% of the patients. (TALTON et al. 1981; RAINE et al. 1982) Other symptoms include otalgia, hoarseness of voice, hemoptysis, and a foreign body sensation in the throat or a neck mass (TALTON et al. 1981, WANG 1970; RAINE et al. 1982). Otalgia is referred pain along the auricular branch of the vagus nerve as previously noted.

The primary lesion has a prediliction to spread vertically and extend into the oropharynx readily. Thus, the majority of the lesions are large, fungating masses easily seen on depressing the tongue on oral exam. Early lesions are seen either as an ulcer or an exophytic mass upon mirror examination (Fig. 9-14).

Submucosal spread can cause a smooth bulge with a normal-appearing overlying mucosa. In advanced lesions, spread occurs circumferentially with extension to the lateral wall of the pyriform sinus or onto the tonsil superiorly. Extension through the pharyngeal wall to invade the para-pharyngeal space may be unsuspected upon physical examination, but is readily detected with CT scans. Posterior extension into pre-vertebral muscles is uncommon. Inferior extension into the esophagus is also uncommon.

The frequency of lymph node involvement is high (50-60%), but slightly lower than that seen in pyriform fossa lesions (75%) (Table 9-1). Bilateral nodal involvement is found in 10-35% (MEOZ-MENDEZ et al. 1978; WANG 1970). MEOZ-MENDEZ et al. (1978) found 22% bilateral nodal involvement in lateral lesions and 35% in posterior lesions. Pharyngeal wall tumors have a high incidence of retropharyngeal nodal involvement. (BALLANTYNE 1964)

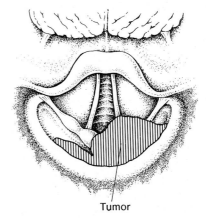

Fig. 9-14. Carcinoma of posterior wall of the hypopharynx

Table 9-8. Distributions by T-staging

Total No of %	T_1	T_2	$T_{3/4}$
99	42 (42%)	33 (33%)	20 (20%)

Pooled data from TALTON et al. (1981), WANG (1971), RAINE et al. (1982).

Table 9-9. Distribution by N-staging

Total No of %	N_0	N_1	N_2	N_3
99	42 (42%)	34 (34%)	8 (8%)	5 (5%)

Pooled data from TALTON et al. (1981), WANG (1971), RAINE et al. (1982).

The Distribution of patients at presentation by T and N staging are shown in Tables 9-8 and 9-9. As in both AJC and UICC staging, the T staging is done by the number of sites involved, large lesions can still be staged as T_1. For this reason, several authors (MARKS et al. 1978; MEOZ-MENDEZ et al. 1978) have based their staging system on size.

9.5.2 Treatment Selection

The majority of patients with carcinoma of the posterior pharyngeal wall are treated with curative radiation therapy. This is due to the difficulties in performing extirpative procedures with acceptable morbidity.

A variety of surgical procedures have been done alone or in combination with irradiation. Local excision, either through mandibulotomy-glossotomy or lateral pharyngotomy is one of the procedures used. The resultant defect is closed either primarily or with a split thickness skin graft. Partial or total laryngo-pharyngectomy can be done with reconstruction by visceral transposition or delta pectoral flaps. Comparative evaluation is difficult because of the multitude of surgical procedures used and the differences in size and location of the tumors.

9.5.3 Radiation Treatment Techniques

Because of the extensive submucosal spread, the field margins should be generous around the visible primary. Extending the field superiorly to the base of the skull is necessary to give adequate margins

around the primary lesion and to treat the retropharyngeal lymph nodes. Inferiorly, the upper cervical esophagus is included. Anteriorly, the base of the tongue is included to obtain adequate margins. The posterior border of the field should include the lymph nodes in the posterior cervical triangle. Opposed lateral fields are most commonly used. Directing the fields inferiorly by couch angulation might be necessary to avoid the shoulders in the tratment fields. Field sizes are reduced at 4400 cGy to avoid the spinal cord. Posteriorly located positive lymph nodes might pose a problem after reduction of the field size. Posterolateral oblique fields with reversed wedges (ELKON et al. 1978) are not preferred in posterior pharyngeal wall lesions due to the proximaty of the tumor to the spinal cord. Electron boosts with 9–12 MeV electrons are preferred. If the lymph nodes are negative clincially, high energy photon beam radiation of 18–22 MeV can be used. This will deliver an adequate dose to both the primary and microscopic disease in the superficial nodes. If the nodes are positive, low energy photons with 4MeV or Co^{60} beams are preferred.

As these lesions have a significant incidence of lower neck nodal involvement, an anterior lower neck field is always used. Matching of the lateral fields to anterior field is done as discussed previously. Five-thousand cGy are given to the anterior lower neck field. The dose given to the primary is 7000 cGy to the gross disease in 7 weeks at 200 cGy per fraction with a shrinking field technique. In older and more debilitated patients, 180 cGy per fraction is preferred to the same total dose. Radiation mucositis of the pharyngeal mucosa often necessitates a rest period of a week during the course of the treatment. Careful monitoring of the patient's nutrition is important as described previously.

9.5.4 Treatment Results

Results of treatment of posterior pharyngeal wall carcinomas are poor. An overall survival rate of 17% to 46% at 3 years and 14% to 33% at 5 years has been reported (MARKS et al. 1978; TALTON et al. 1981; MEOZ-MENDEZ et al. 1978; INOUE et al. 1972; MILLION 1984; RAINE et al. 1982; WANG (1971); PUHAKKA et al. 1980). The major cause of death is loco-regional failure. Loco-regional control is achieved in 30% to 60%. (MAKRS et al. 1978; TALTON et al. 1981; MEOZ-MENDEZ et al. 1978; INOUE T et al. 1972; HORWITZ et al. 1979). Second primaries as the cause of death have been reported in as high as 16% (MEOZ-MENDEZ et al. 1978) and distant metastases as high as 23% (TALTON et al. 1981).

Loco-regional control is dependent on the size of the primary and dose delivered. TALTON et al. (1981) reported a 50% local control in $T_{1,2}$ N_0 lesions as opposed to 0% in T_3 and T_4 lesions. Similarly, 39% achieved local control in N_0 patients whereas 14% of N+ patients had local control. MEOZ-MENDEZ et al. (1978) reported local controls of 100%, 78%, 71% and 41% in T_1, T_2, T_3 and T_4 lesions at 1 year. PENE et al. (1978) reported 70% local control in lesions less than 4 cm and 10% in lesions greater than 4 cm in size. WANG (1971) reported 12.5% local control at doses less than 6000 cGy and 53% in patients receiving greater than 6000 cGy.

Results with surgery even when feasible are about the same as with radiation therapy alone. GUILLAMONDEGUI et al. (1978) reviewed results in 94 patients treated with the surgical approach at M. D. Anderson Hospital between 1954 and 1974 and compared the results with radiation therapy by MEOZ-MENDEZ et al. (1978) from the same institution for the same time period. Control rates were found to be similar for comparable stages.

Combining surgery and radiation therapy when feasible might improve local control of larger lesions. MEOZ-MENDEZ et al. (1978) reported a 66% local control in patients with T_3 and T_4 lesions receiving combination therapy as opposed to 42% with radiation therapy alone for similar lesions.

Similarly, MARKS et al. (1978) reported 48% local control with low dose pre-operative radiation vs. 38% lcoal control with radiation alone.

9.5.5 Complications

When surgery has been used alone or as part of the treatment, fatal complications are as high as 14%. (MARKS et al. 1978; WANG 1971) Pharyngo-cutaneous fistula resulting in carotid rupture was the most common complication. Radiation therapy complications have included carotid rupture (associated with surgical salvage) (MEOZ-MENDEZ et al. 1978), laryngeal and pharyngeal edema needing tracheostomy, aspiration pneumonia (MARKS et al. 1978; MEOZ-MENDEZ et al. 1978) and osteo-radionecrosis and radiation myelitis. MEOZ-MENDEZ et al. (1978) reported a 5% incidence of fatal complications in patients with radiation therapy alone.

9.6 Post-Cricoid Carcinoma

9.6.1 General Remarks

Post cricoid carcinoma is quite uncommon in the United States. This disease comprises 3–6% of all hypopharyngeal lesions diagnosed in this country (EL BADAWI et al. 1982; SHAH et al. 1976; CARPENTER et al. 1976). However, higher incidences have been reported in Japan (INOUE et al. 1972) Britain (STELL et al. 1981; PEARSON 1966) Canada (LORD et al. 1973; KEANE et al. 1983) and Sweden (JACOBSSON 1981).

Unlike hypopharyngeal carcinomas in other sites, post-cricoid lesions are more common in women than men, with M:F ratios of 1:4–5. There is also an association of Plummer-Vinson syndrome with carcinoma of the post-cricoid region (AHLBOM 1974). Post-cricoid lesions arise from the anterior mucosa covering the cricoid lamina. (Fig. 9-15) These lesions have a tendency to spread inferiorly involving the wall between the trachea and esophagus. (MACBETH 1971)

In the vast majority of patients the presenting symptom is dysphagia. (LEDERMAN 1958) The majority of these lesions extend into the esophagus. Advanced cervical esophageal lesions can extend superiorly to involve the postcricoid region. Because the exact origin of the tumor cannot often be determined, any lesion involving the post-cricoid region with esophageal involvement has been considered as a post-cricoid lesion in the literature (PEARSON 1966).

9.6.2 Treatment Selection

The best type of treatment for post-cricoid carcinoma is not clear. As the surgery for these lesions would entail total pharyngolaryngectomy or total

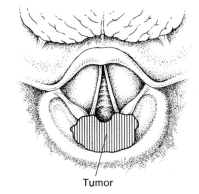

Fig. 9-15. Carcinoma of post-cricoid region

laryngo-esophagectomy with viscus transposition, with high morbitdity, the treatment of choice for smaller lesions would be radical radiation therapy.

9.6.3 Treatment Techniques

As these tumors have a tendency to spread inferiorly into the esophagus as well as the paratracheal lymph nodes, the inferior margin of the fields need to be generous. Thus, treatment techniques for post-cricoid carcinomas are more akin to cervical esophageal treatment techniques rather than to other hypopharyngeal cancers. A 3-field technique with an anterior and 2 posterior obliques is the most common treatment technique used. Anterior and posterior opposed fields can be combined with various spinal cord sparing techniques (3-field or crossing firing 4 field obliques). Contours can be taken at multiple levels for treatment planning. Inhomogeneity correction of lung transmission should be used whenever possible for determination of dose distribution. To compensate for the position of the spinal cord at the thoracic inlet, the collimator angle can be rotated. This can also be accomplished with custom made blocks.

9.6.4 Treatment Results

Post-cricoid carcinomas have a poor prognosis due to the advanced stages at the time of presentation. STELL et al. (1981) found that 41 of 141 patients seen between 1965 and 1978 were not treated because of poor general health and extensive disease. Twenty-three patients were treated with radiation therapy. Only tumors less than 5 cm in vertical length with no palpable nodes were selected for radiation therapy. Five year survival for these highly selected group of patients was 38%. Surgery for larger tumors with or without lymph node involvement resulted in a 20% 5-year survival. Similarly, PEARSON (1966) reported a 25% 5-year survival in 43 patients with post-cricoid carcinoma treated with radical radiotherapy, MACBETH (1971) reported a 36% 5-year survival in 39 post-cricoid lesions under 5 cm in length and without cervical node involvement.

Combined treatment philosophies have not had wide enough acceptance and need exploration at the present time.

References

Ahlbom H (1941) Results of radiotherapy of hypopharyngeal cancer at Radiumhummet; Stockholm, 1930-1939, Acta Radiol 22: 155-177

Ahmad K (1984) High-dose radiation therapy in carcinoma of the pyriform sinus, Cancer 53: 2091-2094

Andrew JW, Eapen L, Kulkarni NS (1984) Homogenous irradiation of the "short-necked" laryngeal cancer patient, Int J Rad Oncol Biol Phys 10: 549-553

Atkinson D, Fleming S, Weaver A (1982) Triple endoscopy – a valuable procedure in head and neck surgery, Am J Surg 144: 416-419

Ballantyne AJ (1964) Significance of retropharyngeal nodes in cancer of the head and neck, Am J Surg 108: 500-504

Bataini P, Brugere J, Bernier J, Jaullery CH, Picot C, Ghossein NA (1982) Results of radical radiotherapeutic treatment of carcinoma of the pyriform sinus: experience of the Institut Curie, Int J Rad Oncol Biol Phys 8: 1277-1286

Bradshaw RB, Van Nostrand AW (1971) Fibrosarcoma of the hypopharynx, J Laryngol Otol 85: 113-124

Bryce D (1967) Pharyngectomy in the treatment of Carcinoma of the hypopharynx. "In": John Conley, M.D. (ed) Cancer of the Head and Neck – Papers Presented at the International Workshop on Cancer of the Head and Neck, Session VI, Kingsport Press, Inc., Kingsport, Tenn, pp. 341-346

Byhardt RW, Cox JD (1980) Patterns of failure and results of preoperative irradiation vs radiation therapy alone in carcinoma of the pyriform sinus, Int J Rad Oncol Biol Phys 6: 1135-1141

Carpenter RJ III, DeSanto LW, Devine KD, Taylor WF (1976) Cancer of the hypopharynx – analysis of treatment and results in 162 patients, Otolaryngol 102: 716-721

Chiang TC, Culbert H, Wyman B, Cohen L, Ovadia J (1979) The half-field technique of radiation therapy for the cancers of head and neck, Int J Rad Oncol Biol Phys 5: 1899-1901

Damiani JM, Damiani KK, Hauck K, Hyams VJ (1981) Mucoepidermoid-adenosquamous carcinoma of the larynx and hypopharynx: a report of 21 cases and a review of the literature, Otolaryngol Head Neck Surg 89: 235-243

Datta R, Mira JG, Pomeroy TC (1979) Dosimetry study of split beam technique using megavoltage beams and its clinical implications – I ^{60}Co beam, head and neck tumors, Int J Rad Oncol Biol Phys 5: 565-571

Donald PJ, Hayes RH, Dhaliwal R (1980) Combined therapy for pyriform sinus cancer using postoperative irradiation, Otolaryngol Head Neck Surg 88: 738-744

Doppke K, Novack D, Wang CC (1980) Physical considerations in the treatment of advanced carcinomas of the larynx and pyriform sinuses using 10 Mv X rays, Int J Rad Oncol Biol Phys 6: 1251-1255

Driscoll WG, Nagorsky MJ, Cantrell RW, Johns ME (1983) Carcinoma of the pyriform sinus: analysis of 102 cases, Laryngoscope 93: 556-560

El Badawi SA, Hoepfert H, Fletcher GH, Herson J, Oswald MJ (1982) Squamous cell carcinoma of the pyriform sinus, Laryngoscope 92: 357-363

Eisbach KJ, Krause CJ (1977) Carcinoma of the pyriform sinus - a comparison of treatment modalities, Laryngoscope 87: 1904-1909

Elkon D, Kartha PKI, Hendrickson RF (1978) A radiotherapy treatment technique for cervical lymph node metastases, Int J Rad Oncol Biol Phys 4: 509-513

Fletcher GH (1973) Textbook of Radiotherapy. Lea & Febiger, Philadelphia

Fletcher G (1984) Irradiation of subclinical disease in the draining lymphatics, Int J Rad Oncol Biol Phys 10: 939–942

Freeman RB, Marks JE, Ogura JH (1979) Voice preservation in treatment of carcinoma of the pyriform sinus, Laryngoscope 89: 1855–1863

Goepfert H, Lindberg RD, Jesse RH (1981) Combined laryngeal conservation surgery and irradiation: Can we expand the indications for conservation therapy? Otolaryngol Head Neck Surg 89: 974–978

Gofinet DR, Fee WE Jr, Goode RL (1984) Combined surgery and postoperative irradiation in the treatment of cervical lymph nodes 110: 736–738

Guillamondegui OM, Meoz R, Jesse RH (1978) Surgical treatment of squamous cell carcinoma of the pharyngeal walls 135: 474–476

Harrison DF (a) (1979) Pathology of hypopharyngeal cancer in relation to surgical management, J Laryng 84: 349–367

Harrison DF (b) (1979) Surgical management of hypopharyngeal cancer - particular reference to the gastric "pull up" operation, Arch Otolaryngol, 105: 149–152

Hirano M, Kurrita S, Kuratomi K, Mihasi S (1982) Carcinoma of the hypopharynx and cervical esophagus - A retrospective investigation of 67 patients, Kurume Medical Journal, 29: 97–111

Horwitz SD, Calderelli D, Hendrickson FR (1979) Treatment of carcinoma of the hypopharynx, Hypopharyngeal Carcinoma 2: 107–111

Inoue T (a), Hata K, Chatani M, Sato T, Suzuki T (1983) Revaluation of treatment result fo carcinoma of the hypopharynx using quantification II of multivariate analysis, Strahlentherapie 159: 203–207

Inoue T (b), Shigamatsu Y, Sato T (1972) Treatment of carcinoma of the hypopharynx, Cancer 31: 649–655

Jacosson F (1951) p.25 "1981" Carcinoma of the Hypopharynx; a clinical study of 322 cases treated at Radiumhenmet from 1939 to 1947, Acta Radiol 35: 1–21

Keane TJ (1982) Carcinoma of the hypopharynx, J. Otolaryng 11: 226–231

Keane TJ et al. (1983) p. 9, 20

Keane TJ (1982) Carcinoma of the hypopharynx - results of primary radical radiation therapy, Int J Rad Oncol Biol Phys 9: 659–664

Kirchner JA, Owen JR (1977) Five hundred cancers of the larynx and pyriform sinus - results of treatment by radiation and surgery, Larynx and Pyriform Cancers, 1288–1302

Lam KH, Wong J, Lim STK, Ong GB (1981) Pharyngogastric anastomosis following pharyngolaryngoesophagectomy - analysis of 157 cases, World Journal of Surgery 5: 509–516

Larsson S, Mancuso A, Hoover L, Hanafee W (1981) Differentiation of pyriform sinus cancer from supraglottic laryngeal cancer by computed tomography, Radiology 141: 427–432

Lederman M (1958) Post-cricoid carcinoma, carcinoma of the phyopharynx, J. of Otolaryn 72: 397–411

Levitt SH (1984) Technologic basis of radiation therapy - Practical clinical applications. In: du V Tapley N (ed) Lea & Febiger, Philadelphia, Pa., pp 29–130

Lord IJ, Briant TDR, Rider WD, Bryce DP (1973) A comparison of pre-operative and primary radiotherapy in the treatment of carcinoma of the hypopharynx, Br J of Rad 46: 175–179

Lore JM, Klotch DW, Lee KY (1982) One-stage reconstruction of the hypopharynx using myomucosal tongue flat and dermal graft, Am J Surg 144: 473–476

McGuirt WF, Matthews B, Koufman JA (1982) Multiple simultaneous tumors in patients with head and neck cancer - a prospective, sequential panendoscopic study, Cancer 50: 1195–1199

Macbeth R (1971) Malignant disease of the hypopharynx, J Laryng Otol 85: 1215–1226

Mantravadi R, Katz AM, Skolnik EM, Becker S, Freehling D, Friedman M (1981) stomal recurrence: a critical analysis of risk factors. Arch Otolaryngol 107: 735–738

Marcus RB, Million RR, Cassissi NJ (1979) Postoperative irradiation for squamous cel carcinomas of the head and neck: analysis of time-dose factors related to control above the clavicles, Int J Radiation Oncol Biol Phys, 5: 1943–1949

Marks JE, Freeman RB, Lee F, Ogura JH (1978a) Pharyngeal wall cancer: an analysis of treatment results complications and patterns of failure, Int J Rad Oncol Biol Phys 4: 587–593

Marks JE, Kurnik B, Powers WE, Ogura JH (1978b) Carcinoma of the pyriform sinus - an analysis of treatment results and patterns of failure, Cancer 41: 1008–1015

Martin SA, Marks JE, Lee JY, Bauer WC, Ogura JH (1980) Carcinoma of the pyriform sinus: predictors of TNM relapse and survival, Cancer 46: 1974–1981

Meoz-Mendez RT, Fletcher GH, Guillamondegui OM, Peters LJ (1978) Analysis of results of irradiation in the treatment of squamous cell carcinomas of the pharyngeal walls, Int J Rad Oncol Biol Phys 4: 479–585

Million RR (1984) Management of head & neck Cancer: a multidisciplinary approach. In: Million RR, Cassissi J (Eds.) Management of Head Head & Neck Cancer: A Multidisciplinary Approach. (Lippincott, Philadelphia, Pa.)

Million RR, Cassisi NJ (1984) Hypopharynx: pharyngeal walls, pyriform sinus, and postcricoid pharynx (Lippincott, Philadelphia, Pa.) Management of Head and Neck Cancer (Eds.) Million RR, Cassissi J, pp 373–391

Nathan MD, El Gammal T, Hudson JH, Jr. (1980) Computerized axial tomography in the assessment of thyroid cartilage invasion by laryngeal carcinoma: a prospective study, Otolaryngol Head Neck Surg 6: 726–733

Ogura JH (a), Biller HF, Wette R (1980) Elective neck dissection for pharyngeal and laryngeal cancers - an evaluation, Otol 80: 646–651

Ogura JH (b), Marks JE, Freeman RB (1980) Results of conservation surgery for cancers of the supraglottis and pyriform sinus, Laryngoscope 90: 591–600

Ong GB, Wong J (1979) Jejunal replacement after pharyngolaryngo-esophagectomy for carcinoma of hypopharynx, World J Surgery 3: 381–386

Paradelo JC, Ucmakli A, Schiller B, Sternick E, Mower H (1981) Mid-saggital plane dosimetry in patients with extensive head and neck malignancy, Int J Rad Oncol Biol Phys 7: 115–120

Pene F, Avedian V, Eschwege F, Barrett A, Schwabb G, Marandas P, Vandenbrouck C (1978) A retrospective study of 131 cases of carcinoma of the posterior pharyngeal wall, Cancer 42: 2490–2493

Pearson JG (1966) The radiotherapy of carcinoma of the esophagus and post-cricoid region in south east scotland, Clin Radiol 17: 242–257

Persky MS, Daly JF (1981) Combined Therapy vs. curative radiation in the treatment of pyriform sinus carcinoma, Otolaryngol Head Neck Surg 89: 87–91

Pezner RD, Findlay DO (1981) A simplified alternative to orthogonal field overlap when irradiating a tracheostomy stoma or the hypopharynx, Int J Rad Oncol Biol Phys 7: 1121–1124

Puhaka H, Nordman EM (1980) Radiotherapy of carcinoma of the hypopharynx, Strahlentherapie 156: 315–317

Rabuzzi DD, Chung CT, Sagerman RH (1980) Prophylactic neck irradiation, Arch Otolaryngol 106: 454–455

Raine CH, Stell PM, Dalby J (1982) Squamous cell carcinoma of the posterior wall of the hypopharynx, J of Laryngology and Otology 96: 997–1004

Razack MS, Sako K, Kalnins I (1978) Squamous cell carcinoma of the pyriform sinus, Head & Neck Surg 1: 31–34

Russell EJ (1985) The radiologic approach to malignant tumors of the head and neck, with emphasis on computed tomography, Clinics in Plastic Surgery 12: 343–374

Sagerman RH, Chung CT, King GA, Yu WS, Cummings CW, Johnwon JT (1979) High dose preoperative irradiation for advanced laryngeal-hypopharyngeal Cancer, Ann Otol 88: 178–182

Shah JP, Shaha AR, Spiro RH, Strongt EW (1976) Carcinoma of the hypopharynx (1976) Am J Surg 132: 439–443

Silverman PM, Bossen EH, Fisher SR, Coile TB, Korobkin M, Halvorsen RA (1984) Carcinoma of the larynx and hypopharynx: computed tomographic-histopathologic correlations. Radiology 151: 697–702

Spiro RH, Shah JP, Strong EW, Gerold FP, Bains MS (1983) Gastric transposition in head and neck surgery - indications, complications and expectations, Am J Surg 146: 483–487

Stell et al. (1971) p. 25 (1981) p. 26

Talton BM, Elkon D, Kim J, Fitz-Hugh GS, Constable WC (1981) Cancer of the posterior hypopharyngeal wall, Int J Rad Oncol Biol Phys 7: 597–599

Terz JJ, Lawrence W (1983) Ineffectiveness of combined therapy (radiation and surgery) in the management of malignancies of the oral cavity, larynx and pharynx, In: Head and Neck Oncology - Controversies in Cancer Management. Eds. Kagen and Milos (G. K. Hall) pp. 111–126

Tom LWC, Wurzel JM, Wetmore RF, Lowry LD (1981) Mucoepidermoid carcinoma of the hypopharynx, Otolaryngol Head Neck Surg 89: 753–757

Wang CC (1971) Radiotherapeutic management of carcinoma of the posterior pharyngeal wall, Cancer 27: 894–896

Wang (1970) p. 4, 20

Yates A, Crumley RL (1984) Surgical treatment of pyriform sinus cancer: A retrospective study, Laryngoscope 94: 1586–1590

Yeager VL, Lawson C, Archer CR (1982) Ossification of the laryngeal cartilages as it relates to computued tomography, Invest Radiol 1: 11–19

10 Larynx

GEORGE E. LARAMORE

CONTENTS

10.1 Introduction

The ability to communicate is one of the major distinguishing characteristics between man and the lower animals. "Speaking" developed long before the invention of writing and in all human societies, continues to be the major vehicle for social intercourse. The loss of the ability to "speak" always causes significant changes in one's lifestyle and the consequences of this can be devastating. Cancer of the larynx directly threatens the main communication organ and in evaluating the various treatment alternatives, it is important to take into consideration the ability of the various treatments to preserve a functional voice. The patient needs to be brought into the decision making process when the various treatment options are being formulated as he may well decide that he would prefer to "lose" a few percentage points in terms of survival probability in return for having a higher probability of preserving his voice if the chosen treatment is successful.

Laryngeal cancer constitutes approximately ⅓ of all head and neck cancers. In 1987 the American Cancer Society (SILVERBERG and LUBERA 1987) estimates that there will be 12,100 new cases of laryngeal cancer and 3,800 deaths due to this disease in the United States alone. It represents 1–2% of all cancers in males (excluding non-melanoma skin cancer) with the incidence being about 8.1 per 100,000. The incidence is lower in females being only about 0.9 per 100,000. It occurs mainly in the 5th and 6th decades of life and has an equal predilection in Whites and Blacks. There is a definite causal relationship with cigarette smoking (WYNDER et al. 1976; WYNDER et al. 1977) with the relation between the number of cigarettes smoked each day and the risk of developing laryngeal cancer being almost linear. For about 30 cigarettes smoked each day, the risk is approximately 18 times that of the nonsmoker; while for 41+ cigarettes smoked a day, the risk is approximately 32 times that of the nonsmoker. Cessation of smoking reduces the risk of developing larnygeal cancer, but the effect is not instantaneous. It takes about 15 years for the risk factor to reduce to that of someone who has never smoked. Moreover, patients who continue to smoke after being successfully treated for larnygeal cancer, both have an increased risk of developing a second malignancy and also have shorter life expectancies than their counterparts who stop smoking. Alcohol consumption alone does not appear to cause an increased incidence of larnygeal cancer but clearly

GEORGE E. LARAMORE, Ph.D., M.D., Department of Radiation Oncology, RC-08, University Hospital, University of Washington, Seattle, Washington 98195, USA

acts as a "co-promoter" in synergism with smoking. Other possible risks include industrial exposure to asbestos and nickel and various air pollutants although these agents have not as yet been well studied.

10.2 Anatomical and Histological Considerations

10.2.1 General Anatomy

The larynx connects the lower portion of the pharynx with the trachea. It serves three major functions: (1) it is a valve that guards the air passages during swallowing, (2) it aids in the maintenance of a patent airway, and (3) it is the organ for vocalization. In choosing a form of treatment one most often focuses on preservation of voice, but it must be recognized that loss of the other functions can be fatal. In the adult male the larynx is about 5 cm long and is located anteriorly to the cervical vertebrae generally lying between C3 and C6. The anterior aspect of the larynx lies within 1.0 cm of the anterior surface of the neck and this must be taken into account in designing radiation therapy treatment portals. In particular, lateral fields need to "flash" over the anterior portion of the neck.

The various regions of the larynx are shown in Fig. 10-1. The larynx is generally divided into three regions - the supraglottis, the glottis, and the subglottis. Tumors arising in these regions behave differently in regards to their presentation, propensity to spread, and prognosis.

The supraglottis consists of the epiglottis, the aryepiglottic folds, the arytenoids, the false vocal cords, and the laryngeal ventricles. This region is richly endowed with lymphatics and tumors arising here are prone to spread via the regional nodes.

Positive nodes most commonly occur in the anterior or cervical chain. The primary lesion is generally confined to the pre-epiglottic space but can penetrate the epiglottic cartilage superiorly. However, the hypoepiglottic and thyroepiglottic ligaments and the hyothyroid membranes serve as secondary containment barriers. Approximately 30-35% of laryngeal tumors arise in supraglottic sites.

The glottis consists of the true vocal cords and the anterior commissure. It extends to a distance of 1 cm below the true cords. It is contained within the thyroid cartilage and is sparsely endowed with lymphatics. Glottic tumors spread superiorly and inferiorly in the paraglottic space but generally are contained by the cricothyroid membrane and the thyroid cartilage until they are very advanced. In general, they do not spread via the regional lymphatics until these barriers are breached. The glottis is the most common site of origin for laryngeal cancers and accounts for 60-65% of such tumors.

The subglottis starts 1 cm below the true cords and extends to the inferior border of the cricoid cartilage. These tumors spread through the lymphatics that penetrate the cricothyroid membrane to involve the pretracheal nodes and the lower nodes in the anterior cervical chain. Tumors that arise in the subglottic region are rare and constitute only about 1-5% of reported laryngeal cancers.

Most authors consider a further class of laryngeal cancers - transglottic lesions that involve both the true and false cords. These can spread by the same regional lymphatics as described for the supraglottic lesions.

10.2.2 Tumor Histologies

Diseases of the larynx generally fall into two categories: inflammatory processes or neoplasms. Both benign lesions and malignant lesions can arise from

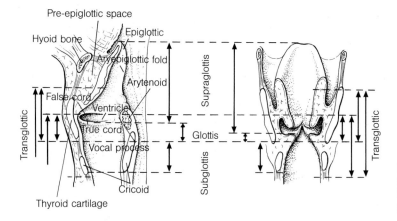

Fig. 10-1. Drawing of larynx with major anatomical sites labeled. The regions defining the supraglottis, the glottis, and the subglottis are also indicated

any cell type found in the larynx. Benign neoplasms include polyps, papillomas, chondromas, leiomyomas, amyloid deposits, and neurofibromas.

At least 95% of all malignant laryngeal tumors are squamous cell in histology and originate in the larynx itself. The most common of the "rarer" tumors are adenoidcystic carcinomas and lymphomas. Other tumors that have been reported are pseudosarcomas (actually a squamous cell carcinoma with a sarcomatous stroma), mucoepidermoid carcinomas, myelomas, granular cell myoblastomas, neurofibrosarcomas, chondrosarcomas, osteosarcomas, malignant melanomas, and chemodectomas. Metastatic tumors to the larynx are quite rare and usually arise from primary malignancies in the gastrointestinal or genitourinary tracts. Lung and breast are other sites that have been known to metastasize to the larynx. The remainder of this chapter will be confined to the squamous cell carcinomas that originate in the larynx although many of the considerations for selecting a given form of treatment and choosing a specific radiotherapy technique apply to other tumor histologies as well.

Local/regional tumor persistence or recurrence constitutes the primary failure mode. About 90% of such failures will occur within two years following therapy. Distant metastases from laryngeal tumors occur primarily from advanced supraglottic lesions. The most common metastatic site is lung followed by bone, gastrointestinal sites, and brain. About 80% of all distant metastases will present within two years following treatment. Distant metastases are the primary cause of death in 20% of patients who present with laryngeal cancers.

10.3 Tumor Staging

The staging system utilized for any given tumor should reflect the known prognostic factors for both local control and survival. For laryngeal tumors the following are important prognostic factors: location, status of cord fixation, disease status of cervical nodes, and presence or absence of distant metastases. These are reflected in the American Joint Committee TMN staging system that is summarized in Table 10-1. There is evidence that impaired cord mobility is a deleterious factor and some authors (HARWOOD et al. 1981; VAN DEN BOGAERT et al. 1983; WANG unpublished) take this into account by further subdividing T_1 and T_2 lesions into the categories "a" (normal cord mobility) and "b" (impaired cord mobility). Classically the

Table 10-1. TNM staging system for cancer of the larynx following the 1978 recommendations of the American Joint Committee for Cancer Staging and End Result Reporting

T-Staging

Supraglottis

TIS: Carcinoma in situ

T_1: Tumor confined to one supraglottic site

T_2: Tumor involving more than one supraglottic site and/or extension to the true cords *without* cord fixation

T_3: Tumor limited to laryngeal structures with fixation of cords and/or extension to involve the postcricoid area, medial wall of piriform sinus or pre-epiglottic space

T_4: Massive tumor extending beyond larynx to involve the oropharynx, soft tissues of the neck and/or destruction of the thyroid cartilage

Glottis

TIS: Carcinoma in situ

T_1: Tumor confined to vocal cord(s) (including the possibility of involvement of the anterior and/or posterior commissures) with normal or impaired cord mobility

T_2: Tumor extends to supraglottic and/or subglottic structures with normal or impaired cord mobility

T_3: Tumor confined to laryngeal structures *with* cord fixat.

T_4: Massive tumor with extension beyond larynx and/or destruction of thyroid cartilage

Subglottis

TIS: Carcinoma in situ

T_1: Tumor confined to the subglottis

T_2: Tumor extends to vocal cord(s) with normal or impaired cord mobility

T_3: Tumor confined to larynx *with* cord fixation

T_4: Massive tumor extending beyond the larynx and/or destruction of thyroid or cricoid cartilages

N-Staging

NX: Nodes cannot be assessed

N_0: Clinically negative nodes

N_1: One clinically positive homolateral node $\varnothing$ 3 cm or less

N_2: A single clinically positive homolateral node more than 3 cm but less than 6 cm in diameter or multiple clinically positive homolateral nodes none of which are more than 6 cm in diameter

    N_{2a}: Single homolateral node between 3 and 6 cm in diameter

    N_{2b}: Multiple homolateral nodes none of which are more than 6 cm in diameter

N_3: Massive homolateral node(s), bilateral nodes or contralateral node(s)

    N_{3a}: One clinically positive homolateral node greater than 6 cm in diameter

    N_{3b}: Bilateral clinically positive nodes. Each side of neck should be separately staged

    N_{3c}: Clinically positive contralateral node(s)

M-Staging

MX: Metastatic disease not assessed

M_0: No known distant metastases

M_1: Distant metastases present

Stage Grouping

Stage I: $T_1 \, N_0 \, M_0$

Stage II: $T_2 \, T_0 \, M_0$

Stage III: $T_3 \, N_0 \, M_0$

           $T_1 \, T_2 \, T_3 \, N_1 \, M_0$

Stage IV: $T_4 \, N_0 \, M_0$

           Any T-stage, $N_2 \, N_3 \, M_0$

           Any T-stage, any N-stage, M_1

TNM staging was thought to correlate with general prognosis through the general stage grouping shown at the bottom of Table 10-1. Age and sex of the patient are also significant prognostic indicators with females living longer than males and younger patients living longer than older patients (LEDERMAN 1970; SHAW 1965). Some measure of the baseline medical status of the patient (such as Karnofsky performance status) is also felt to be important.

More recently with the advent of sophisticated computer techniques, it has been possible to analyze large patient data bases and to factor together the major variables to obtain a quantitative representation of tumor control probability with conventional radiotherapy techniques. This work is still in its infancy but results from the Radiation Therapy Oncology Group (GRIFFIN et al. 1984) give the following equation for the probability of achieving local control with definitive radiotherapy for tumors of the supraglottic and glottic larynx.

$$P = \exp(F)/[1+\exp(F)] \tag{1}$$

where

$$F = 2.100 - 0.960(T - 2.072) - 0.245(N - 0.622)$$
$$+ 0.855(S - 1.854) + 0.761(K - 1.613) \tag{2}$$

In Eq. (2) T is the T-stage [1, 2, 3, 4]; N is the N-stage [0, 1, 2, 3]; S is the site of tumor origin [1 = oral cavity, 2 = hypopharynx, supraglottic larynx, and glottic larynx, 3 = nasopharynx]; and K is the patient's Karnofsky performance status [0 = less than 70, 1 = 70-80, and 2 = 90-100]. This model was developed on the basis of data for approximately 1000 patients and its validity has been checked for several independent data sets. For those patients predicted to have a 90% or better probability of tumor clearance, 87% remained with a controlled primary at 2 years after treatment.

It is particularly instructive to see the effect of different Karnofsky performance status on the local control probability. Table 10-2 shows this as a function of T and N stages for the different Karnofsky status categories. There are two main things to note from this table. First, for a given T and N stage, there is a major dependence of primary tumor control probability on the patient's Karnofsky status and this is most pronounced for the more advanced tumors. It is important to keep this in mind when comparing the results of nonrandomized studies from different institutions. It is also important when comparing the results of surgical series with radiation series as in general, patients treated with surgery often have better Karnofsky status than those

Table 10-2. Probability of controlling the primary tumor with radiotherapy for squamous cell cancers of the supraglottic and glottic larynx. (After GRIFFIN et al. 1984)

		K = 90-100 T			
		1	2	3	4
N	0	0.98	0.94	0.87	0.76
	1	0.96	0.92	0.82	0.72
	2	0.96	0.90	0.78	0.66
	3	0.95	0.74	0.74	0.61
		K = 70-80 T			
		1	2	3	4
N	0	0.95	0.88	0.74	0.53
	1	0.94	0.86	0.69	0.47
	2	0.92	0.82	0.64	0.41
	3	0.90	0.78	0.58	0.35
		K < 60 T			
		1	2	3	4
N	0	0.91	0.79	0.59	0.35
	1	0.88	0.74	0.53	0.30
	2	0.86	0.69	0.46	0.25
	3	0.82	0.64	0.41	0.21

referred for primary radiotherapy. Secondly, note that T-stage tends to be a stronger prognostic factor than N-stage when the Karnofsky status is fixed. This table might be useful in evaluating a given patient for primary radiotherapy but the reader should be cautioned that it is by no means the final word on this subject and variables such as degree of tumor infiltration and tumor grade will almost certainly be important as well.

10.4 Evaluation of the Patient

10.4.1 Presentation

10.4.1.1 Supraglottic Tumors

The most common symptoms are dysphagia and odynophagia. There is often a "tickling" sensation as if there is a foreign body lodged in the throat. Pain, if present, tends to be of a "sore throat" nature. Hoarseness, if it occurs, is intermittent in nature. A large tumor is generally required to produce dyspnea which is a rare presenting symptom for tumors of the supraglottis. Emergency tracheostomy is necessary in only about 7% of patients (MARKS and SESSIONS 1985). Hemoptysis is also uncommon. The median duration of symptoms before diagnosis of tumor is approximately 3 months (MARKS and SESSIONS 1985). The presenting sign is most commonly a "neck mass" - particularly, for tumors that arise in the epiglottis.

10.4.1.2 Glottic Tumors

The most common presenting symptom is hoarseness of a chronic and progressive nature which may progress to complete aphonia. It precedes tumor diagnosis by a median time of about 6 months (SHAW 1965). Dyspnea is uncommon but can occur - particularly, if there is subglottic extension of tumor. Hemoptysis is uncommon and, generally, there is no odynophagia if the lesion is confined to the endolarynx. Local pain, if present, is generally due to cartilage invasion. An emergency tracheostomy is necessary in about 14% of lesions that are *transglottic* in nature (MARKS and SESSIONS 1985).

10.4.1.3 Subglottic Tumors

Dyspnea is the most common presenting symptom and occurs because of tumor growing in a confined space. There are generally minimum symptoms until the orifice is sufficiently narrowed that the air flow becomes turbulent and then dyspnea and stridor develop rapidly. Hoarseness, odynophagia, and hemoptysis are uncommon. A dry cough occurs occasionally.

10.4.2 Patient Workup

The key to the evaluation of a patient with laryngeal cancer is the history and physical examination. The history should be directed to elucidate the presence or absence of the symptoms discussed above. The physical examination requires careful palpation of the neck and supraclavicular fossa and both direct and indirect visualization of the oral cavity, pharynx, and larynx. Laryngeal crepitus (thyrovertebral crackle) is normally present. If it is absent, it may mean that there is tumor (or perhaps only edema) present in the postcricoid region. Sometimes adequate visualization of the larynx is difficult with the standard mirror examination and utilization of a fiberoptic device is necessary. It should always be remembered that most patients with head

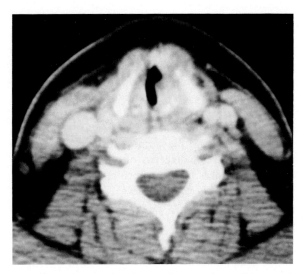

Fig. 10-2. CT scan of patient having an advanced laryngeal tumor that has caused destruction of the thyroid cartilage

and neck cancer will have the multiple risk factors of tobacco and alcohol abuse. For these patients, in particular, the incidence of synchronous "second" primaries is appreciable and other lesions must be ruled out before embarking on a definitive course of therapy directed at the laryngeal lesion alone. A direct examination under anesthesia by a qualified otolaryngologist is mandatory and obviously the diagnosis of cancer must be established via a biopsy.

Routine laboratory tests include liver function tests, serum alkaline phosphatase, serum calcium, and a chest x-ray to rule out metastatic disease. Followup studies such as liver and bone scans are needed if the screening tests are abnormal. A CBC is also recommended since there is some evidence for uterine cervical cancer that an adequate hematocrit improved tumor control with radiotherapy (BUSH et al. 1978). Many radiotherapy departments use transfusions, if necessary, to maintain the patient's hematocrit above 30 during radiotherapy. Certainly, the amount of bone marrow irradiated in the treatment of head and neck cancer is minimal, but patients are often debilitated from other medical problems and increasing numbers of patients receive marrow-toxic chemotherapy as part of their overall management.

Today there is increasing use of the CT scan, rather than the laryngogram, to further evaluate the more advanced lesions. A barium swallow with fluoroscopy to study the pharyngoesophageal junction and the status of the esophagus is sometimes helpful. These radiographic investigations can assess the extent of the primary lesion by evaluating the mobility of the involved region, whether or not carti-lage destruction is is present, and whether or not there is tumor extension into the pre-epiglottic space or subglottic region. Fig. 10-2 shows a CT scan of a patient with gross destruction of the thy-roid cartilage by a laryngeal tumor. This finding au-tomatically upstages the patient to a "T_4" status. CT scans also may show the presence of adenopathy, particularly behind the sternocleidomastoid muscle that has not been detected on clinical exam. The cost effectiveness of these ancillary tests is low for early T_1 and T_2 glottic cancers.

10.5 Supraglottic Tumors

10.5.1 Regional Lymphatics

As previously described, positive regional nodes are not uncommon at the time of presentation. Fletch-er's classic data from M.D. Anderson (FLETCHER 1978) showed that for 267 patients treated between 1948 and 1965, there was a 55% incidence of nodal involvement by tumor. The ipsilateral subdigastric nodes were involved 37% of the time and the ipsi-lateral midjugular nodes were involved 26% of the time. The overall incidence of contralateral nodal involvement was 16%.

In a survey of patients with N_0 necks treated sur-gically at the Mallinckrodt Institute, MARKS et al. (1985) found the incidence of occult lymph node metastases to be in the range of 20-38% for tumors arising in the "marginal larynx". The "marginal lar-ynx" was defined as the glossoepiglottic area, the suprahyoid epiglottis, the aryepiglottic fold, the arytenoids, and the free margins of the epiglottis. They defined the "central larynx" as the false cords and the infrahyoid epiglottis and found a 16% inci-dence of occult nodal metastases for tumors arising in these areas. The patients, in many cases, had received "low dose" preoperative radiotherapy to 3000 cGy in 3 weeks prior to the surgery. Although patients with keratin debris in the nodes were clas-sified as having had occult disease, this may not have taken into account all of the potential down-staging since some tumors are nonkeratinizing. Hence, the above numbers may somewhat underes-timate the true situation.

It is important to include the neck nodes in the radiation fields. LINDBERG and FLETCHER (1978) have shown that the incidence of neck failures was 33% for patients with N_0 necks treated only with surgical resection of the primary. It was only 1% in those patients treated with surgery and radiation if adequate doses in the range of 5000-6000 cGy were given. MARKS et al. (1979), describe a series of 129 patients treated with low-dose preoperative ir-radiation in the range of 2500-3000 cGy at 200 cGy per fraction for 5 days-per-week. Twenty seven pa-tients (21%) exhibited ultimate neck failures with 20 of these having a failure component in the contra-lateral neck that was initially clinically negative. They now recommend using higher radiation doses to eliminate this problem.

10.5.2 Definitive Radiotherapeutic Management

Definitive radiotherapy is recommended for early stage T_1, T_2, N_0, and N_1 lesions. It is also recom-mended for the very advanced lesions where sur-gery may not be an option. The trade-offs between definitive radiotherapy with surgery held in reserve for salvage vs. a combined surgical-radiotherapeu-tic approach for moderately advanced lesions will be discussed elsewhere in the chapter as will the possible applications of chemotherapy in this class of tumors.

The design of the radiation portals must be tai-lored to the specific patient and tumor but some general statements can be made. A "typical" port design is shown in Fig. 10-3. The upper border of the field should include approximately one cm of the mandible in order to adequately cover the sub-mandibular and subdigastric nodes. If the posterior pharyngeal wall or the piriform sinus apex or later-al wall is involved with tumor, then one needs to treat the pharyngeal wall up to the level of the base of the skull in order to adequately cover the retro-pharyngeal nodal drainage as shown in Fig. 10-4. The upper portion of the field is eliminated after 5000 cGy unless there is gross disease in this region. The posterior cervical nodes on the ipsilateral side should be covered for N_+ patients and probably should be treated for N_0 patients having extensive primary lesions (T_3 or T_4). The spinal cord should be shielded after 4500 cGy and the posterior cervi-cal nodes boosted with electrons of properly chosen energy. Recommended total doses are in the range of 6600-7200 cGy at 180-200 cGy per daily frac-tion to areas that are grossly involved by tumor. The dose to areas at risk for microscopic disease is 5000 cGy at the same fractionation schedule. A typ-ical lower neck and supraclavicular fossa treatment field is shown in Fig. 10-5a. The dose to the anterior supraclavicular fossa is generally calculated at a 3 cm depth. However, in cases where the lower

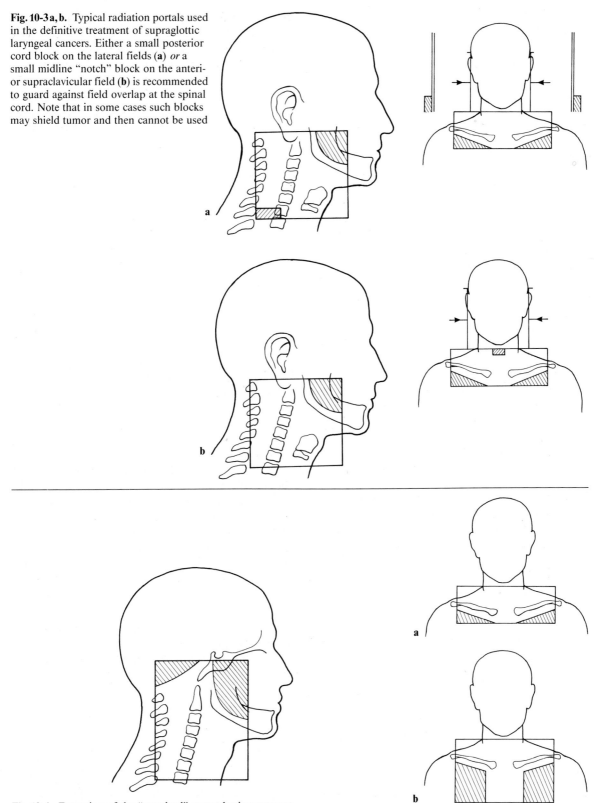

Fig. 10-3a, b. Typical radiation portals used in the definitive treatment of supraglottic laryngeal cancers. Either a small posterior cord block on the lateral fields (**a**) *or* a small midline "notch" block on the anterior supraclavicular field (**b**) is recommended to guard against field overlap at the spinal cord. Note that in some cases such blocks may shield tumor and then cannot be used

Fig. 10-4. Extension of the "standard" supraglottic treatment field to encompass the retropharyngeal nodes to the base of the skull for situations where the apex or lateral wall of the piriform sinus or the pharyngeal wall is involved with tumor

Fig. 10-5a, b. Typical radiation fields used to treat the lower neck and supraclavicular regions (**a**). A "T" field that includes the upper mediastinal nodes is shown in (**b**)

neck and/or the supraclavicular nodes are clinically positive, then the upper mediastinal nodes are at risk and need to be treated in the lower neck field. This can be accomplished by modifying the supraclavicular field into a "T" field as shown in Fig. 10-5b. The radiation dose is then calculated to a depth of ⅓ the AP dimension along the central axis or in some cases a parallel opposed AP/PA configuration may be used.

Isodose calculations are highly desirable and in most cases "wedged" compensator filters are required because of the anatomical configuration of the human neck being thin anteriorly and much wider posteriorly. Gross residual disease in the posterior nodal region should be boosted with electrons of appropriate energy such that the spinal cord dose is kept to within acceptable levels. If electrons are not available, PA neck photon fields can be used but this technique may give rise to increased dose inhomogeneity.

The results of primary radiotherapy for supraglottic lesions is summarized for some series in Tables 10-3 and 10-4. This information is meant to be representative and not all-inclusive. Also, the data summarizes results for various nodal status and thus smears out the effect of this important prognostic variable. Local control rates for T_1 lesions generally run between 80–90% with radiation alone. For the more advanced T_3 and T_4 lesions, one can

do fairly well for selected exophytic lesions as demonstrated by GOEPFERT et al. (1975). For more typical patients local control rates run between 25–45%. For the intermediate T_2 lesions, local control rates run between 60–80% depending on the particular series. Survival rates are lower than local control rates because of deaths from second primaries and other intercurrent diseases. Nevertheless, definitive radiotherapy with surgery held in reserve as a salvage procedure is still a preferable option to a total laryngectomy for advanced T_2 lesions. The difficulty in the decision process comes in the situation where the initial surgical procedure is a voice-preserving partial laryngectomy and the "salvage" procedure will likely be a total laryngectomy.

10.5.3 Combined Surgery-Radiation Approach

For advanced lesions that are still resectable, a combined approach utilizing surgery with planned preoperative or postoperative radiotherpy offers improved local control rates and survival when compared to the results of definitive radiotherapy. MIRIMANOFF et al. (1985) show local control rates of 90% for T_3 lesions and 42% for T_4 lesions. The T_3 results are better than shown in Table 10-3 for definitive radiotherapy but the T_4 results are not noticeably different. Survival data is shown in Table 10-5. Comparing the data of VERMUND (1970) between Tables 10-4 and 10-5 shows noticeable improvement in survival for T_3 and T_4 lesions with the addition of surgery. While this was not a randomized comparison, hopefully, the two series were not too dissimilar. Also, the data of WANG et al. (1972, 1973) from the Massachussetts General Hospital shows a similar survival benefit to a combined approach for resectable T_3 and T_4 lesions. MARKS and SESSIONS (1985) summarize data from different series and show a 74% rate of tumor control with adequate voice preservation for T_1 and T_2 lesions treated both primarily with radiotherapy and also with a voice conserving surgical procedure and adjuvant

Table 10-3. Local control rate for patients with supraglottic tumors treated with definitive radiotherapy

	T_1 (%)	T_2 (%)	T_3 (%)	T_4 (%)
FLETCHER et al. (1975)	80	91	73	33
GOEPFERT et al. (1975)[a]	89	81	72	60
GHOSSEIN et al. (1974)	82	69	—	—
HARWOOD et al. (1983)[b]	71	68	56	52
WANG (1973)	94	80	35	33

[a] With preservation of normal voice; T_3 and T_4 highly selected

[b] N_0 patients only

Table 10-4. Survival rate for patients with supraglottic tumors treated with definitive radiotherapy

	T_1 (%)	T_2 (%)	T_3 (%)	T_4 (%)
HARWOOD et al. (1979)	—	63	55	49
WANG (1973)	89	66	21	23
WANG (unpublished)[a]	73	50	37	23
with surgical salvage	80	58	46	26
VERMUND (1970)[b]	65	61	36	14

[a] NED survival at 5 years

[b] N_0 patients only

Table 10-5. Survival rate for patients with supraglottic tumors treated with planned surgery and adjuvant radiotherapy

	T_1 (%)	T_2 (%)	T_3 (%)	T_4 (%)
MIRIMANOFF et al. (1985)[a]	—	—	66	34
VERMUND (1970)[b]	73	61	45	56
WANG et al. (1972)	90	79	63	32
MARKS et al. (1979)	46	69	63	43

[a] Series contains some glottic tumors

[b] N_0 patients only

radiotherapy. For T_3 and T_4 lesions, on the other hand, the success rate increases for 40% to 67% when a combined surgical-radiotherapeutic approach is used.

In a combined approach the adjuvant radiotherapy can be given either preoperatively or postoperatively. Preoperative radiotherapy has the advantage of shrinking the primary tumor as well as sterilizing microscopic disease in the lymph nodes. Some authors (OGURA and BILLER 1970; KAZEM et al. 1982) advocate a relatively low dose of 1500–2500 cGy given in 1–2 weeks followed by immediate surgery while others (WANG 1973; GOLDMAN et al. 1972) advocate higher doses of 5000–5500 cGy in 5–6 weeks with the surgery following after 3–6 weeks. There is no clear evidence that one approach is better than the other in terms of demonstrated patient survival but the higher dose in principle should offer a higher rate of sterilization of microscopic disease. Also a longer delay between the radiotherapy and the surgery should allow for better tumor shrinkage provided that cellular repopulation does not dominate the tumor kinetics during this time interval.

Postoperative radiotherapy is felt better than preoperative radiotherapy by many workers since it allows one to specifically target the patient subgroup requiring radiotherapy on the basis of the pathological findings at the time of surgery. For example many clinical N_0 necks contain microscopic foci of metastases and conversely some clinically N_+ necks in reality contain only reactive nodes. Furthermore, the radiotherapist has the option of boosting to higher doses any areas of postoperative residual disease in a continuous, planned course of radiotherapy. In addition, many surgeons feel that there are fewer wound healing complications with postoperative radiotherapy.

In an attempt to address the question of whether preoperative or postoperative radiotherapy was better, the RTOG performed a randomized study (KRAMER, 1985; KRAMER et al. 1987) that compared 5000 cGy preoperative radiotherapy with 6000 cGy postoperative radiotherapy for various head and neck sites. The postoperative dose was higher because of the increased risk of hypoxic tumor cells in the post surgical treatment field. For supraglottic lesions the 4-year local control rate was 53% for the preoperative treatment and 77% for the postoperative treatment. The 4-year survival was 41% in the preoperative arm and 47% in the postoperative arm. While the patient numbers were such that these differences were not statistically significant, they are suggestive. Part of the difference in local control between the two arms is due to some preoperatively irradiated patients refusing the planned surgery after an apparent "complete response" to radiotherapy. Most of these patients subsequently failed as might be expected from the moderate dose of radiation that was given. Also, it should be noted that there was no difference in overall morbidity between the two arms. At the present time it appears that postoperative radiotherapy is more widely accepted than preoperative radiotherapy in the United States but certain institutions strongly favor the preoperative approach.

As in the case of definitive radiotherapy, radiation treatment fields must be specifically tailored to the individual patient. The same general considerations as to the regions covered as a function of specific sites of tumor involvement apply as indicated in Section 10.5.2. Normally 5000–6000 cGy is given to areas at risk for microscopic disease and an additional 1000–1200 cGy is given via small "boost" fields to areas of gross residual disease. The uses of "wedged" compensator filters and electrons are the same as in the case of definitive radiotherapy. Similarly, an anterior supraclavicular field or a mediastinal "T" field is used to treat the lower neck as circumstances warrant.

Postoperative radiotherapy is recommended for T_3 and T_4 lesions regardless of the surgical findings and for all lesions where positive nodes are found in the operative specimen. Most institutions in the United States treat the contralateral posterior triangle nodes to 5000 cGy and the ipsilateral posterior triangle nodes to the full 5000–6000 cGy dose using electrons of appropriate energy after the spinal cord dose of 4500 cGy is reached with the primary photon fields. Specific indications for irradiating the tracheostoma will be discussed in Section 10.9.

10.6 Glottic Tumors

10.6.1 Regional Lymphatics

For tumors that arise in the glottic larynx, regional nodes are uncommon at the time presentation – particularly, for early stage lesions. The risk of lymphatic involvement increases when tumors extend beyond the confines of the larynx and so elective treatment of the neck is recommended for T_3 and T_4 lesions. Some authors advocate treating the anterior neck nodes for advanced T_2 lesions – especially if the histology is poorly differentiated. On occasion the tumor metastasizes to the Delphinian node at the thyroid isthmus but this is certainly included in any normal larynx field.

10.6.2 Definitive Radiotherapeutic Management

Definitive radiotherapy is recommended for T_1, T_2, and early T_3 lesions. Although a vertical hemilaryngectomy yields equal cure rates for T_1 and early T_2 lesions, the quality of the speaking voice is generally thought to be better with radiotherapeutic management.

Carcinoma-in-situ may be managed with vocal cord stripping but it should be noted that if enough serial sections are examined, foci of invasive carcinoma are often found (BAUER, 1974). It is interesting to note that the majority of recurrences after definitive radiotherapy tend to be invasive carcinoma while the recurrences after a vocal cord stripping procedure tend to be divided with about half being again carcinoma-in-situ and half being frankly invasive.

PENE and FLETCHER (1976) report on a series of 79 patients with the diagnosis of carcinoma-in-situ and 7 patients with the diagnosis of leukoplakia/atypical hyperplasia that were treated with radiation therapy. They staged the patients as T_1 or T_2 using the same systems as for frankly invasive lesions and furthermore, used the same radiation therapy techniques. The ultimate failure rates were the same as for invasive lesions – 11% for T_1 and 26% for T_2. However, only 2/12 failures were on the initially involved cord suggesting that most of the failures were *not* true recurrences but rather new disease developing on dysplastic epithelium. Also, it took about 5 years for approximately 80% of the failures to occur which further suggests a "second primary" rather than a true recurrence. The 12 patients who failed required a partial or a total laryngectomy for salvage. Sixty-six patients were cured with a normal speaking voice and 7 patients exhibited some residual hoarseness. The remaining patient was treated with orthovoltage during the early years of the study and developed complications that ultimately required a laryngectomy.

For early stage T_1 lesions the radiation ports cover just the larynx and are approximately 5 cm × 5 cm in size. The upper border of the field is located at the thyroid notch and the anterior border flashes across the skin. The posterior border of the field includes the anterior portion of the posterior pharyngeal wall. Normally, a simple parallel opposed pair of fields incorporating wedged compen-

sators is used as indicated in Fig. 10-6 a. In general, wedge filters must be used to avoid overdosing the anterior part of the neck and increasing the risk of thyroid cartilage necrosis. The particular choice of wedges used must be individualized to the given patient's anatomy. Note the large relative volume included in the 100% ± 5% region. For unusual anatomical configurations, the usefulness of the "standard" wedge set can be extended by using different ones on alternate treatment days. C. C. WANG (1983) advocates a four field technique, as illustrated in Fig. 10-6 b. This reduces, somewhat, the dose to the anterior neck and to the lateral subcutaneous tissues but it is not clear that the benefits are commensurate with the added complexity of setup in most instances. Typical doses are in the range of 6500–7000 cGy in 180–200 cGy increments over 6.5–7.5 weeks.

Results of treatment for early lesions are shown in Tables 10-6 and 10-7. For T_1 lesions, local control rates run between 85–95% with at least half of the failures being surgically salvageable. Except for the series by VERMUND (1970), the survival rates are also between 85–95% at 5 years. For T_2 lesions local control runs between 65–75% and survival rates run between 60–85%. The fact that the survival figures are comparable to the local control figures reflects the effectiveness of surgical salvage and the fact that few patients with early stage glottic cancer die of their disease. Impaired cord mobility adversely impacts local control and survival for T_2 lesions. WANG (unpublished) notes for T_2 lesions that the

Table 10-6. Local control rate for patients with glottic tumors treated with definitive radiotherapy

	T_1 (%)	T_2 (%)	T_3 (%)	T_4 (%)
FLETCHER et al. (1975)	86	—	—	—
HARWOOD et al. (1979)	86	—	—	—
HORIOT et al. (1972)	88	75	—	—
MILLION et al. (1982)	93	66	20	—
KARIM et al. (1978)	92	69	37	25

Table 10-7. Survival rate for patients with glottic tumors treated with definitive radiotherapy

	T_1 (%)	T_2 (%)	T_3 (%)	T_4 (%)
HARWOOD et al. (1979)	95	—	—	—
VERMUND (1970)[a]	78	63	50	8
WANG (unpublished)[a] with surgical salvage	91 / 97	71 / 85	36 / 57	—
NASS et al. (1976)	89	76	—	—
CONSTABLE et al. (1975)	91	—	—	—
FLETCHER et al. (1975)[a]	86	—	—	—

[a] N_0 neck disease only

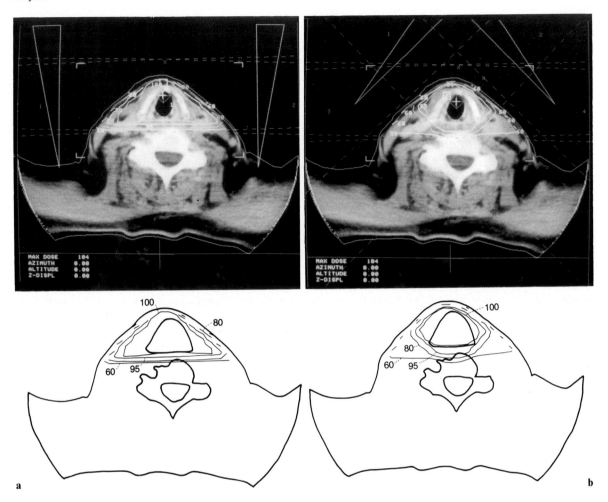

Fig. 10-6a, b. Typical radiation isodose distributions for the treatment of T_1 lesions of the glottic larynx. **a** A simple, parallel-opposed set of lateral fields utilizing wedge compensators. **b** A four-field configuration as advocated by WANG (1985)

5 year NED actuarial survival drops from 79% to 61% when there is impaired cord mobility. HARWOOD et al. (1980) evaluated 164 patients with T_2 N_0 M_0 glottic carcinoma and noted a 5 year actuarial survival of 75% for patients with impaired cord mobility compared with 87% for patients with normal cord mobility. The local control rates were, respectively, 51% vs 77%.

Field size is important, particularly, with the larger penumbra present on ^{60}Co fields. OLSZEWSKI et al. (1985) reviewed 137 patients treated for T_1 glottic cancer on ^{60}Co units and found a 15% increase in the failure rate for field sizes less than or equal to 30 cm^2. They also noted that patients had a higher risk of local recurrence if their lesions were either poorly differentiated or involved the anterior commissure.

For the more advanced T_3 and T_4 lesions, the field sizes used are more akin to those used for supraglottic lesions. It is important to treat the neck nodes using the same criteria as noted in Section 10-5. If the neck is N_0, then, the nodal drainage on both sides of the neck should receive 5000 cGy with the spinal cord dose being limited to 4500 cGy. Electrons of appropriate energy can be used to treat the posterior neck nodes beyond 4500 cGy. If the apex of the piriform sinus or the posterior pharyngeal wall is also involved, then, the retropharyngeal nodes to the level of the base of the skull should be treated to 5000 cGy.

The radiation ports are then limited to the areas of gross disease and these areas taken to 7000–7500 cGy. The lower neck and supraclavicular nodes are treated with an anterior neck field or a mediastinal "T" field depending upon whether or not there are clinically positive nodes in the lower neck and whether or not there is subglottic extension of tumor.

The local control rates for T_3 and T_4 lesions run between 20–35%. Survival rates for T_3 lesions run between 36–57%, while the data of VERMUND (1970) shows a survival rate of only 8% for T_4 lesions. Surgical salvage of uncontrolled primary disease will almost certainly entail a total laryngectomy. There tends to be a direct correlation between the local failure rate and the pathologic grade of the tumor. MILLS (1979) reviewed 96 patients with T_1, T_2, and T_3 glottic cancers and found a failure rate of 24% for the well-differentiated lesions, 41% for the moderately-differentiated lesions, and 67% for the poorly-differentiated lesions. However, it should be noted that there was a correlation with stage of tumor in that a greater percentage of the poorly differentiated lesions were T_3. Hence, tumor grade and stage may not be totally independent variables.

A final point relates to the treatment of a well-differentiated "verrucous" variant of squamous cell carcinoma that may arise in the glottis as well as other head and neck sites. It constitutes 1–4% of all laryngeal tumors and most commonly arises in the glottis (FERLITO and RECHER 1980; BATSAKIS et al. 1982). The majority of reported cases treated with radiotherapy have exhibited a persistence/recurrence of the neoplasm with the summed local control rate being only 29% (26/90) (FERLITO and RECHER 1980). This would argue that this type of tumor should be treated primarily with surgery. There is also some feeling that such tumors have the propensity to transform to a more malignant nature if treated with radiation. SCHWADE et al. (1976) have reviewed the data and find that this is not the case. Hence, in selected cases it would be reasonable to use primary radiation therapy with surgery held in reserve for salvage.

Side effects of radiotherapy often include arytenoid edema which can cause a vocal hoarseness. Usually, this is temporary but there may be some permanent alteration in vocal quality – particularly, for the more advanced lesions. Edema that persists more than 6 months after completion of therapy is an ominous sign as in approximately 50% of cases, it is associated with persistent or recurrent tumor (KAGAN et al. 1974; MILLS 1979; FU et al. 1982). Unfortunately, this edema often makes the diagnosis of recurrent tumor difficult since the recurrences are generally submucosal in nature and so a biopsy may simply return inflammatory tissue. Multiple biopsies may be necessary to confirm the presence of tumor before a salvage surgery is performed. How-

ever, this must be tempered by increased risk of cartilage necrosis in the patients who do not ultimately prove to have active tumor. If there is no visible lesion on direct laryngoscopy and if the edema is mild and primarily limited to the arytenoids, then close observation after the first negative biopsy is the recommended approach.

10.6.3 Combined Surgery–Radiation Approach

It is generally possible to make only a crude comparison between radiation and combined surgery/radiation series because of different treatment policies at the various reporting institutions. VERMUND (1970) shows a 5-year survival of 83% for T_1 N_0 lesions, 57% for T_2 N_0, 61% for T_3 N_0 lesions and 32% for T_4 N_0 lesions. The T_3 N_0 results are only marginally improved compared to the radiotherapy results shown in Table 10-7, but the improvement for the T_4 N_0 lesions is more marked. MIRIMANOFF et al. (1985) describe a "mini-mantle" technique for delivering postoperative radiotherapy for advanced cancers of the hypopharynx and larynx. They show 3-year survival rates of 46% for T_3 glottic cancers and 20% for T_4 glottic cancers. They noted that a similar group of patients treated at the Massachusetts General Hospital with primary radiotherapy and surgery held in reserve for salvage had a 3-year survival of 57%. KIRCHNER and OWEN (1977) found a 3-year NED survival of 72% for T_3 glottic lesions treated with surgery alone.

KAZEM et al. (1982) describe a series of 110 patients with advanced laryngeal cancer of whom 26 had lesions originating in the glottis, who were treated with 2500 cGy preoperative irradiation given in 500 cGy fractions over a 5 day period. Surgery was performed 2 days later. The 5-year survival of this subgroup of patients was approximately 70%. The short time interval between the completion of the radiation and the surgery does not allow for repopulation of the tumor cells but also does not allow for significant tumor shrinkage due to the radiation treatments. Thus this treatment regimen would not be likely to convert an inoperable lesion to an operable one. The treatment-related morbidity appeared to be minimal.

The overall pattern is somewhat confusing, but if the required surgical procedure is a total laryngectomy, it seems reasonable to attempt a curative course of radiotherapy and hold surgery in reserve as a salvage for T_3 lesions while a combined approach seems the better choice for the more advanced T_4 lesions that are still operable.

10.7 Transglottic Tumors

10.7.1 General Considerations

The term "transglottic carcinoma" was first used by McGavran et al. (1961) to describe tumors that cross the laryngeal ventricle to involve both the true and false cords. Hence, their specific site of origin is uncertain. These lesions typically spread in the paraglottic space and tend to be difficult to accurately stage. The use of CT and/or NMR scans may help in this regard. The more advanced stages tend to spread outside the larynx.

Lymph node metastases are fairly common – particularly for the more advanced stages. Mittal et al. (1984) reviewed a series of 152 patients with transglottic lesions. The incidence of positive nodes showed a clear association with T-stage. It was 15% for T_2 lesions, 25% for T_3 lesions, and 40% for T_4 lesions. A total of 53 patients in the series had N_0 necks and did not have either a neck dissection or radiotherapy to the neck. The overall incidence of subsequent failure in the neck was 19% – 13% in the ipsilateral neck and 6% in the contralateral neck. Thus it appears that this lesion behaves more like a supraglottic lesion in its propensity to metastasize to the lymph nodes.

10.7.2 Treatment Considerations

Kirchner and Owen (1977) report on 61 patients with transglottic tumors who were primarily treated with surgery (total laryngectomy) with or without adjuvant radiotherapy. A total of 25/61 (41%) exhibited local tumor control at times greater than 3 years post treatment. A total of 12/61 failed at the primary site alone and 18/61 had distant metastases (with or without failures at the primary site). Three patients were treated with radiation alone and all were local failures.

Mittal et al. (1984) discuss several treatment procedures for their series of patients. Patients with early lesions were treated with voice conserving surgery with or without a neck dissection. Thirty patients fell into this category. Patients with advanced lesions generally were treated with a total laryngectomy with or without a neck dissection. Ninety-eight patients fell into this category. Twenty four patients who were either inoperative for medical reasons or refused surgery were treated with radiation alone. This group thus included patients with early and advanced lesions. Low dose preoperative irradiation was used in 93 of 128 patients treated primarily with surgery. As with other head and neck cancers, 90% of the patients exhibiting a local/regional failure did so within the first two years after treatment. However, about ⅓ of the distant metastases (22/152) occurred after 2 years post therapy. The local/regional control rate was 74% for the patients treated with voice conserving surgery, and 67% for patients treated with definitive radiotherapy. The local/regional control rate was thus somewhat higher in the subgroup of patients treated with more radical surgery although the difference probably would not have been significant even if the study were randomized. After salvage procedures, the ultimate local/regional control rate was 75% in the total laryngectomy subgroup, 80% in the voice-conserving surgery subgroup and 88% in the definitive radiotherapy subgroup. However, the survival was markedly different in the three subgroups which probably reflects patient selection biases more than treatment effectiveness. At two years patient survival was 70% in the total laryngectomy subgroup, 85% in the voice-conserving surgery subgroup, and only 40% in the definitive radiotherapy subgroup. The overall incidence of successful voice preservation was 60% for the voice-conserving surgery subgroup and 67% for the definitive radiotherapy subgroup. The incidence of significant major complications was 10% in the total laryngectomy subgroup, 47% in the voice-conserving surgery subgroup and 17% in the definitive radiotherapy subgroup.

It thus appears reasonable to treat patients with smaller transglottic lesions – T_2 or T_3 – with either voice-conserving surgery or definitive radiotherapy and hold a total laryngectomy in reserve as a salvage procedure. Radiation fields and doses should be as discussed for supraglottic lesions.

10.8 Subglottic Tumors

10.8.1 Regional Lymphatics

Tumors arising in the subglottic larynx can spread to the upper paratracheal nodes as well as to the nodes in the cervical chain. The overall incidence of clinically positive nodes at the time of presentation is approximately 10-20%. The incidence of positive nodes tends to be higher for the more advanced lesions which have breached the thyroid cartilage and extended into the soft tissues of the neck. Radiation treatment fields must be designed to cover the nodes at risk in either a definitive or an adjuvant form of radiation treatment. In general, this means "covering" the upper mediastinal nodes via a "T" field as shown in Fig. 10-5b.

10.8.2 Treatment Considerations

Many subglottic tumors are quite advanced at the time of presentation and so in reality may simply be glottic tumors with subglottic extension. The principles of treatment are, nevertheless, the same. The numbers of patients in reported series tends to be small and therefore it is difficult to compare the results of alternative forms of therapy.

Early forms of treatment were primarily surgical. NORRIS (1969) reports on a series of 50 patients with N_0 tumors treated by a total laryngectomy but without an associated neck dissection. His cure rate was 66%. For a group of 15 patients with N_0 tumors treated by a total laryngectomy with an accompanying neck dissection, the cure rate was 73%. However, in another surgical series of 5 patients SESSIONS et al. (1975) found a survival rate at 5 years of only 20%.

VERMUND (1970) reports on a large series of patients with subglottic tumors. The 5-year survival in a group treated with primary radiotherapy was 36% (46/127) while for a group treated primarily with surgery it was 42% (24/58).

It certainly appears reasonable to utilize primary radiotherapy with surgery held in reserve as a salvage procedure for early T_1 or T_2 lesions and to reserve a laryngectomy for the larger lesions with either destruction of the thyroid or cricoid cartilage and/or vocal cord fixation. Postoperative irradiation is generally in order and it is important to adequately irradiate the tracheal stoma as discussed in the following section.

10.9 Irradiation of the Tracheal Stoma

10.9.1 Background

Many surgical procedures for carcinoma of the larynx involve the creation of a tracheal stoma. This is an area oftentimes at significant risk for tumor recurrence. Once a stomal recurrence is clinically evident, the prognosis is very grave in spite of aggressive treatment.

SISSON et al. (1975) have devised a surgical technique for treating a recurrence by extending the dis-

Table 10-8. High risk factors for a tracheal stomal recurrence. (After TONG et al. 1977)

Extensive primary lesion (T_3 or T_4)
Subglottic tumor extension
Preliminary emergency tracheostomy for airway obstruction
Inadequate tumor margins on the pathological specimen
Tumor involvement of the paratracheal lymphatics
Large, fixed nodes or multiple involved cervical nodes
Perineural or venous invasion by tumor

---

section into the upper mediastinum. The tracheal aperture is relocated to a position in the upper chest wall. They report on a series of 28 patients of whom 14 required more than one operative procedure. Only 48% of the 27 patients at risk for one year were still alive and 8 had died within the first 2 months after the last surgery. The 5-year survival was 17%.

Radiotherapy for a stomal recurrence does not produce better results. GUNN (1965) reports on a series of 12 patients treated with radiotherapy. All had palliation of local pain and/or bleeding but no survival data is given. SCHNEIDER et al. (1975) noted only 2/31 (6%) of patients receiving radiotherapy for stomal recurrences were alive at 2 years.

With these poor salvage results it is clearly better to prevent the recurrence in the first place. Various authors have attempted to identify the high risk factors for a stomal recurrence. These are nicely discussed in a paper by TONG et al. (1977) and are summarized in Table 10-8. If any of these factors are present, then the tracheal stoma should be irradiated as part of the overall plan of medical management.

10.9.2 Treatment Considerations

If high risk patients are to receive preoperative radiotherapy, then the radiation fields should encompass the stomal site and 5000 cGy delivered to this region. A midline shielding block should not be used on the anterior lower neck field. Similar considerations hold for patients treated postoperatively. It is usually not necessary to bolus the stomal site if either ^{60}Co, 4 MeV x-rays, or 6 MeV x-rays are used since a brisk local reaction usually develops without bolus. If higher energy x-ray sources are used, then consideration should be given to bolusing the site every other treatment. Although the stomal reactions may cause the patient considerable discomfort, they are temporary and are not life-threatening. The tradeoff is reasonable, given the ominous prognosis of a frank recurrence.

If a stomal recurrence develops in an unirradiated patient, Tong et al. (1977) recommend treating more than the palpable mass plus a small margin because their experience indicated the high probability of subsequent metastases developing in the upper cervical and/or mediastinal nodes. They recommend treating the upper cervical nodes, supraclavicular region, and upper mediastinum to 5000 cGy at a 3 cm depth using an extended version of the "T" field shown in Fig. 10-5b. Then an additional 1500 cGy is given to the initially palpable mass plus a 1-2 cm margin using an electron beam. While there is no definite evidence that this procedure improves survival, it is a reasonable approach.

If a stomal recurrence develops in a previously irradiated field, then low to moderate doses of local radiation may be effective in palliating symptoms but it is doubtful that this will be of much survival benefit.

10.10 Tracheal Carcinoma

Primary carcinoma of the trachea is an extremely rare entity. In most centers it is treated primarily by surgery with radiotherapy given in an adjuvant setting. However, most of the early reports on the "ineffectiveness" of primary radiotherapy for this tumor date back to the orthovoltage era and both the poor local control results and excessive treatment related morbidity may be due to the use of equipment that would be inadequate by today's standards. Also, 3-dimensional treatment planning techniques coupled with CT scanning information make it possible to now deliver reasonably high doses of radiation to selected regions of the mediastinum.

Rostom and Morgan (1978) describe a series of 19 patients treated with radiation doses between 5000-7000 cGy. Eight of these were either disease free at last followup or died free of disease. However, no local control was achieved for patients whose tumor extended beyond the trachea. Birt (1970) controlled tumors less than 3.5 cm in diameter in 2 of 3 patients who received 6500 cGy but was not able to control the tumor in 11 patients with lesions greater than 4 cm in diameter. Green et al. (1985) were able to sterilize the tumors in 3/3 patients with doses of 5000-7000 cGy. All three lesions were less than 3.5 cm in diameter.

However, the treatment morbidity still remains appreciable if doses in excess of 6500 cGy are used.

Two patients treated by Green et al. (1985) had upper tracheal lesions and after receiving 7000 cGy, developed esophageal strictures, bilateral vocal cord paresis, and tracheal stenosis. No complications were reported by Birt (1970) and the complication rate reported by Rostom and Morgan (1978) was only 3/44. Hence, it appears reasonable to use 6500 cGy to treat patients with small tracheal lesions in lieu of surgery. The larger lesions should still be primarily managed with surgery unless there are medical contra-indications.

10.11 Dose Response and Treatment Morbidity

10.11.1 General Considerations

There is a general feeling in the radiotherapy community that any tumor can be sterilized if only sufficient radiation doses could be given. The problem is that normal tissue side effects limit this dose. Above a given level, treatment morbidity outweighs any presumed benefit to improved tumor control. Moreover, even within the dose range that can be given with acceptable morbidity, there is some evidence that above a certain dose there is little benefit to increasing the amount of radiation given for a given stage of tumor. This data is very site-specific and will be summarized for laryngeal tumors in the following sections. The analyses are generally based upon the Ellis NSD formulation (Ellis 1967). This is admittedly fraught with errors but nevertheless is a schema for comparing different treatment regimens. As a point of general reference the reader should note that a "typical" conventionally-fractionated treatment of 180 cGy/fraction 5-days-a-week to 7020 cGy corresponds to about 1850 ret using the Ellis formula.

10.11.2 Primary Sites

Ghossein et al. (1974) used Ellis's NSD approach to analyze the doses given to 203 patients with tumors of the supraglottic larynx treated at the Curie Institute with ^{60}Co irradiation $\pm$ an electron beam. They found a dose response curve for T_1 and T_2 lesions but not for T_3 and T_4 lesions. Approximately 90% of T_1 and T_2 lesions were controlled if more than 2300 rets were given. This corresponded to 7700 cGy given in 6 weeks with treatments being given 6 days-a-week. The overall incidence of major complications (either death or a tracheostomy required) was approximately 7% and did not increase for patient groups receiving more than 2300 rets compared with patient groups receiving 2100–2300 rets. The apparent lack of a dose response curve for the larger tumors was attributed to associated features such as inflammation, necrosis, and connective tissue reaction. By these features the authors may have meant "an increased hypoxic cell population" which is a reasonable hypothesis in light of current radiobiological knowledge.

KARIM et al. (1978) analyzed 119 consecutive patients with glottic carcinomas who were treated at the Free University in Amsterdam from 1965 through 1974. From 1965–1969 the policy was to deliver a "short course" of orthovoltage radiation consisting of 5500 cGy in 4 weeks. Thirty-one patients were treated in this manner. In 1970 the same orthovoltage equipment was used but the 5500 cGy was given in 30 fractions over a 6 week period and a total of 52 patients were treated. From 1971–1974, a 4 MeV linear accelerator was used and 36 patients treated to 6600–7400 cGy using 200 cGy daily fractions. The relative biological effectiveness (RBE) of megavoltage x-rays to orthovoltage x-rays was taken to be 0.85 and the Ellis NSD formula used to compare the three dose schedules. For T_1 tumors no dose response curve was found. For T_2 tumors a rather steep dose response curve was found with approximately 2000 rets needed for a 75% local control rate. Two of the patients treated with orthovoltage radiation had thyroid cartilage necrosis and 8 patients had severe laryngeal edema with one of these requiring surgery. No such problems occurred in the patients treated with megavoltage radiation.

HARWOOD and TIERIE (1979) compared patients with early glottic tumors treated at the Princess Margaret Hospital in Toronto with a similar group of patients treated at the Antoni van Leeuwenhook hospital in Amsterdam. For T_1 lesions the dose-response curve was essentially flat from 1700–2100 rets but there was a sharp increase in the incidence of major complications when more than 2050 rets were given. A total of 14/202 patients had major complications consisting of necrosis of the laryngeal tissues (10 cases), laryngeal edema requiring a tracheotomy (3 cases), and severe arytenoid edema (1 case). Four patients died of these complications.

OLSZEWSKI et al. (1985) reviewed 137 patients with T_1 glottic tumors treated with megavoltage radiation between 1966–1980. Some patients were treated with 180 cGy fractions for 5 days-a-week while some patients were treated with 225 cGy frac-

tions for 4 days-a-week. The patients were not randomized but were treated according to individual physician preference. The Ellis NSD formulation was used to analyze the data. No dose response curve was found out to 1950 rets.

HARWOOD et al. (1981) reviewed 110 patients at the Princess Margaret Hospital for T_3 N_0 M_0 glottic carcinomas. The logrank method was used to analyze the various prognostic factors. Radiation dose had a great effect on the adjusted *relative* recurrence rate. This ranged from 1.59 for doses less than or equal to 1675 ret, to 0.99 for doses between 1675–1699 ret, to approximately 0.80 for doses between 1700–1750 ret, and to 0.61 for doses greater than or equal to 1750 rets. Approximately ⅔ of the radiation failures were successfully salvaged with surgery. Radiation field size within the range of 25–100 cm² was not found to be an important factor affecting local/regional recurrence.

Similar analyses were carried out for a group of 244 patients with T_2 N_0 M_0 lesions (HARWOOD et al. 1981) and for a group of 56 patients with T_4 N_0 M_0 lesions (HARWOOD et al. 1981). For the T_2 lesions a local control rate of 53% was obtained for a NSD of less than 1650 ret was used compared with a local control rate of 81% for doses between 1650–1699 ret. Improved local control occurred for both normal cord mobility and impaired cord mobility subgroups. An increase in field size from less than 36 cm² to more than 36 cm² improved local control from 57% to 70%, thus indicating the importance of adequate tumor margins. For the T_4 lesions the local control rate was 42% for patients receiving less than 1700 ret compared with 82% for patients receiving doses greater than 1700 ret. Patients who were classified as T_4 on the basis of thyroid cartilage destruction had a local control rate of 67% compared to 19% in a subgroup of patients with piriform sinus involvement.

Analysis of 410 patients with various stage supraglottic cancers showed no obvious dose response curve over the range 1650–2300 ret for any stage lesion (HARWOOD et al. 1983). Field size did not greatly influence control at the primary site but did markedly affect regional control in necks that were initially N_0. Field sizes less than 49 cm² resulted in an 18% neck failure rate compared with a 3% failure rate for larger field sizes.

In a review course MARKS and SESSIONS (1985) note that the treatment related complications depend critically on the fraction size, the total dose given, and the overall time of treatment. They state that significant laryngeal edema and/or cartilage necrosis are seldom seen for doses below 1900 ret.

LOEFFLER (1974) studied the influence of daily fraction size with orthovoltage radiation. Patients were treated 5 days-a-week using one of the following treatment schedules: a) 200 R/fraction to 6000 R, b) 180 R/fraction to 6300 R, c) 170 R/fraction to 7140–7310 R, and d) 160 R/fraction to 6800 R. In group (a) *all* patients developed moderate to severe aryepiglottic edema which was either permanent or persisted for years. In group (c) only half the patients had any development of aryepiglottic edema and only in about 10% of cases was it of a long term nature. In no case did the edema persist more than 2.5 years. None of the patients in group (d) had any edema at any time. Although the patient numbers in each subgroup were small, there were no obvious differences in local control for comparably staged patients among the 4 groups. Loeffler used the Ellis NSD formulation with a conversion factor of 1 R = 0.89 cGy but could not find a correlation between this parameter and the incidence of complications. His work does show the increased morbidity that can occur when the daily dose fraction is increased.

10.11.3 Nodal Sites

SCHNEIDER et al. (1975) analyzed 344 patients with positive neck nodes from various head and neck primaries who were definitively treated with external beam irradiation. Unfortunately, only 28 of these patients had tumors originating in the supraglottic larynx but hopefully the nodal disease response is roughly site-independent for squamous cell primaries. They found a plateau in the dose-response curve for N_1 disease starting at about 6500 cGy (conventional fractionation schema) with approximately 90% of nodes being controlled with this dose. For N_2 disease there were a significant number of failures even for doses as high as 8000 cGy.

10.12 New Treatment Approaches

10.12.1 Altered Radiation Fractionation

Although there is considerable evidence that simply increasing the size of the radiation dose fraction causes increased morbidity, this argues only against a hypofractionation approach. Accelerated or hyperfractionation schemes use fraction sizes smaller than the "standard" of 180–200 cGy and either shorten or maintain the overall duration of a course of treatment by giving multiple daily treatments.

The RTOG is currently investigating a continuous treatment regimen consisting of 120 cGy fractions given twice daily with there being at least 4 hours between fractions to allow for sublethal damage repair. A randomized dose-searching study is currently in progress and the larynx will likely be a site for a future phase III clinical trial.

WANG et al. (1986) have reported on a series of 106 patients with supraglottic carcinomas who were treated with an accelerated fractionation scheme. Their program consisted of giving 160 cGy per fraction, twice-a-day, 5 days-a-week, to a total of 6400 cGy with a 2 week break in treatment after 3200 cGy. The treatment break was required in order to allow the acute mucositis reaction to resolve. WANG et al. (1986) compared the results of this form of therapy with the results for patient with similar lesions treated in previous years at their institution using a conventional fractionation scheme. If one assumes that the two patient groups were indeed comparable, then the authors claim that the results are statistically different in favor of the accelerated fractionation treatment method. For patients with T_1 and T_2 lesions at 3 years the respective local control rates were 88% and 63%. For patients with the more advanced T_3 and T_4 lesions the respective local control rates at 3 years were 66% and 33%. The authors found minimal late radiation effects and state that surgical salvage was feasible for many of the primary radiation failures. These results are intriguing but need to be tested in the context of a randomized clinical trial.

10.12.2 Adjuvant Chemotherapy

Recently there have been numerous reported trials on the use of adjuvant and neoadjuvant chemotherapy in the treatment of head and neck cancers. The current status of this approach is summarized in Chapter 16. At present there is only one ongoing major clinical trial directed at patients with advanced laryngeal tumors and this is being conducted under the auspices of the Veteran's Administration Hospital System (CSP 268). This study is designed to determine whether or not induction chemotherapy with 5-FU and cis-platinum followed by definitive radiotherapy provides an acceptable alternative to the "standard" approach of surgery followed by postoperative radiotherapy. Endpoints of the trial include local/regional control, survival, and quality of life in part measured by voice preservation of post-surgical rehabilitation. Such controlled trials are the proper approach for evaluating the potential role of new methods of cancer treatment.

References

Batsakis JG, Hybels R, Crissman JD, Rice DH (1982) The pathology of head and neck tumors: verrucous carcinoma, part 15. Head and Neck Surg 5: 29–38

Birt BD (1970) The management of malignant tracheal neoplasms. J Laryngol Otol 84: 723–731

Bauer WC (1974) Concomitant carcinoma-in-situ and invasive carcinoma of the larynx. Cand J Otolaryngol 3: 533–542

Bush RS, Jenkin RDT, Allt WEC, Beale FA, Bean H, Dembo AJ, Pringle JF (1978) Definitive evidence for hypoxic cells influencing cure in cancer therapy. Br J Cancer 37: 302–306

Constable WC, White RL, El-Mahdi AM, Fitzhugh GS (1975) Panel discussion on glottic tumors – IX. Radiotherapeutic management of cancer of the glottis, University of Virginia, 1956–1971. Laryngoscope 85: 1494–1503

Ellis F (1967) Fractionation in radiotherapy. In: Modern Trends in Radiotherapy Vol. I (Eds) Dealy, Wood. (Butterworth, London) pp 34–51

Ferlito A, Recher G (1980) Ackerman's tumor (verrucous carcinoma) of the larynx – a clinico-pathologic study of 77 cases. Cancer 46: 1617–1630

Fletcher GH, Jesse RH, Lindberg RD, Westbrook KC (1978) Neck nodes. In. Textbook of Radiotherapy, 3rd edn (Ed). Fletcher GH (Lea & Febiger Philadelphia PA) pp 249–271

Fletcher GH, Lindberg RD, Hamberger A, Horiot JC (1975) Reasons for irradiation failure in squamous cell carcinoma of the larynx. Laryngoscope 85: 987–1003

Fu KK, Woodhouse RJ, Quivey JM, Phillips TL, Dedo HH (1982) The significance of laryngeal edema following radiotherapy of the vocal cord. Cancer 49: 655–658

Ghossein NA, Bataini JP, Ennuyen A, Stacey P, Krishnaswamy V (1974) Local control and site of failure in radically irradiated supraglottic laryngeal cancer. Radiology 112: 187–192

Goepfert H, Jesse RH, Fletcher GH, Hamberger A (1975) Optimal treatment for technically resectable squamous cell carcinoma of the supraglottic larynx. Laryngoscope 85: 14–32

Goldman J, Silverstone S, Roffman J, Birken E (1972) High dose preoperative radiation and surgery for carcinoma of the larynx and laryngopharynx, a 14 year program. Laryngoscope 82: 1869–1882

Green N, Kulber H, Landman M, Pierce M (1985) The experience with definitive irradiation of clinically limited squamous cell cancer of the trachea. Int J Radiat Oncol Biol Phys 11: 1401–1405

Griffin TW, Pajak TF, Gillespie BW, Davis LW, Brady LW, Rubin P, Marcial VA (1984) Predicting the response of head and neck cancers to radiation therapy with a multivariate modelling system: an analysis of the RTOG head and neck registry. Int J Radiat Oncol Biol Phys 10: 481–487

Gunn WG (1965) Treatment of cancer recurrent at the tracheostome. Cancer 18: 1261–1264

Harwood AR, Beale FA, Cummings BJ, Keane TJ, Payne D,

Rider WD (1985) T_4 N_0 M_0 glottic cancer: an analysis of dose-time-volume factors. Int J Radiat Oncol Biol Phys 7: 1507–1512

Harwood AR, Beale FA, Cummings BJ, Keane TJ, Payne DG, Rider WD, Rawlinson E, Elhakim T (1983) Supraglottic laryngeal carcinoma: an analysis of dose-time-volume factors in 410 patients. Int J Radiat Oncol Biol Phys 9: 311–319

Harwood AR, Beale FA, Cummings BJ, Keane TJ, Rider WD (1981) T_2 glottic cancer: an analysis of dose-time-volume factors. Int J Radiat Oncol Biol Phys 7: 1501–1505

Harwood AR, DeBoer G (1980) Prognostic factors in T_2 glottic cancer. Cancer 45: 991–995

Harwood AR, Denboer G, Kazim F (1981) Prognostic factors in T_3 glottic cancer. Cancer 47: 367–372

Harwood AR, Hawkins NV, Rider WD, Bryce DP (1979) Radiotherapy of early glottic cancer I. Int J Radiat Oncol Biol Phys 5: 473–476

Harwood AR, Tierie A (1979) Radiotherapy of early glottic cancer II. Int J Radiat Oncol Biol Phys 5: 477–482

Horiot JC, Fletcher GH, Ballantyne AJ, Lidberg RD (1972) Analysis of failures in early vocal cord cancers. Radiology 103: 663–665

Kagan AR, Calcaterra T, Ward P, Chan P (1974) Significance of edema of the endolarynx following curative irradiation for carcinoma. Amer J Roentgen 120: 169–172

Karim ABMF, Snow GB, Hasman A, Chang SC, Kelhotz A, Hoekstra F (1978) Dose response in radiotherapy for glottic carcinoma. Cancer 41: 1728–1732

Kazem I, Van den Broek P, Huygen PLM (1982) Planned preoperative radiation therapy for advanced laryngeal carcinoma. Int J Radiat Oncol Biol Phys 8: 1533–1537

Kirchner JA, Owen JR (1977) Five hundred cancers of the larynx and piriform sinus: results of treatment by radiation and surgery. Laryngoscope 87: 1288–1303

Kramer S (1985) Combined surgery and radiation therapy in the management of locally advanced squamous cell carcinomas. In: Head and Neck Cancer, Vol. I, (Eds) Chreitien PM, Johns ME, Shedd DP, Strong EW, Ward PH (B.C. Decker, Inc., Philadelphia) pp 48–54

Kramer S, Gelber RD, Snow JB, Marcial VA, Lowry LD, Davis LW, Chandler R (1987) Combined radiation therapy and surgery in the management of advanced head and neck cancer: final report of study 73-03 of the Radiation Therapy Oncology Group. Head & Neck Surg 10: 19–30

Lederman M (1970) Radiotherapy of cancer of the larynx. J Laryngol and Otolaryngol 84: 867–896

Lindberg RD, Fletcher GH (1978) The role of irradiation in the management of head and neck cancer: analysis of results and causes of failure. Tumor 64: 313–325

Loeffler RK (1974) Influence of fractionation on acute and late reactions in vocal cord carcinoma. Am J Roentgen 121: 748–753

Marks JE, Breaux S, Smith PG, Thawley SE, Spector GG, Sessions DG (1985) The need for elective irradiation of occult lymphatic metastases from cancers of the larynx and piriform sinus. Head & Neck Surg 8: 3–8

Marks JE, Freeman RB, Lee F, Ogura JH (1979) Carcinoma of the supraglottic larynx AJR 132: 255–260

Marks JE, Sessions DG (1985) Carcinoma of the larynx – ASTRO Refresher Course (unpublished)

McGavran MH, Bauer WC, Ogura JH (1961) The incidence of cervical lymph node metastases from epidermoid carcinoma of the larynx and their relationship to certain characteristics of the primary tumor. Cancer 14: 55–66

Million RR, Cassisi NJ, Wittes RE (1982) Cancer in the head

and neck. In: Cancer – Principles and Practice of Oncology. (Eds) Devita VT, Hellman S, Rosenberg SA (Lippincott, Philadelphia 1982) pp 301–395

Mills EED (1979) Early glottic carcinoma: factors affecting radiation failure, results of treatment and squelae. Int J Radiat Oncol Biol Phys 5: 811–817

Mirimanoff RO, Wang CC, Doppke KP (1985) Combined surgery and postoperative radiotherapy for advanced laryngeal and hypopharyngeal tumors. Int J Radiat Oncol Biol Phys 11: 499–504

Mittal B, Marks JE, Ogura JH (1984) Transglottic carcinoma. Cancer 53: 151–161

Nass JM, Brady LW, Glassburn JR, Prasasvinichai S, Schatanoff D (1976) Radiation therapy of glottic carcinoma. Int J Radiat Oncol Biol Phys 1: 867–872

Norris CM (1969) Laryngectomy and neck dissection. Otolaryngol Clin N Am 69: 667–683

Ogura J, Biller H (1970) Preoperative irradiation for laryngeal and laryngopharyngeal cancers. Laryngoscope 80: 802–810

Olszewski SJ, Vaith JM, Green JP, Schroeder AF, Chauser B (1985) The influence of field size, treatment modality, commissure involvement and histology in the treatment of early vocal cord cancer with radiation. Int J Radiat Oncol Biol Phys 11: 1333–1337

Pene F, Fletcher GH (1976) Results in irradiation of the in situ carcinomas of the vocal cords. Cancer 37: 2586–2590

Rostom AY, Morgan RL (1978) Results of treating primary tumors of the trachea by irradiation. Thorax 33: 387–393

Schneider JJ, Fletcher GH, Barkely (1975) Control by irradiation alone of nonfixed clinically positive nodes from squamous cell carcinoma of the oral cavity, oropharynx, supraglottic larynx, and hypopharynx. Amer J Radiol 123: 42–48

Schneider JJ, Lindberg RD, Jesse RH (1975) Prevention of tracheal stoma recurrences after total laryngectomy by postoperative irradiation. J Surg Oncol 7: 187–190

Schwade JG, Wara WM, Dedo HH, Phillips TL (1976) Radiotherapy for verrucous carcinoma. Radiology 120: 677–679

Sessions DG, Ogura JH, Fried MP (1975) Carcinoma of the subglottic area. Laryngoscope 85: 1417–1423

Shaw HJ (1965) Glottic cancer of the larynx 1947–1956. J Laryngol and Otolaryngol 79: 1–14

Silverberg E, Lubera J (1987) Cancer Statistics, 1987. Ca – A Cancer Journal for Clinicians 37: 2–19

Sisson GA, Bytell DE, Edison BD, Yeh Jr S (1975) Transsternal radical neck dissection for control of stomal recurrences – end results. Laryngoscope 85: 1504–1510

Tong D, Moss WT, Stevens KR (1977) Elective irradiation of the lower cervical region in patients at high risk for recurrent cancer at the tracheal stoma. Radiology 124: 809–811

Van den Bogaert W, Ostyn F, Van Der Schueren E (1983) The significance of extension and impaired mobility in cancer of the vocal cord. Int J Radiat Oncol Biol Phys 9: 181–184

Vermund H (1970) Role of radiotherapy in cancer of the larynx as related to the TNM system of staging. Cancer 25: 485–504

Wang CC (1973) Megavoltage radiation therapy for supraglottic carcinoma: results of treatment. Radiology 109: 183–186

Wang CC, Schulz MD, Miller D (1972) Combined radiation therapy and surgery for carcinoma of the supraglottis and piriform sinus. Amer J Surgery 124: 551–554

Wang CC (1983) Radiation Therapy for Head and Neck Neoplasms. John Wright, Littleton, MA. Chapt. 11, pp 165–199

Wang CC, Suit HD, Phil D, Blitzer PH (1986) Twice-a-day radiation therapy for supraglottic carcinoma. Int J Radiat Oncol Biol Phys 12: 3–7

Wynder EL, Covey LS, Mauchi K, Mushinski M (1976) Environmental factors in cancer of the larynx – a second look. Cancer 38: 1591–1601

Wynder EL, Mushinski MH, Spivak JC (1977) Tobacco and alcohol consumption in relation to the development of multiple primary cancers. Cancer 40: 1872–1878

11 Nasal Vestibule, Nasal Cavity, and Paranasal Sinuses

Toby S. Kramer

CONTENTS

Toby S. Kramer, M.D., Assistant Professor of Therapeutic Radiology, Department of Therapeutic Radiology Rush Presbyterian St. Luke's Medical Center, 1653 West Congress Parkway Chicago, IL, 60612, USA

11.1 Introduction

Malignant disease of the nose and sinuses accounts for only a small proportion of human cancers. The challenge to the managing physician on the other hand is usually greater than that presented by cancer in many other sites. The advanced stage of disease at presentation and the proximity of critical normal structures mandates a high degree of technical competence in order to produce acceptable results. An interdisciplinary approach is necessary to insure optimal diagnosis, staging, therapy and rehabilitation. The spectrum of malignancies encountered in this region is broad, further confusing the principles of management. In this chapter, major emphasis is placed on the therapy of epithelial neoplasms arising from the mucosal lining of the nasal chambers. Salient features of non-epithelial tumors are mentioned separately where appropriate.

11.2 Nasal Vestibule

11.2.1 Anatomy (See Figures 11-1 and 11-2)

The most anterior portion of each nasal cavity is termed the vestibule. This is a pear-shaped space extending from the nares anteriorly to the limen nasi posteriorly, a distance of about 2 cm. The limen nasi is a crescent shaped infolding of tissue from the lateral wall which demarcates the mucocutaneous junction. There is no anatomic boundary medially or inferiorly between the vestibule and the main body of the nasal cavity.

The vestibule is lined by skin-containing hair follicles and sebaceous glands. The skin overlies a bony and cartilagenous frame work which supports its shape. The lateral wall is formed by the lateral crus of the greater alar cartilage. Medially, the septal cartilage and the medial crus of the greater alar cartilage give support. These medial cartilages are attached to the columella by a fibrous ligament, the

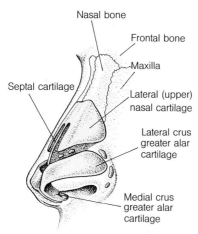

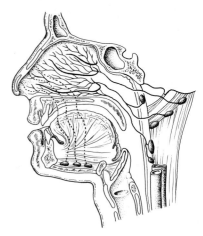

Fig. 11-1. External nasal cartilages. These cartilages and the nasal bones form the support of the nasal vestibule

Fig. 11-3. Lymphatic drainage of the nose and sinuses. Note that the superior nasal cavity drains to deep lymph nodes along the base of the skull and to the pre-auricular region. The anterior, inferior nasal cavity drains to the retropharyngeal and high anterior cervical chains. The vestibule lymphatics *(dotted lines)* end in the submandibular and submental lymph nodes

membranous septum. The vestibular floor overlies the nasal process of the maxilla.

Lymphatic drainage is primarily to the submandibular lymph nodes by way of the facial node (which lies on the buccinator muscle at the level of the oral commissure) (MENDENHALL et al. 1984; GOEPFERT et al. 1974). The submental, preauricular and cervical chain are stations infrequently involved by metastatic tumor (see Figure 11-3). Drainage of the vestibule is continuous with that of the external nose and upper lip and can therefore cause bilateral metastases (GOEPFERT et al. 1974).

The incidence of node involvement by vestibular tumors is considered in section 11.2.4.

11.2.2 Epidemiology

Malignancies in the nasal vestibule are rare. Since tumors arising in this location are generally grouped with the larger category of nasal cavity cancer, the exact incidence in the vestibule is hard to assess. Within the broad category of nasal cavity tumors, 50% arise on the turbinates and the remainder are divided amongst the septum, vestibule, posterior choanae, and the floor in order of decreasing frequency. In seven reported series limited to the vestibule, it took, on the average, 15 years to accumulate 27 cases.

Most document a white male predominance (GOEPFERT et al. 1974; SCHAEFER and HILL 1980; MAK et al. 1979). A smaller number of series show male to female ratios of only 2 or 3 to 1 (MENDENHALL et al. 1984; WANG 1976). The median age at presentation is about 60 years. There is no report of a patient younger than 40 with this condition. There is no known relationship to any environmental carcinogens.

Tobacco usage is very common in these patients (CHASSAGNE and WILSON 1974). All patients in the series of SCHAEFER and HILL (1980) had a history of moderate to heavy cigarette smoking. There is a high risk for developing a second malignant process. In the report of MAK et al. (1979) 5 of 32

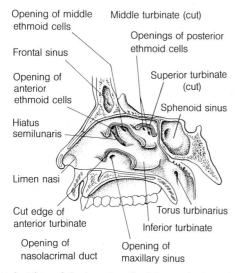

Fig. 11-2. View of the lateral wall of the vestibule and nasal cavity with the superior and middle turbinates removed. The inferior turbinate has been cut to reveal the opening of the nasolacrimal duct. The openings to the other paranasal sinuses are also depicted

patients had a second cancer at some time during their course.

11.2.3 Pathology

The malignant neoplasms arising in the nasal vestibule are squamous cell carcinomas, other histologies being exceedingly rare. Tumors are most often well to moderately well diferentiated. HAYNES and TAPLEY's series (1973) consisted of 4 Grade I, 11 Grade II, and 3 Grade III patients (4 patients ungraded).

The degree of differentiation is related to the risk of recurrence as indicated by the experiences of MAK et al. (1979). Recurrence-free survival at 40 months was 83% for well differentiated tumors as opposed to 20% for Grade II and III malignancies. Although there is no data relating patterns of failure to differentiation, at least two groups recommend elective neck irradiation for patients with highly undifferentiated lesions, implying a high risk of nodal metastases (HAYNES and TAPLEY 1973; MENDENHALL et al. 1984).

11.2.4 Natural History

Tumors begin in the mucosa of the vestibule and spread by direct invasion into contiguous structures. Invasion of the septal or alar cartilages is common. Penetration through the septum can produce perforation. Occasionally the tumor will grow through the cartilaginous skeleton and involve the skin on the surface of the nose. Invasion posteriorly into the nasal cavity may cause confusion as to the exact site of origin of the tumor. Bulky lesions filling the vestibule can cause the same problem. Inferior invasion to involve the columella, membranous septum and upper lip is a frequent pathway of spread. Bone invasion is a late finding usually associated with tumors involving the floor of the vestibule. Lymph node involvement (Table 11-1) at the

time of presentation is seen in 0–10% of cases. Another 10–20% will develop nodes at some time during their course of treatment or follow-up. Most clinicians do not add any regional therapy for patients presenting with N_O disease. Factors associated with a high risk of occult involvement of regional nodes include 1) invasion of the upper lip 2) invasion of the skin of the nasal dorsum 3) multiple site involvement within the vestibule and possibly 4) poorly differentiated histologies. In the report by MAK et al. (1979) 5 patients with local failures also developed nodal metastases suggesting an increased risk with recurrent disease. Distant metastases are reported in a small number of patients in most series, the incidence is 10% (MENDENHALL et al. 1984; WANG 1976).

11.2.5 Diagnosis

Most patients give a history of a persistant nodule in one side of their nose anteriorly. Often this had been considered an inflammatory process by the physician before the true neoplastic nature became evident by progression. GOEPFERT et al. (1974) describe a case where the patient presented with a neck mass and the primary in the vestibule was found only by careful head and neck exam. Physical exam should be oriented toward defining sites of local spread, and neck node status.

Biopsy through the external nares is diagnostic. Posterior and inferior invasion might require tomography to rule out bone involvement. Otherwise, a chest X-ray represents the radiographic work-up.

No formal staging system enjoys widespread use (Table 11-2). WANG proposed a system based on the extent of spread and invasion of tissues. GOEPFERT et al. (1974) and SCHAEFER and HILL (1980) divide cases into those with disease localized to one site within the vestibule and those with multi-site involvement. MENDENHALL et al. (1984) reported results as categorized by the American Joint Committee staging for skin cancer. Each of these sytems

Table 11-1. Lymphatic metastases from carcinomas of the nasal vestibule

Series	Number of cases	Positive nodes at presentation	Lymph node failures	Primary lesion controlled
1. MENDENHALL et al. 1984	13	1 (8%)	2 (16%)	2/2
2. HAYNES and TAPLEY 1973	22	0	5 (23%)	3/5
3. GEOPFERT et al. 1974	26	1 (4%)	8 (31%)	7/8
4. WANG 1976	36	5 (14%)	3 (8%)	?
5. SCHAEFER and HILL 1980	12	2 (17%)	2 (17%)	?
6. MAK et al. 1979	46	4 (9%)	5 (11%)	0/5

Table 11-2. Staging systems for carcinoma of the nasal vestibule

WANG 1976	MENDENHALL et al. 1984	GEOPFERT et al. 1974	SCHAEFER and HILL 1980
T_1: The lesion is limited to the nasal vestibule, relatively superficial, involving one or more sites within	T_1: Tumor ≥ 2 cm in largest dimension, strictly superficial or exophytic	Localized to site of origin	Localized to site of origin
T_2: The lesion has extended from the nasal vestibule to its adjacent structures, such as the upper nasal septum, upper lip, philtrum, skin of the nose and/or nasolabial fold, but not fixed to the underlying bone	T_2: >2 cm but ≤ 5 cm in largest dimension or minimal infiltration of dermis regardless of size	Extension to floor, base of columella or upper lip	Involvement of more than one site
T_3: The lesion has become massive with extension to the hard plate, buccogingival sulcus, large portion of the upper lip, upper nasal septum, turbinate and/or adjacent paranasal sinuses, fixed with deep muscle and bone involvement	T_3: >5 cm or deep infiltration of dermis irrespective of size		
	T_4: Tumor involving other structures such as cartilage, muscle, or bone		

correlates with prognosis and yet major inconsistancies are present. A small nodule involving the vestibular septum would be T_1 according to WANG and yet T_4 if it involved cartilage according to AJC. Likewise, a 3 cm lesion involving the septum and floor of the vestibule would be T_1 by WANG, T_2 by AJC and in the high risk, multi-site category of SCHAEFER and HILL.

11.2.6 Therapy

11.2.6.1 General Comments

Most authors agree; that as single modalities, surgery and radiation are equally effective in controlling the primary lesion (MENDENHALL et al. 1984; GOEPFERT et al. 1974; WANG 1976). Consideration of the expected cosmetic result will probably weigh most heavily in the choice of therapy for early tumors. If surgical excision with adequate margins is likely to produce deformity, then radiation therapy is the appropriate modality. On the other hand, the dryness and crusting that follow radiation therapy can be avoided by use of surgical excision and reconstruction with good cosmetic results in early lesiosn of the septum and lateral wall. Each form of treatment will have advantages in individual cases.

11.2.6.2 Surgery

The utility of surgery is impaired by the need to obtain generous margins around the known extent of tumor. A 1 cm cuff of normal mucosa is recommended as a minimum (LELIEVER et al. 1984). Immediate reconstruction generally requires a split thickness skin graft or rotation of a flap. Involvement of the columella or upper lip pose serious reconstructive challenges. Considering these limitations, surgery would seem most applicable to small primaries involving the vestibular septum or the alar wall.

With larger lesions, control of the cancer takes precedence over the cosmetic outcome. Most clinicians would combine total rhinectomy and radiation for advanced tumors with cartilage and/or bone involvement. The optimal sequence for combining modalities has not been established. The use of a prosthesis will allow more immediate post-operative radiation therapy than would a major reconstruction done at resection.

Another role of surgery is in the management of massive neck disease. Radical neck disection on the side of gross involvement should be combined with radiation to both sides of the neck. Finally, surgery is the treatment of choice for post-radiation recurrences. SCHAEFER and HILL (1980) recommend aggressive surgery and post-operative radiation therapy when the cancer involves more than one site within the vestibule. For operable T_3 lesions, WANG (1976) advocates pre-operative radiation.

11.2.6.3 Radiation Therapy

Due to the anatomy of the nose, small lesions of the vestibule are particularly well suited for radiation by means of interstitial implants. The geometric arrangement of needles or catheters is individualized to the location and extent of disease. Small lesions of the anterior septum, columella, alar wall and upper lip can be treated in this manner. Theoretically, cartilage which has been compromised by prior surgery, infection and tumor invasion is more susceptible to damage by radiation (DEL REGATO and VUKSANOVIC 1961).

This admonition has prompted most radiotherapists to restrict interstitial therapy as the sole modality to small tumors only. Several reports however indicate that even moderate sized lesions can be effectively treated with only minimal risk to the normal cartilage (MENDENHALL et al. 1984; CHASSAGNE and WILSON 1984; HAYNES and TAPLEY 1973; WANG 1976).

Relatively small, superficial lesions confined to one side of the vestibule are suitable for intracavitary therapy. Due to the limited depth of penetration of the radiation, invasive lesions are not appropriately treated in this fashion. Suitable molds or carriers are required for accurate placement of the radiation sources.

External beam therapy with supervoltage radiation or electrons form the mainstay of treatment for more advanced lesions. For large, inoperable cancers, this is the only effective means of therapy. For limited lesions, the target volume should include the entire vestibule with wide margins. Laterally, the eyes limit the width of the field. The inferior margin should include most of the upper lip, stopping just short of the muco-cutaneous junction. The placement of the upper border is dictated by the location of the tumor within the vestibule: Low-lying and anteriorly placed lesions can be treated by ports up to the bridge of the nose. The more superiorly placed septal lesions can invade the ethmoids and the port should be extended to the level of the glabella. If the tumor extends into the nasal cavity or adjacent paranasal sinuses, the treatment volume should be similar to that used for primary lesions arising in those structures.

Another role of radiation therapy is the elective treatment of the clinically uninvolved neck under certain circumstances. WANG (1976) states that small, limited lesions present approximately a 10% incidence of nodal mets and therefore elective neck irradiation is not warranted. MENDENHALL et al. (1984) treat the ipsilateral, clinically negative neck

when the primary lesion is advanced. SCHAEFER and HILL (1980) recommend irradiation of the bilateral necks and intervening facial lymphatics when the disease involves more than one site of the vestibule. The concensus of opinion is that the small lesions suitable for brachytherapy management do not require elective neck irradiation. The high risk factors which indicate some form of therapy to the neck include massive tumors, invasion of the upper lip, multi-site involvement within the vestibule, poorly differentiated lesions and those which have recurred after a first attempt at treatment. Gross metastatic disease in the neck is a dangerous condition whether found at presentation or during the subsequent course of the disease. Most authors would recommend combined radical neck dissection with pre or post operative irradiation.

Dose is dictated by the amount of tumor, the modality of radiation employed, and the size of the target volume. Small lesions treated by implant should receive a tumor dose of between 6000 and 7000 cGy in 144 to 168 hours (HAYNES and TAPLEY, 1973). Larger tumors treated with external beam should be given 6500 to 7000 cGy. An interstitial boost of 1000 to 2000 cGy could be considered. The neck should be given 5000 cGy when treated electively or preoperatively for gross disease. Higher doses may be given post-operatively.

11.2.7 Prognosis

Radiation and surgery produce equivalent local control rates for early lesions. CHASSAGNE and WILSON (1984) report 13 of 13 patients with T_1 and 13/14 patients with T_2 lesions locally controlled at 4 years by brachytherapy alone. HAYNES and TAPLEY (1973) had 9/9 implant cases and 4/4 intracavitary patients controlled locally at 2 years. MENDENHALL et al. (1984) controlled 4/4 cases with implant alone. As expected, larger lesions are harder to contain. Only 6 of 9 external beam treated patients were controlled by HAYNES and TAPLEY (1973).

As previously mentioned, about 1/3 of patients will have neck disease at some point in their clinical course. Control of neck disease is poor when the primary is recurrent or residual. GEOPFERT et al. (1974) controlled 9/10 involved necks by surgery alone or surgery and radiation therapy. Salvage of patients who fail only in the submandibular region is very good leading some authors to recommend no primary therapy to the uninvolved neck. WANG's (1976) 3 year disease free survival rates were 83, 71 and 50% respectively for T_1, T_2 and T_3 lesions.

In conclusion, squamous cancers of the nasal vestibule resemble skin cancer in appearance. Their behavior on the other hand is characterized by invasion of cartilage and adjacent structures along with a propensity for spread into the regional lymphatics. The results of surgery or radiation for early lesions should produce cures in 90-100% of cases. More advanced disease requires early aggressive treatment.

11.3 Nasal Cavity and Septum

11.3.1 Anatomy (See Figure 11-2)

As mentioned in the previous section, the nasal cavities are continuous with the vestibule anteriorly and with the nasopharynx through the posterior choanae. The two cavities are separated from each other by the septum. Each cavity can be divided into a superior, olfactory region and an inferior respiratory region. The special sense of smell resides in part in the chemoreceptors of the olfactory epithelium. This is a thick, pseudostratified epithelium containing sustentacular cells and bipolar neuronal cells. The respiratory mucosa is lined by a pseudostratified ciliated, columnar epithelium which is interspersed with abundant mucin producing glands. These glands produce approximately one pint of secretions each day. This mucous blanket traps dust particles and bacteria. The blanket is propelled posteriorly into the pharynx at a rate of 5 mm per minute by the coordinated action of the cilia. When tumors, surgery or radiation disrupt this orderly flow, stasis and subsequent infection is the result.

The nasal septum is composed of cartilage anteriorly and bone posteriorly. The perpendicular plate of the ethmoid forms the upper bony portition and the vomer forms the inferior portion. The maxilla and palatine bones contribute small processes inferiorly. These bones form the floor of the nasal cavity.

The lateral nasal wall bears the turbinates (also called conchae). These are scroll shaped bony processes covered with respiratory epithelium. There are usually three turbinates on each lateral wall dividing the cavity into channels termed meati. Each meatus is named after the turbinate which it lies under; i.e. the inferior meatus is the channel under the inferior turbinate. The inferior turbinate is the largest and longest. The middle turbinate is almost as

long while the superior turbinate is only one third the length of the middle. The turbinates increase the amount of nasal surface available for warming and filtering the air before it enters the lower respiratory passageways.

The roof of the cavity is formed by the cribriform plate of the ethmoid which allows tumors of this region access to the sub-arachnoid space. The nasal cavity receives drainage from the adjoining sinuses and lacrimal system. The various connections between the nasal cavity and paranasal sinuses will be elaborated in section 11.4.1 of this chapter.

The lymphatic drainage is via three main channels. 1) The superior turbinate drains to the retropharyngeal nodes. 2) The middle and lower turbinates drain to the medial, deep jugular nodes at the base of the skull. 3) The lymphatics of the floor and septum end in the anterior jugular chain in the neck.

11.3.2 Epidemiology

Tumors of the nasal cavity and septum represent approximately one third of the neoplasms arising in the sino-nasal region (Table 11-3). Given an estimated incidence of 1300 new cases of sino-nasal cancer in the United States per year (REDMOND et al. 1982), this means about 430 cases will be diagnosed nationwide. In LEWIS and CASTRO's (1971) series of 237 cases of nasal cavitiy cancer, not one arose from the septum. In contrast to this is the series by BADIB et al. (1969) in which 16 of 50 nasal cancers were located on the septum. The bulk of literature regarding septal cancers would support the view that they are extremely rare. Age and sex incidence for cavity tumors and septal tumors are similar. The average age at presentation is 60 years. The great majority of cases are seen between the fifth and eighth decades of life. The male to female ratio is 3 to 2. There is no evidence of racial predilection.

Table 11-3. Anatomic distribution of epithelial sino-nasal cancers

Reference	Nasal cavity and septum	Paranasal sinuses
LEDERMAN 1970	122	532
JACKSON et al. 1977	19	96
BOONE et al. 1968	28	93
LEWIS and CASTRO 1972	237	535
HOPKIN et al. 1984	147	414
REDMOND et al. 1982	174	185
Total	727 (28%)	1,855 (72%)

Several etiologic agents have been identified. Occupational risks are known in nickel refinery workers, boot and shoe makers and wood workers. Nickel workers stand an 800 fold increase in relative risk for developing squamous and anaplastic tumors in the nose and ethmoids as compared to the general population. The number of reported cases has already begun to fall in areas affected due to improved safeguards.

11.3.3 Pathology

The majority of neoplasms arising from the respiratory mucosa are squamous cell carcinomas and adenocarcinomas. Of the 237 cancers of the nasal cavity reported by LEWIS and CASTRO (1971) 52% were squamous and 16% adenocarcinoma. Lymphoma, melanoma and sarcomas accounted for 20% of the cases in approximately equal proportion. In a series of 85 septal cancers (BEATTY et al. 1982), 68% were squamous, 14% adeno, 8% melanoma with the remaining 10% consisting of assorted single cases of other histologies. Esthesioneuroblastoma is derived from the olfactory nerve involving the roof of the nasal cavity. The epithelial neoplasms will be described in the following sections. Esthesioneuroblastomas, melanomas, sarcomas and lymphomas will receive individual attention elsewhere in this chapter.

11.3.4 Natural History

These tumors originate from the mucosal surface. They generally reach an advanced state before causing vague symptoms such as nasal stuffiness (40% from bulky tumor obstructing the airway), facial pain and swelling (29% due to bone destruction and infection) and epistaxis (29% by erosion of small mucosal vessels) (HOPKIN et al. 1984). Even then, symptoms are often treated conservatively under an incorrect diagnosis of chronic sinusitis or nasal polyps. The average delay in diagnosis is 6 to 9 months (FRAZELL and LEWIS 1963; LEDERMAN 1970). There is early spread into the adjoining paranasal sinuses and then into adjacent soft tissue compartments ie, orbit, brain, face, base of skull and infratemporal fossa. Tumors originating in the narrow roof of the cavity have direct access into the anterior cranial fossa by way of the lymphatic drainage which passes through the cribriform plate to join the subarachnoid lymphatic vessels. Ethmoid and orbit involvement are frequently seen.

The lymphatic drainage has already been described in section 11.3.1. Frequency of nodal metastases at the time of diagnosis is from 8 to 15% (HOPKIN et al. 1984; BADIB et al. 1969; LEWIS and CASTRO 1971). The histology of the primary lesion does not particularly influence the incidence of lymph node metastases. Distant disease is found in less than 1% of cases at presentation. Metastases were present more often in non-carcinomas than in carcinomas (ROBIN and POWELL 1980). In the largest series of septal cancers, 20% of patients had synchronous or metachronous second primary cancers the majority of which were head and neck cancers. BOSCH et al. (1976) found 11/40 (28%) of nasal cavity cases with second primaries.

11.3.5 Diagnosis

The nasal cavity is subject to direct inspection through the nares anteriorly and via the posterior chonae. A fungating mass is seen in 20% of cases and an ulcerative lesion in 52% (BOSCH et al. 1976). Biopsy is the definitive diagnostic procedure. Physical examination alone is inadequate for defining the extent of disease, extensive radiographic evaluation being required for this purpose. Since the adjacent sinuses are so commonly involved, the workup is identical to that used for tumors originating in the sinuses. This will be described in detail in section 11.4.6 (diagnosis of maxillary antrum malignancies).

LEWIS and CASTRO (1971) have stated that classification is of statistical interest but is of limited value as an aid to treatment. This statement is valid in that current ability for precise localization of all tumor extensions is limited thereby necessitating treatment of the entire region regardless of staging.

There is no generally agreed upon staging system in use for this site. Several clinical classifications have been utilized. BOONE et al. (1968) divided nasal cavity tumors into a superior group arising above the superior turbinate and an inferior group below this plane. This correlates to a division between respiratory and olfactory region lesions with the subsequent ability to predict patterns of local extension. BADIB et al. (1969) proposed the following staging: T_1 less than 1 cm, limited to the mucosa; T_2 mucosal lesions 1 cm; T_3 bone or cartilage involvement; T_4 extension outside the nose. Overall survival was predicted by this system. The system with the most widespread acceptance is that of LEDERMAN (1969). This classification of tumors of the upper jaw will be described in detail in section 11.4.4.

11.3.6 Therapy

The optimal therapy for nasal fossa tumors has not been defined. Several factors are responsible for this: 1) These are rare lesions. 2) Most series have included other sites such as the paranasal sinuses or the vestibule in their analysis. 3) Most series considered epithelial as well as non-epithelial neoplasms together. 4) A wide range of therapeutic approaches have been considered together. 5) No randomized trials have been done. 6) Absence of a generally accepted staging system allowing comparison of results.

Most sources agree that surgery and radiation therapy offer equivalent results for early lesions, ie those limited to a single site in the nasal cavity without extension to adjacent sinuses or node metastases. Regardless of which agent or combination of modalities is chosen, the surgeon plays an important role. Biopsy is the first procedure and is usually performed through the nares. Exploratory procedures such as Caldwell-Luc or trans-palatal fenestration assist in staging and can provide drainage of the antrum thereby reducing radiation morbidity (CHUNG et al. 1980). These procedures can also create a cavity for the application of radium if indicated.

The surgeon can cure the patient with septal cancer if it is small enough to be excised with wide margins. BEATTY et al. (1982) recommend this as the treatment of choice. They also advocate using frozen section sampling of the surgical margins to ensure completenes of resection.

POPE (1978) has described a procedure whereby moderately advanced lesions of the lateral nasal wall may be cured. This involves the removal of the nasoantral-ethmoid complex and is suitable for lesions which are localized therein. As this approach affords excellent exposures of the septum for inspection and possible resection, it is advocated when there is question whether the lesion arises from the septum or the lateral wall.

Radiation produces equivalent results for these same small, early cancers. Treatment for anterior lesions can be accomplished with a single AP field or a heavily-wedged, anterior-oblique pair. Lesions extending posteriorly require high energy photons from anterior fields or wedged lateral fields to increase the dose posteriorly. A minimum tumor dose between 6000 and 6500 cGy is indicated. Details of

therapy are covered insection 11.5 (technique of radiation).

When dealing with advanced cancer in this region, the exact site of origin is often impossible to determine. Aggressive surgery consists of radical maxillectomy with extensions to include the ethmoids, orbit, cribriform plate, or base of skull as indicated.

Surgery can be combined with radiation given either pre- or post-operatively. Pre-op dosage is in the range of 4500 to 5000 cGy. Post-op dosage 6000 cGy with an additional 1000 cGy boost to any area of gross residual. Dosage is delivered at a rate of 180 to 200 cGy per day.

Often disease is advanced to the state of inoperability. Combination of radiation and intra-arterial chemotherapy has been tried in this setting (GOEPFERT et al. 1973).

Most authors do not recommend any form of therapy for a clinically uninvolved neck. Most of the patients who develop disease in the neck can be salvaged by surgery and radiation if the primary has been controlled. When patients present with neck nodes, surgery is usually combined with pre- or post-op radiation assuming that the primary is operable.

11.3.7 Results

11.3.7.1 Nasal Septum

BEATTY et al. (1982) reported 67% five year survival in a series of 58 patients with squamous cell cancer of the septum. Over 70% of this series was treated by wide local excision alone. WEIMERT et al. (1978) treated 10/14 pts with squamous cancers by surgery only; 80% of the whole group survived 5 years. MC GUIRT et al. (1984) advocate combined wide excision and post-operative irradiation. Amongst 18 patients with squamous histology treated by LE LIEVER et al. (1984), 66% survived 5 years. This team treated nearly half the patients with surgery alone and another half with surgery and radiation. Local control was achieved in 17/18 patients.

The disparity between the overall survival rate and the local control rate is accounted for by the fact that 8/18 pts. (44%) failed in the lymph nodes. This led the authors to recommend wide excision and post-op radiation including treatment of the neck with subclinical disease. There were however, too few patients in each treatment group for valid comparison between them. YOUNG (1979) treated 18/23 patients with squamous cell cancers using radiation alone. Local control was achieved in 74% of the cases and five year survival was 77%. Lymph node involvement was present in only one of these patients at presentation. When other histologies were also considered, 8/43 presented with node metastases. Neither histology or neck status were found to be prognostic predictors.

11.3.7.2 Nasal Cavity (See Table 11-4)

LEWIS and CASTRO (1971) found that surgery yielded a 40% cure rate in nasal cavity cancers as opposed to 32% for the whole group which included paranasal sinus tumors. In a series of 32 patients with epithelial and non-epithelial cancers limited to the infrastructure of the nasal cavity, BARTON (1980) found only 4 failures after resection of the naso-antral ethmoid complex.

The great majority of nasal cavity lesions are advanced at presentation. Combined therapy with surgery and either pre- or post-operative radiation has the widest support. This is most likely due to the practice of grouping nasal cavity cancers with those of the maxillary antrum where the treatment of choice is surgery, with or without radiation. Several reports however show excellent control by radiation alone. ELLINGWOOD and MILLION (1979) rendered 14/15 patients disease free at two years. BOONE et al. (1968) achieved local control in 22/28 patients. Survival rates were 93% at 2 years in the former series and 65% at 5 years in the latter. CHUNG et al. (1980) controlled 12/12 T_1 and T_2 lesions (Lederman staging). Eleven of 12 remained disease free. Nine of 13 patients with more advanced disease were controlled yielding an overall local control rate of 21/25 or 84%. Actual survival at 3 years was 76%.

These results not withstanding, the majority of authors recommend combined surgery and radiation. The results from the Royal Marsden Hospital are typical. The two-part paper by HOPKIN et al. (1984) and MC NICOLL et al. (1984) incorporates earlier data reviewed by LEDERMAN (1970). One hundred sixteen patients had disease in the nasal cavity arising from sites other than the septum. Determinate 5 year survival in this group was 48% as opposed to 79% for the 31 septal lesions. When all 147 patients with nasal fossa primaries were compared by treatment, 5 year NED survival was 57% in the radiotherapy alone group versus 62% in the combined therapy group. The majority of surgical procedures were local excision indicating early lesions. The two groups are therefore probably not comparable with respect to stage of disease. Only 38% of 13 patients presenting with neck node involvement were alive at 5 years.

It would appear that contrary to popular belief,

Table 11-4. Treatment results cancer of the nasal cavity

Reference	Total No Nas. Cav. Cases in Series	No at Risk for Survival Time	Non-Epithelial Histologies	TX Mode	No by Tx	Local Control (%)	NED	Survival Rate (%)	Survival Time Year
BADIB et al. (1969)	57	39	Yes	RT	20	41/57 (72)	10	50	5
				RT + Sx	9		7	78	
				Sx	10		5	50	
BOSCH et al. (1976)	40	23	Yes	RT	34	10/18 (56)	9	50	
				Sx	6	2/5 (40)	4	80	5
ELLINGWOOD and MILLION (1979)	15	15	No	RT	15	14/15 (93)	7	54	5
CHUNG et al. (1980)	25	25	No	RT	25	21/25 (84)	16	76	3
LEDERMAN (1960)	105	75	Yes	RT	48		18	37	
				RT + Sx	29		9	31	5
MCNICOLL et al. (1984)	130	128	Yes	RT	75		43	57	
				RT + Sx	46		28	62	5
BOONE et al. (1968)	28	28	Yes	Not defined but in general RT alone	22/28 (79)	18	65	5	

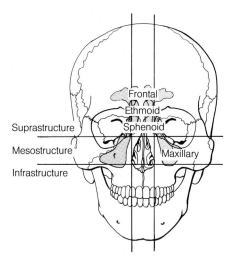

Fig. 11-4. Frontal projection of the sinuses with Lederman lines showing division of the sino-nasal region into supra-, meso- and infrastructures

radiation therapy as a sole modality is efficacious in patients with early and intermediate stages of disease. Combined surgery and radiation are advocated when disease is advanced but operable. There was no local failure in 11/23 patients completing intraarterial 5 FU infusion and radiation in the study by GOEPFERT et al. (1973). Adding this third modality in the treatment of more limited disease may improve the results in this group as well.

11.4 Paranasal Sinuses

11.4.1 Anatomy (See Figures 11-2 and 11-4)

The paranasal sinuses develop as diverticula from the nasal cavity. They invade the surrounding bones and replace the diploe there. The frontal sinuses are the most variable in size and position. They are not fully aerated until after puberty. A vertical extension occupies the space between the outer table of the frontal bone and the inner table which forms the anterior-most wall of the brain case. A horizontal extension is intercalated between the floor of the anterior cranial fossa and the roof of the orbit. These large, paired sinuses communicate with the nasal cavity via ostia in the middle meatus anteriorly.

The ethmoid cells are variable in number. The small but numerous anterior cells open into the middle meatus close to the frontal and maxillary ostia. The larger middle cells open into the middle

meatus often each through its own ostium. There are typically about three cells on each side of the nasal cavity. The thin bone forms the common wall of the ethmoid cells and the lateral nasal cavity. Posteriorly, a highly variable number of small cells enter the superior meatus and sometimes even the space above the superior turbinate, the spheno-ethmoidal recess. As opposed to the frontal sinuses, the ethmoid cells are well developed at birth. Besides the main body of the labyrinth, the ethmoid bone also forms the perpindicular plate and the cribriform plate.

The sphenoid sinuses are paired structures situated deep in the head. They communicate anteriorly by openings into the sphenoethmoidal recess of the nasal cavity. Many critical structures surround this sinus. The pituitary is immediately superior to the sphenoid with the optic chiasm just in front of this gland. On either side is the cavernous sinus which also transmits the carotid artery and the ophthalmic and maxillary divisions of the trigeminal nerve. The nerve of the pterygoid canal runs along the floor of the sinus. The nasopharynx is inferior to the floor. The sphenoids are developed within the first 8 years of life.

The largest sinuses are the maxillary antra which are not fully developed until the permanent teeth are grown. The antrum is roughly a pyramidal cavity whose base is formed by the lateral nasal wall with the apex directed toward the zygoma. Inferiorly the antrum is related to the teeth and palate. Superiorly it shares a common wall with the floor of the orbit. Anteriorly it is associated with the canine fossa and cheek while posteriorly it approximates the pterygomaxillary fossa. Its communication with the nasal cavity is located two thirds up the medial wall entering the middle meatus (see Figure 11-2).

As in the other sinuses, the maxillary antrum is lined by pseudostratified, ciliated, columnar epithelium. The antrum however contains the largest number of mucous glands within its epithelium. As one can imagine by recalling the location of the various drainage openings of these sinuses, gravity plays an appreciable role only in the frontal sinus. The rest of these cavities depend on the ciliary action to drain them.

Lymphatic drainage is via vessels which merge with the lymphatics of the nasal cavity. Patterns of lymph node metastases therefore are to the retropharyngeal, submandibular and jugular nodes.

11.4.2 Epidemiology

The exact figures for incidence and prevalence of these tumors are not available for the subsites within the sinonasal region. Data from the Third National Cancer Survey (REDMOND et al. 1982) which sampled 10% of the U.S. population between 1969–1971 showed 48% of incident cases arising in the nasal cavity and the remainder distributed among the various paranasal sinuses. This is in contradiction to the distribution of cases as reported by the larger treatment series in the literature (see Table 11-5). These series would indicate that 73% of sinonasal cancer originates in the sinuses. Most would agree that sinus cancer is more prevalent than nasal cavity tumors and that maxillary antral tumors form the preponderance of malignant sinus disease.

Maxillary antral cancer accounts for 80% of sinus malignancies and 3% of cancers in the respiratory system. The male to female ratio is approximately 2:1. It is a disease of advanced age with 95% of patients beyond 40 years and 75% in the sixth, seventh and eight decade of life (TABB and BARRANCO 1971). In this country, blacks and whites exhibit equal incidence of the disease.

Tumors of the frontal sinus are extremely rare with little more than a hundred cases in the literature. Of these, many have questionable origin in the ethmoid sinuses. Ethmoid cancers comprise between 5 and 25% of sinus malignancies. The lower figures originate from series with disease limited only to the ethmoid cells while the larger number represents series where site of origin was determined by the location of greatest tumor bulk. There is a slight male preponderance and the peak age is in the mid-fifties. Incidence of sphenoidal primaries is difficult to estimate due to the fact that the great majority present only after invasion of the nasal cavity or nasopharynx with which they are commonly grouped.

Japan and sections of Africa have two to three times the incidence of sinus tumors than is seen in this country. No specific genetic factor has been implicated. Various environmental agents are known to increase the risk of these diseases. As mentioned, nickle refinery workers suffer a relative increase in risk of squamous and anaplastic carcinomas of the ethmoids. Wood dust may led to adenocarcinomas of the ethmoids and antrum. Other environmental dusts have been implicated in sinus adenocarcinomas seen in boot and shoe manufacture, chrome pigment workers, textile workers, flour millers and bakers. Laboratory proven carcinogens are found in the manufacture of isopropyl alcohol, hydrocarbon gas and mustard gas. Radium dial painters had high rates of squamous cell cancers of the antrum. Children treated with radiation for retinoblastoma are at a higher risk for developing tumors in the sinuses than the general population (ROWE et al. 1980). The use of thorium dioxide (thorotrast) has caused squamous and mucoepidermoid carcinomas of the antrum when used as an imaging agent in this area. Cigarrette smoking has not been adequately studied as a causative agent although many clinical series report a high incidence of tobacco and snuff users in their material.

11.4.3 Pathology

A variety of neoplasms, both benign and malignant, originate in the paranasal sinuses. Benign masses such as inflammatory polyps and papillomas are more commonly seen in the nasal cavity. Squamous cell carcinoma is the most prevalent malignant tu-

Table 11-5. Sinonasal cancer – site involvement

Reference	Antrum	Ethmoid	Sphenoid	Frontal	Nasal	Total
LEDERMAN (1970)	367	176	–	4	168	715
BOONE et al. (1968)	70	20	2	1	28	121
LEWIS and CASTRO (1971)	451	75	3	6	237	772
SAKAI et al. (1975)	830	33	1	8	31	903
JACKSON et al. (1977)	77	15	1	3	19	115
BUSH and BAGSHAW (1982)	27	6	–	1	4	38
Subtotal	1,822 (68%)	325 (12%)	7 (0.3%)	23 (0.9%)	487 (18%)	2,664
CHENG and WANG (1977)	50	11	4	1		66
SHIDNIA et al. (1984)	94	17	4	1		116
Total	1,966 (83%)	353 (15%)	15 (0.6%)	25 (1%)		2,846

mor in the sinuses (see Table 11-6). Other epithelial neoplasms include adenocarcinomas and salivary gland tumors (mixed, adenoid cystic, and muco-epidermoid). Lymphoepitheliomas more frequently arise from the nasopharynx and invade the sinuses secondarily. Solitary plasmacytomas and lymphomas may also originate in these structures. Mesodermal tumors including chondrosarcomas, osteosarcomas, fibrosarcomas and various tumors of dental origin are occasionally seen in the paranasal sinuses. The remainder of this section will deal with the epithelial neoplasms leaving consideration of other histologies to section 11.7.

11.4.4 Classification and Staging

The lack of a generally accepted classification system for sinonasal cancer has contributed to our inability to compare the experience of one center with that of another. Due to the scarcity of case material, such comparison is necessary in order to achieve the goal of improved methods of management. This not withstanding, there are several useful systems which have been developed (HARRISON 1978; RUBIN 1972; SAKAI et al. 1976). LEDERMAN (1969) modified the 1906 system of Sebileau, adapting it to a TNM staging. His classification is as follows: Two horizontal, parallel lines are drawn across a frontal section of the skull at the level of the floor of the nose and at the inferior rim of the orbits (see Figure 11-4). These lines define a) Suprastructure containing the ethmoids, frontal sinuses and the olfactory portion of the nasal cavity. b) Mesostructure with the maxillary antra, nasal vestibule and the remaining nasal cavity. c) Infrastructure including the floor of the antra, hard palate and alveolar ridges. Two additional vertical lines at the medial aspect of the orbits separate the ethmoids and nasal fossa from the maxillary sinuses. The T-staging associated with this system is: T_1 tumor limited to one sinus or the tissue of origin, T_2 limited horizontal spread within the same region or spread to two adjacent, vertically related regions, T_3 tumor involving three regions or extension of the tumor beyond the upper jaw (ie to nasopharynx, cranial cavity, skin, buccal cavity or palatine fossa).

The American Joint Committee on Cancer (AJCC) offers a staging strictly for tumors of the maxillary antrum. This system makes use of Ohngren's line, a theoretic plane joining the medial canthus of the eye with the angle of the mandible. As originally devised by OHNGREN (1933) this "plane of malignancy" separated the resectable anterior, inferior tumors from the unresectable lesions posteriorly and superiorly. The AJCC system describes four T-Stages: T_1 tumor confined to the antral mucosa of the infrastructure with no bone erosion or destruction; T_2 tumor confined to the suprastructure mucosa without bone destruction or to the infrastructure with destruction of the medial or inferior bony walls only; T_3 more extensive tumor invading skin of cheek, orbit anterior ethmoid sinuses, or pterygoid muscle; T_4 massive tumor with invasion of the cribriform plate, posterior ethmoids, sphenoid, nasopharynx, pterygoid plates, or base of skull.

HOPKIN et al. (1984) are in agreement with HARRISON (1978) that, granted the known difficulty of clinically assessing this region, staging would be simple, practical, and more useful if it were based on a) presence or absence of spread into danger areas (ie orbit, skull base, pterygopalatine fossa, etc.) b) presence or absence of lymph node metastases.

11.4.5 Natural History (see Table 11-7)

RUBIN (1972) has described four phases in the natural history of these tumors. In phase I, the tumor masquerades as an inflammatory process. In

Table 11-6. Sinonasal cancer pathology

	Squamous	Anaplastic	Transit	Adeno	Salivary	Melanoma	Lymphoma	Sarcoma	Plasma	Other	Total
HOPKIN et al. (1984)	198	92	61	40	34	39	35	25	8	29	561
JACKSON et al. (1977)	61	11	2	9	8	7	3	7	2	5	115
LEWIS and CASTRO (1971)	496			129		34	40	23	13	26	761
LEDERMAN (1970)	323	104	62	28	26	31	47	31		34	686
BOONE et al. (1968)	79			8	7			3		24	121
Total	1,157 (51%)	207 (9%)	125 (6%)	214 (10%)	75 (3%)	111 (5%)	125 (6%)	89 (4%)	23 (1%)	118 (5%)	2,244

Table 11-7. Maxillary antrum cancers symptoms and signs at presentation

	Oral				Facial			Ocular					Nasal					Other			
	Swelling	Pain	Ulcer	Dental NOS	Swelling	Pain	Numbness	Diplopia	Pain	Visual Change	Proptosis	Epiphora	Mass	Obstruction	Epistaxis	Rhinorrhea	Swelling	Trismus	H/A	Pain NOS	Neck Swelling
Hopkin (1984)	58	16			126	83	7	11			28	25		99	64			5			25
Lederman (1970)	←———— 51 ————→				←— 143 —→			←———— 35 ————→					←———— 125 ————→					←— 13 ——→			2
Tabb & Barranco (1971)	22			22	22		4		2	27	21	17	35	52	38	57		2		45	
Schechter & Ogura (1972)	6	4	6	2	7	6	2	1	2	1	2	5	8	11	5	28				1	1
Total	86	20	6	24	155	89	13	12	4	28	51	47	43	162	107	85		7	1	46	27
1,380	187 (13%)				400 (29%)			177 (13%)					522 (38%)					94 (7%)			

phase II, a dull ache becomes manifest as the bone is eroded. Phase III is accompanied by patches of hypesthesia and deep pain secondary to nerve invasion. Phase IV is characterized by major deformity with gross local and distant spread.

CHAUDHRY et al. (1960) divided the most important signs and symptoms into five groups. Group I includes oral signs and symptoms. Invasion of antral tumors inferiorly into the alveolar process and palate produces swelling which may first present as poorly fitting dentures. Toothache, pain and eventually ulceration follow. Teeth may loosen and the socket fails to heal after extraction leading to oral-antral fistula. Trismus results from invasion into the pterygoid fossa. Group II is related to medial extension into the nasal cavity. Unilateral nasal obstruction is the most common symptom followed by epistaxis and rhinorrhea. Purulent discharge is also common in this situation. Occasionally a nasal polyp or mass visible in the nasal cavity is the first sign of disease. Group III is related to orbital invasion. Proptosis, lacrimation and changes in visual acuity are the most common symptoms with occasional orbital pain or diplopia. Group IV is composed of facial symptoms from anterior extension into the cheek. The first sign is usually loss of the nasolabial fold on the involved side followed by obvious swelling and bulging. This can be quite painful and signs of local inflammation are common. If the infraorbital nerve is involved, hypesthesia of the cheek develops. Group V includes the

neurologic symptoms secondary to superior extension involving the base of the skull, meninges and cranial neves. Headache, anosmia and deficits related to the VIIth and VIIIth nerves are included in this group. Approximately 2% of patients will have a neck mass as their presenting symptom.

Early cancers of the antrum are invariably discovered accidentally because the above listed signs and symptoms develop only after the tumor has escaped the bony confines of the sinus (HARRISON 1972).

Lymph node metastases are present at diagnosis in 13–15% of cases. They subsequently develop during follow-up in 14–26% of patients (KENT and MAJUMDAR 1984; ROBIN and POWELL 1980; LEWIS and CASTRO 1972; LEE and OGURA 1981). Invasion into the cheek allows access into the facial lymphatics and increases the risk for neck disease.

Distant metastases were seen in 12% of KENT and MAJUMDAR's (1984) series. Sites involved in order of decreasing frequency are bone, lung, liver, brain, and kidney. Four per cent of the series by HOPKIN et al. (1984) developed second malignancies.

The majority of patients with this disease will eventually die from its manifestations. HARRISON (1972) tabulated the cause of death in his series. He found death from hemorrhage, 3%; intracranial extension, 18%; systemic metastases, 8%; bronchopneumonia and cachexia, 71%. This latter category was referred to as "morphine toxicity" because it develops in patients who are bedridden from the in-anition of severe bone pain. The fact that most pat-ients die a lingering, painful death has engendered a pessimistic attitude in the majority of clinicians. It is important that this attitude not interfere with the identification and aggressive treatment of the sub-group of patients who are curable.

11.4.6 Diagnosis

The majority of the mucosa lining the paranasal si-nuses is inaccessible to direct inspection rendering diagnosis of the malignancies which arise from this mucosa extremely difficult. Physical examination should nevertheless be done with special care given to evaluate potential areas of spread. The anterior cheek and malar region can be palpated for masses. The orbital floor can be palpated by inserting the fingertip between the globe and the inferior orbital rim. The hard palate and gingivobuccal gutter are also subject to examination by the palpating finger. Anterior and posterior rhinoscopy are important to rule out origin of the tumor from the nasopharynx. Cranial nerve exam and palpation of the lymph node bearing areas are part of the complete assess-ment.

Radiography is one of the most useful diagnostic tools. Plain films taken in the occipito-mental, oc-cipitofrontal, lateral and sub-mento vertical projec-tions give the first indication of extent of the dis-ease by showing clouding of the sinuses, soft tissue masses and bone destruction. Polytomography in the frontal and sagittal planes is a more sensitive procedure for defining spread. At present, the most useful investigation is computed tomography (CT). This imaging modality can detect bony destruction with the same accuracy as plain tomograms and has replaced plain tomography in many centers.

Comparison of sinus roentgenography, polytom-ography and CT has been done by JEANS et al. (1982). They found that plain films do not detect the presence of bone destruction in half of patients. CT and polytomography detected bone involve-ment in equivalent proportions of cases. When con-sidering sinus films alone, 40% of patients were found to have LEDERMAN T_1 lesions. When these patients underwent CT scanning, no patient had T_1 disease. The proportion of patients with stage T_3 tu-mors after sinus films, tomograms, and CT were 23%, 31%, and 63% respectively.

The particular strength of CT is in the evaluation of the extent of soft tissue disease (JUNG et al. 1978). Invasion of soft tissue masses into the orbit, pterygopalatine fossa, infratemporal fossa, and the brain can be detected and evaluated best by CT. In-fusion of contrast agents is necessary when exten-sion through the cribriform plate or into the middle cranial fossa is suspected. In these instances, the tu-mor will enhance while the brain tissue does not. It is important to scan in both the frontal and axial planes. The regions of the cribriform plate and the infero-medial quadrant of the orbit may only be adequately evaluated in the coronal plane (LUND et al. 1983).

Although CT is a definite advance in diagnosis and staging, it is still subject to drawbacks and shortcomings. The large contrast in tissue density between the air in the sinus and the dense bone of the hard palate and base of the skull produces arti-facts which limit accurarcy in these areas. Often, poorly vascularized, intracranial extensions of tu-mor will be isodense with brain tissue, even after in-fusion, thus defying diagnosis by CT. ROBIN and POWELL (1981) found that 89 of 282 cases (32%) un-dergoing surgical exploration had underestimates of tumor extent after CT. It remains to be seen whether magnetic resonance imaging (MRI) will exceed the ability of CT scanning in defining extent of invasion. Certainly the ability of MRI to image in the saggital and coronal planes offers advantages in evaluating the thin plates of orbital bone. It is widely accepted however that the final decision to exenterate the orbit can only be made at surgery (LUND et al. 1983).

Prior to major explorations or resections, tissue must be obtained for histopathologic examination. The maxillary antrum is best approached through a Caldwell-Luc antrotomy although medial extension of maxillary tumors may be biopsied through the nasal cavity. Ethmoid tumors are also biopsied by their extension into the nasal cavity. A frontal oste-otomy allows access to the frontal sinus. Sphenoid tumors are usually biopsied transnasally taking samples of nasal or nasopharyngeal extensions. Oc-casionally a lateral rhinotomy is required for access to these lesions. Other procedures useful in staging include chest x-ray laryngoscopy, bronchoscopy and esophagoscopy. Suspicious neck nodes should also be biopsied prior to deciding management.

11.4.7 Therapy of Paranasal Sinus Cancers

11.4.7.1 Surgery

Total maxillectomy is the oldest of all monobloc operations for cancer dating back to Gensoul of Lyons in 1827 (LEDERMAN 1970). This procedure is rarely used because it is suitable only for the rare, early lesion mainly of the infrastructure. Extensions of tumor into suprastructure, or the nasal cavity require radical maxillectomy for complete extirpation. This operation removes the hard palate, teeth and alveolar ridge on the involved side along with the lateral nasal wall, all 3 turbinates and the orbital floor. Function and cosmesis are maintained by the use of an obturator/prosthesis which is made from pre-op dental impressions. This prosthesis preserves the contour of the face in the event that much of the zygoma is removed. It also supports the eye when this structure is not removed. The obturator seals the defect in the palate allowing speech and swallowing to be restored.

Various extensions of the radical maxillectomy are possible. These include the addition of orbital exenteration, removal of the nasal septum and contralateral nasal wall and turbinates, removal of the pterygoid plates and ethmoidectomy. The introduction of craniofacial techniques in 1954 and the subsequent development of this procedure by KETCHAM et al. (1963) allowed surgical attack on the previously unresectable areas of the cribriform plate, posterior ethmoid cells, anterior wall of the sphenoid and the floor of the middle cranial fossa (TERZ et al. 1980). The net result of these procedures is to transform the sinus system into a single epithelial-lined cavity. Due to the proximity of unresectable vital structures in this region, wide surgical margins are rarely if ever obtained even with the most radical operations. It is this inability to obtain wide margins coupled with the propensity for local recurrence that causes the majority of oncologists to recommend aggressive combinations of surgery and radiation therapy.

11.4.7.2 Radiation Therapy

The discovery of radium led to a period in which partial maxillectomy was performed in conjunction with intra-cavitary applications. This combination was routine during the 1930's and 40's until external radiation with orthovoltage beams supplanted radium therapy. Although the orthovoltage pioneers reported fairly good results, they were limited by the tolerance of the normal tissues and they were therefore inclined to be less aggressive, giving non-cancerocidal doses. With these limitations of radiation, and continuing surgical improvements, the management of this disease became mostly surgical. The emergence of megavoltage equipment and high energy electron beams made more aggressive irradi-

ation possible. As a result, there have emerged reports of primary radiation management of resectable lesions (BATAINI and ENNUYER 1971; ELLINGWOOD and MILLION 1979; FRICH 1982; AMENDOLA et al. 1981). The introduction of radiosensitizing chemotherapeutic agents and particle beams such as fast neutrons may lead to an increasing number of patients being managed primarily with radiation.

At present, radiation is most widely used as a surgical adjuvant. There are proponents on each side of the pre-op vs. post-op radiation issue.

The advantages and disadvantages of either sequence have been thoroughly discussed in basic texts on radiotherapy. The arguments are as applicable to the sinuses as to other sites in the body and will not be detailed here. Most reported series utilized pre-op doses greater than 5500 cGy the average being 6000 cGy. Post-operative doses range from 6000 cGy to 7500 cGy based on the presence of gross residual tumor. The volume of tissue included is individualized to the extent of the tumor in question. Techniques for adequate coverage of areas at risk are given in section 11.5. Prophylactic neck irradiation is not recommended.

11.4.7.3 Chemotherapy

Several drugs have shown effect upon sinonasal tumors. Most notable among these are bleomycin, methotrexate, 5-fluorouracil, and cis-platinum (BLACKSTEIN and CHAPNIK 1976). These drugs have been used for systemic disease, refractory local recurrences, and as part of a combined modality attack on the initial localized tumor. In 1970, SATO et al. reported a series of 57 patients with various stages of sinus carcinoma treated by triple therapy. This consisted of regional 5-FU infusion via a catheter in the internal maxillary artery combined with daily radiation and suction curettage through a canine fossa antrostomy. Patients with residual tumor one month after 7000 cGy had been delivered went on to partial maxillectomy. A 5 year survival rate of 88% was reported. This experience has not been duplicated in any other center despite the increasing use of regional chemotherapy. Given the known ability of these agents to act as radiation sensitizers it will not be surprising to see them used more commonly in combination with radical radiation therapy and lesser surgical procedures (SHAFIR and RAVENTOS 1983; GEOPFERT et al. 1973; SAKAI et al. 1983).

Table 11-8. Results of therapy for maxillary sinus cancer

Reference	Non-Epithl. Histol.	Treatment Modality	No Tx.	Local Control (%)	No NED No at risk	Surv. Rate (%)	Time (yrs)
LEDERMAN (1970)	Yes	R/S	124		26/99	26	5
		S/R	60		19/55	35	5
		R	77		4/53	8	5
McNICOLL et al. (1984)	Yes	R	91		16/91	18	5
		R/S	154		53/154	34	5
BOONE et al. (1968)	Yes	R			43/70	35	5
		S			(61)		
		R/S or S/R					
FRAZELL and LEWIS (1963)	No	R	59		5/59	8	5
		S	163		47/163	29	5
BARLEY et al. (1976)	No	R/S/Intracavitary	37	17 (46)	14/49	29	5
		R/S	12	2 (17)			
BATAINI and ENNUYER (1971)	No	R	31	21 (68)	12/31	39	3
BEALE and MALONEY (1982)	No	R/S	55		18/50	36	5
FRICH (1982)	No	R	18	10 (56)	7/18	39	5
MOSELEY et al. (1981)	No	RegC + R/S	10	9 (90)	6/10	60	2
SAKAI et al. (1983)	Yes	R/S	282			20	5
		R + RegC	191	(16)		25	5
		R + RegC + Curettage	166	(35)		39	5
		R + RegC + Cryosurgery	134	(45)		54	4
SHIBUYA et al. (1984)	No	R	178			21	10
		S/R	78				
		R/S	42			34	10
		Trimodal	56			49	5
		S/Trimodal	55			68	5
WEYMULLER et al. (1980)	No	Massive S/R	13	3 (23)			
		Limited S/R	6	4 (66)			
		R	13	3 (23)			
AMENDOLA et al. (1981)	S	19	8 (45)	7/19	31	5	
	R	20	13 (66)	10/20	35	5	
HU et al. (1982)	No	S/R	14		4/14	29	5
		R/S	36		23/36	64	5
AHMAD et al. (1981)	No	R	47	15 (32)		39	5
		S/R	9	6 (67)			
TABB and BARRANCO (1971)	Yes	R	17		0/17	0	5
		R + C	10		1/10	10	5
		S	19		10/19	62	5
		R/S	35		11/35	32	5
		S/R	19		2/19	12	5
SCHECHTER and OGURA (1972)	Yes	R	7				
		R/S	31				
		S/R	10		20/50	40	4
		No Tx.	2				
LEE and OGURA (1981)	Yes	R/S	61	42 (69)	18/47	38	5
		R	35	5 (14)	0/23	0	5
CHENG and WANG (1977)	No	R	27		6/27	22	3
		R/S	12	28 (56)	7/12	58	3
		S/R	11		4/11	36	3
PEARLMAN and ADABIR (1974)	No	R/S	19	10 (53)	7/19	37	3.5
SHIDNIA et al. (1984)	No	R/S	30		9/30	30	2.5
		S/R	18		7/18	39	2.5
		R	40		3/40	7	2.5

R = Radiation Therapy, S = Surgery, C = Chemotherapy, $RegC$ = Regional Chemotherapy

11.4.8 Results (see Tables 11-8 and 11-9)

Surgery has allowed 29 to 60% of patients with resectable disease to live for five years (FRAZELL and LEWIS 1963; TABB and BARRANCO 1971; AMENDOLA et al. 1981). The majority of failures are due to local recurrence. Most series reported in the 1960's and 70's used radiation as the primary treatment modality only for disease too advanced for surgical resection, or for patients too debilitated to withstand such procedures. It is not surprising that results ranged from zero to 20% 5 year survivorship (FRAZELL and LEWIS 1963; LEDERMAN 1970; TABB and BARRANCO 1971; CHENG and WANG 1977). In 1971, BATAINI and ENNUYER used a combination of Cobalt-60 and 35 MeV electron beam radiations. This series of 31 patients with mostly advanced epithelial neoplasms of the antrum (10 had positive neck nodes) had a 39% 3 year disease-free survival. AMENDOLA et al. (1981) compared craniofacial resection in 19 cases to radical irradiation in 20. Survival at 3 years was 37% and 50% respectively. These results and others (ELLINGWOOD and MILLION 1979; WEYMULLER et al. 1980; FRICH 1982; BUSH and BAGSHAW 1982) show that modern radiation therapy is a powerful weapon against this disease. CATTERALL et al. (1984) using a fast neutron beam generated with the Hamersmith cyclotron induced complete remissions in all but 2 of 31 patients with very advanced maxillary sinus cancers. These 2, and 4 of the complete responders subsequently died from local disease leaving 69% with local control.

Although FRICH (1982) was able to control the primary tumor in 80% of patients with extensive tumors of the suprastructure with radiation alone, 75% of patients with infrastructure tumors failed. He concluded that combined surgery and radiation were required in that site.

In similar fashion, the great majority of reports in the literature deal with combined modality therapy prompted by the high recurrence rates usually seen when single agents are employed. This large experience with combined surgery and radiation has not yet confirmed any advantage of pre-op radiation over post-op or vice versa. JESSE (1965) made a comparison of the two showing the local control rate and 3 year survival for 22 patients treated preoperatively to be 64 and 45% respectively. The corresponding figures for the 18 patients in the post-op group were 66 and 39%. The average figures for local control and 5 year survival after combined radiation and surgery as generally reported are 115/188 (61%) and 90/239 (38%). The discrepancy is due to distant failure, and intercurrent deaths.

The extent of the primary lesion and the presence or absence of nodal disease are among the recognized prognostic indicators independent of the mode of therapy. The results of CHENG and WANG (1977) are representative. Three year disease free survival was 6/13 (46%) in T_1 and T_2 lesions as opposed to 11/37 (30%) in T_3 and T_4 tumors. Node negative patients enjoyed 3 years NED survival in 14/39 (35%) as compared to 3/11 (27%) of node positive patients.

Some authors feel that the addition of chemotherapeutic agents to the treatment regimen improves the survival rate. SHIBUYA et al. (1984) reported a five year survival of 68% among 55 patients treated with trimodal therapy. SAKAI et al. (1983) used radiation, regional chemotherapy and

Table 11-9. Results of therapy for paranasal sinus cancer

Reference	Non-Epith. Histol.	Treatment Modality	No Tx.	Local Control (%)	No NED No at Risk	Surv. (%)	Time (yrs)
SATO et al. (1970)	No	RegC + R + / − S	57	22 (38)	35/57	61	2
SHAFIR and RAVENTOS (1983)	No	RegC + R + S	12	3 (25)	3/12	25	5
GOEPFERT et al. (1973)	No	RegC + R	23	11 (48)	4/15	26	5
JESSE (1965)	No	R/S	22	14 (64)	10/22	45	3
		S/R	18	12 (66)	7/18	39	3
		R	11		2/11	18	3
		S	20		9/20	45	3
BUSH and BAGSHAW (1982)	No	R	22	18 (47)	5/22	23	5
		Limited S/R	8		4/8	50	5
		Extensive S/R	6		2/6	33	5
		R/S	2		1/2	50	5

cryosurgery to produce a 4 year survival of 54% in 134 patients. Their local control rate was 45%. Small series of patients treated with regional chemo have been reported from this country; however, the 5 year results are not as good averaging about 25% (GOEPFERT et al. 1973; CRUZ et al. 1974; MOSELEY et al. 1981; SHAFIR and RAVENTOS 1983). It is yet to be proven by randomized clinical trials which form of therapy is optimal for this disease.

The patient with recurrent disease has a low probability of salvage. Reoperation, electrocoagulation, curettage and cryosurgery are all effective means of palliating recurrences which are beyond hope of salvage (BLACKSTEIN and CHAPNIK 1976). High-dose-rate intracavitary radiation in this setting has been reported by AKANUMA (1977). Complete responses were achieved with 3000 cGy surface doses administered in a matter of a few minutes with highly active Cobalt 60 sources. Nine of 16 patients were temporarilly controlled in this fashion.

11.5 Techniques of Radiation

The first step in planning radiation therapy for a patient takes place before the patient enters the simulation suite. This consists of defining the known areas of disease extent and areas at risk for containing disease. In post-operative situations, the surgical findings will aid in this process. Computed tomography is the single greatest aid for this purpose when radiation treatment is pre-op or definitive.

With the above information in mind, the therapist may then decide on the appropriate positioning of the patient on the treatment couch. Patients are treated supine. If the head is flexed, anterior fields will necessarily cover an excessive amount of frontal lobe and exit through brain stem and spinal cord. Extension, on the other hand will cause the inclusion of too much oral cavity mucosa. The head should therefore be immobilized in a neutral position, the hard palate assuming a position perpendicular to the treatment couch. Oral cavity mucosa can be removed from fields by means of a tongue depressor taped to a cork, a 30 cc syringe barrel, or custom acrylic resin prostheses (CHENG et al. 1982). Bolus material should be used to provide buildup when the skin of the anterior cheek is involved. The patient is instructed to stare into the beam when the eye is treated so as to reduce the surface dose to the cornea. A lid retractor may be necessary.

Treatment planning is done from orthogonal sim-

ulation films and a contour or from a CT slice through the plane of the central axis of the simulation. CT planning in the treatment position represents the state of the art. It allows the therapist to define the anatomic relationship between the critical normal tissues and the extensions of the tumor. It further allows the input of density information which can be put to use with currently available programs for calculating the effects of inhomogeneities within the treatment volume.

Given the juxtaposition of bone and air cavities in the sinonasal region, these inhomogeneities of density will significantly affect the dose distribution. Whether this capability will result in an improved result from radiation therapy is yet to be determined.

Many therapists will set up standard fields to treat tumors in this region however the prevalent recommendation is to individualize the treatment plan to the case at hand. Several generalizations can however be made. Anterior lesions in the midline (frontal sinuses, anterior ethmoids, nasal cavity) can be treated by anterior fields alone (see Figure 11-5). Combinations of Cobalt-60 high energy X-rays, and electrons are used for this approach. Lateral fields (see Figure 11-6) must be added for tumors extend-

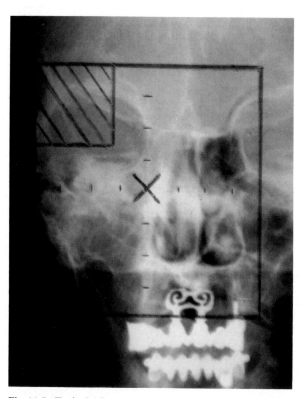

Fig. 11-5. Typical AP treatment port for a tumor of the maxillary antrum

ing more posteriorly in the midline (sphenoid, posterior ethmoids, posterior nasal cavity). Usually the lateral fields will require wedges with the heels directed anteriorly. Weighting is in favor of the anterior field usually 2:1 or 3:1. Angulation of lateral fields with a 5 degree tilt posteriorly reduces the dose to the contralateral eye. Computer calculation of dose distribution is essential to the selection of the right combination of fields, wedging and weighting (Figures 11-7 and 11-8). Shielding of the lacrimal gland from the anterior field is essential to reduce the incidence of dry-eye syndromes. The decision to shield the ipsilateral orbital contents is made on the basis of tumor extent. Ethmoid tumors involving the medial orbital wall and antral tumors invading the floor of the orbit mandate treatment of the eye. In cases where the eye may be excluded, care must be taken not to shield sinus structures with the eye block. It is now widely recognized that the antrum slopes cephalad from the orbital rim to the apex and from lateral to medial. Therefore, an eye block can shadow the postero-medial corner of the antrum unless this is strictly watched for.

Figures 11-5 and 11-6 are illustrative of typical AP and lateral ports. Anterior fields should extend at least 2–3 cm across the midline to the limbus of

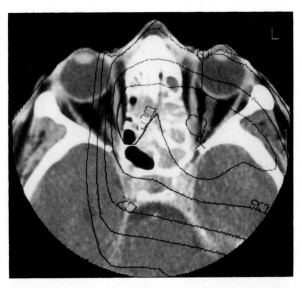

Fig. 11-7. Treatment plan for anterior ethmoid cancer utilizing only anterior fields. In this plan, 18 MV photons are set up to a depth of 4 cm. 20 MeV electrons are set up at the skin surface. The field sizes are 9×9 cm. The weighting is 2:1 in favor of the electrons

the contralateral eye (with the patient gazing straight ahead). This insures complete coverage of the ethmoidal cells and medial wall of the contralateral orbit. The superior border should be placed so as to cover the cribriform plate and frontal sinus. This border is extended upwards 2–3 cm when there is involvement of the frontal sinus or intracranial extensions of tumor. The lower border is placed to include the hard palate and alveolar ridges when the maxillary sinus or nasal cavity are involved. If the tumor is limited to the ethmoids, frontal, or sphenoid sinuses or the olfactory portion of the nasal cavity; the lower border may be raised to the level of the nasal floor. When only midline structures are involved, the lateral border bisects the maxillary sinus. Involvement of the maxillary sinus or orbit requires a wider field completely encompassing these structures. Anterior field sizes may be reduced after 6000 cGy in order to boost areas of gross disease to higher doses.

The commonly utilized borders for lateral fields are as follows; 1) posteriorly to the auditory meatus in order to adequately radiate the sphenoid, base of skull, pterygopalatine fossa and infratemporal fossa; 2) anteriorly to the lateral bony rim of the orbit; 3) superior and inferior to match the anterior field. A block is used to protect as much brain as possible in the postero-superior corner of the field. Care should be taken not to cover the sphenoid or floor of the middle cranial fossa with

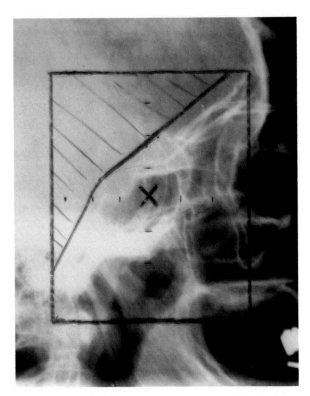

Fig. 11-6. Lateral port for treatment of the maxillary antrum

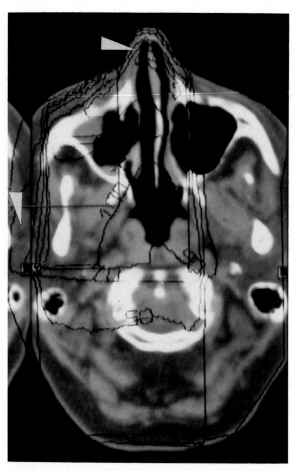

Fig. 11-8. Wedged pair treatment plan for anterior lesion of the maxillary-ethmoidal complex. 4 MV photons. Anterior field: field size 8 × 8 cm, set-up depth 7 cm, wedge 15 degrees. Lateral field: field size 7 × 8 cm, depth 6 cm, wedge 60 degrees. The fields are weighted 3 : 1 anterior to lateral

this block. It should be modified or dispensed with altogether in the event of CNS invasion.

HINTZ et al. (1984) evaluated technical factors leading to radiation failure. They noted that the majority of failures were posterior and medial. This is the region that can be inadvertently shielded by careless eye blocking. It is also the area at highest risk for underdosage by wedge pair techniques. Their recommendations include careful eye blocking when indicated, use of three field technique as opposed to wedged pairs and adequate extension of the medial border of anterior fields across the midline to include convex bowing of the contralateral lamina papyracea.

Various prosthetic devices have been used as source carriers for intracavity applications (CHENG et al. 1982; DEUTCH et al. 1981; GHALICHEBAF et al. 1984). The requirement of very superficial lesions limits the usefulness of this approach.

11.6 Complications of Radiation Therapy

11.6.1 General Commments

Patients are prone to developing complications for a variety of reasons, including; 1) advanced stage of tumors at diagnosis 2) poor nutritional status 3) high radiation dose employed 4) proximity of sensitive and critical normal structures 5) frequent prior use of aggressive chemotherapy and/or surgery.

Complications of a major nature are reported in 15 to 25% of patients. The commonly encountered complications are categorized in this section.

11.6.2 Eye

11.6.2.1 Macular and Retinal Degeneration

This process produced blindness in 7 eyes of 15 patients by SHUKOVSKY and FLETCHER (1972). This complication is seen from 1½ to 3 years after therapy. Clinically it resembles diabetic retinopathy with microaneurysms, cotton-wool spots, hemorrhages and hard exudates seen on funduscopic exam. This problem is dose related with a maximal probability after doses of 5000 cGy have been given to the retina (WARA et al. 1979). Prevention is accomplished by utilization of high energy beams (GALBRAITH et al. 1985) or other technical methods such as conformation moving fields (MORITA and KAWABE 1979) which lower the retinal dose. This complication is seen more frequently in patients receiving chemotherapy agents (CHAN and SHUKOVSKY 1976). Neovascular glaucoma may develop as a complication of retinopathy. This condition may become so painful as to warrant enucleation.

11.6.2.2 Optic Nerve Atrophy

This problem can be subdivided into ischemic optic neuropathy (seen at the distal end of the nerve) and retrobular optic neuropathy (secondary to proximal nerve injury). In the former, changes in the optic disc include papielledema, pallor and splinter hemorrhages while the latter condition produces no visible changes. The risk is related to dose per fraction. PARSON et al. (1983) reported 8% incidence in patients treated with fraction sizes ≤ 190 cGy and 41% with higher daily dose. Usage of smaller fraction size and reduction of fields after 5000 cGy to exclude as much optic nerve as possible may prevent this complication.

11.6.2.3 Central Retinal Artery Thrombosis

This accounts for sudden and complete loss of vision in the affected eye between 9 months and 1 year after therapy. This was reported in 2/15 patients in the series of SHUKOVSKY and FLETCHER (1972) and occurred with doses less than those required for retinal or optic nerve damage.

11.6.2.4 Cataract

This complication was reported in 4/30 patients reported by NAKISSA et al. (1983). Dose response data was not available due to the utilization of corneal shields. Most patients developing this problem will not have significant reduction in useful vision. Extraction is not recommended for patients with good sight in the contralateral eye due to difficulties with correction using an aphakic spectacle or contact lens. Lens implantation may be contraindicated.

11.6.2.5 Lacrimal System

Injury to these tissues result in vision loss secondary to corneal ulceration, opacity or vasualization. Dry-eye syndrome (keratoconjunctivitis sicca) consists of a red, scratchy eye accompanied by photophobia. This develops within a few months of radiation treatment and can progress to blindness within a year. Prevention is possible with proper radiation technique. The eye is treated with the lids opened either voluntarily or by lid retractor. This allows maximal surface sparing and also elevates the accessory lacrimal tissue in the superior conjunctival fornix out of the fields. The major lacrimal gland is shielded by an appropriate block. Doses to the entire eye and lacrimal tissue of greater than 5000 cGy will cause this complication in the majority of patients.

The nasolacrimal duct will not be affected unless previously traumatized by surgery or tumor invasion.

11.6.3 Central Nervous System

Brain necrosis was reported in 3 patients treated by BOONE et al. (1968). This usually will be located in a portion of the frontal lobes. Although this dramatic complication is uncommon, many patients will manifest less severe injuries to nervous tissue. Hypothalamic dysfunction was identified in 76/110 patients terated by SAMAAN et al. (1982). They also described pituitary endocrine abnormalities in 43 patients. ELLINGWOOD and MILLION (1979) experienced injuries ranging from Lhermitte's syndrome to delayed transitory CNS syndrome in 5 of their 32 patients. Aseptic meningitis is a potentially lethal complication that can be ascribed to radiation therapy.

11.6.4 Nose

Cartilage necrosis is rarely seen (even after very high radiation doses) provided adequate fractionation has been employed. Occasionally, septal perforations or deviations are noted. Synechiae and stricture have been described as possible sequellae. Most patients will at least experience dryness and crusting. Many therapists will advise water-pik irrigation, and dilation/lubrication with petroleum jelly coated cotton tipped applicators as preventive measures.

11.6.5 Bone and Soft Tissue

Most series will report one or two cases of osteo-radionecrosis. ELLINGWOOD and MILLION (1979) described two patietns who experienced bone necrosis following tooth extraction. A third patient developed an ethmoid-cutaneous fistula. BOONE et al. (1973) reported two patients in their series with osteonecrosis and a third with exposure of the maxilla. Post-operative healing was delayed in four other patients. Chronic purulent sinusitis can develop in these patients although this is probably only indirectly related to the radiation. Even so, ethmoiditis of this type may extend into the orbit producing blindness if not controlled.

11.6.6 Induction of Second Malignancies

The role of radiation induced neoplasia was mentioned in the section on epidemiology. These are usually sarcomas although epithelial tumors have also been reported (ROWE et al. 1980; COIA et al. 1980; STEEVES and BATAINI 1981). The latent period is from 10 to 15 years.

11.7 Other Histologies

11.7.1 Esthesioneuroblastoma

This tumor was 1st reported by BERGER in 1924, however the 1st English language report did not appear until 1951 (KADISH et al. 1976). Since that time, approximately 150 cases have been described. Synonyms include olfactory neuroblastoma, and olfactory esthesioneuroma. All of these terms reflect the origin of the tumor in the specialized sensory neuroepithelium which covers the superior nasal turbinates and septum. Microscopically, one or more of the following is seen: 1) round, oval, or slightly fusiform cells the size of lymphocytes, 2) neurofibrils, 3) true rosette or pseudo rosette formation, 4) perivascular pallisading of cells, 5) interstitial calcification (ELKON et al. 1979; OBERMAN and RICE 1976). Much effort has been made to subdivide these tumors based on which of the above listed elements is most prominent. Several reviews however are unable to demonstrate any consistant relationship between the morphologic subtype and the clinical behavior of the neoplasm (JENSEN et al. 1976; OBERMAN and RICE 1976).

The derivation from the olfactory epithelium accounts for the common location in the antero-superior portion of the nasal cavity. From this site the tumor can invade the cribriform plate and extend intracranially. Like tumors of the respiratory epithelium, it can also invade the orbit and extend through the nasal cavity to involve adjacent sinuses. KADISH et al. (1976) have suggested the following staging system which predicts the outcome of therapy and has thus gained acceptance. Stage A disease confined to the nasal cavity; stage B disease confined to the nasal cavity and one or more paranasal sinuses; stage C disease extending beyond the nasal cavity or paranasal sinuses.

Because of the scarcity of material, no one author has compiled a large personal series. Collecting case reports from the literature has allowed some principles to be delineated. Esthesioneuroblastoma readily invades adjacent structures and metastasizes to nodal and distant sites. Therefore, therapy must be aggressive. Radiosensitivity is variable and unpredictable. This fact not withstanding, there are many reported cases either cured primarily with radiation or salvaged after post-operative recurrence. ELKON et al. (1979) culled 97 cases from 13 series reported in the literature. They conclude that radiation was as good as surgery (each being as good as combined therapy) for the initial therapeutic attack on stage A and B cases. Although the initial recur-

rence rate in stage A and B trated by any single modality or combination was 50%, ultimate disease free status after salvage therapy was obtained in 23/24 patients. Determinate 5 years survivals were 90% for stage A and 70% for stage B.

Patients with stage C disease fared better when radiation and surgery were combined. All survivors in this group were stage C due to orbital involvement or neck node involvement indicating the grave prognosis for those with invasion of cribriform plate or cranium. Determinate 5 year survival was 47%. Despite this data suggesting the efficacy of radiation therapy, the majority of authors recommend either initial surgery or combined therapy. Most suggest pre-operative radiation (KADISH et al. 1976; BAILEY and BARTON 1975; JENSEN et al. 1976).

Lymph nodes are a site of recurrence in 10% of cases. Therapy for the clinically uninvolved neck is not recommended since salvage therapy, consisting of radiation followed by radical neck dissection, is very effective. The major cause of failure is an inability to control the local tumor. Radiation technique and dosage should be selected in accordance with the recommendations for therapy of respiratory epithelial tumor. Greater than 75% of the failures are apparent by 3 years. Patients must be followed closely.

11.7.2 Lymphoma of Nose and Sinuses

Malignant lymphomas are the most common nonepithelial cancers arising in the nose and sinuses (FU and PERZIN 1979) comprising about 8% of all cancers in this region (SOFFERMAN and CUMMINGS 1975). The majority of tumors are histologically of diffuse pattern with large cells (diffuse histiocytic lymphoma or reticulum cell sarcoma). Other histologies are seen rarely. Two recent reports document a relatively high proportion of diffuse large cell immunoblastic lymphoma (FRIERSON et al. 1984; ROBBINS et al. 1985).

Clinically, these tumors mimic the more common conditions of sinusitis, granulomatous disease, and carcinoma. The diagnosis may be difficult to determine unless a sizeable amount of tissue is obtained and transported to the lab without delay. DUNCAVAGE et al. (1983) found initial histology to be indeterminate in 6/15 patients. Four patients required re-biopsy for diagnosis while the lymphomatous nature of the other two patients was subsequently discovered by cell surface marker studies.

In addition to the usual work-up for a sinonasal tumor, the following studies are recommended to rule out systemic involvement: 1) bone marrow aspirates and biopsies, 2) CT of the abdomen with lymphangiogram if negative, and 3) lumbar puncture for CSF cytology. Most patients will be found to have disease localized to the head and neck region. Of these patients, greater than 85% will have local disease in the sinuses only, ie. Ann Arbor stage IE (ROBBINS et al. 1985). Two recent reports have applied to lymphomas the criteria used by the American Joint Commission for epithelial tumors of the maxillary antrum (ROBBINS et al. 1985; JACOBS and HOPPE 1985). ROBBINS found 66% of cases in the T_3 and T_4 categories while JACOBS and HOPPE reported 75% of their series with these T-stages. Apparently this disease presents with bulky, locally invasive lesions usually without lymph node spread.

11.7.3 Melanoma

Melanomas may arise from the epithelium of the nasal passages. A review by BERTHELSON et al. (1984) quotes in incidence of 1 case in every thousand melanomas. The nasal cavity is the most common site with sinus origin being extremely rare. Thirtythree of 36 patients in the series of LUND (1982) arose from the nasal cavity while 2 were in the ethmoids and 1 in the maxillary sinus. As with melanomas in other sites, the natural history of the tumor and its response to therapy are highly unpredictable. Some patients die of fulminant disease in 3 or 4 months while others will have long dormant periods after initial therapy followed by recurrence up to 20 years later. This fact is reflected in the graphic plot of survival data which shows a continuous downward curve indicating a constant risk of death from disease at all time intervals subsequent to diagnosis.

While optimal therapy has not been defined, the unpredictable radiosensitivity of these lesions has caused most clinicians to elect surgery as the primary modality. Radiation is added in the event of inadequate surgical margins or as a salvage therapy. Although local control is a problem, the cause of death in 22/27 patients in LUND's series was melanomatosis. This fact should not dissuade the physician from recommending aggressive local therapy in that patients with known lung metastases have been followed from five to seven years (BERTHELSON et al. 1984).

11.7.4 Sarcomas

A variety of sarcomas arise from the nasal passages. Fibrosarcomas have the best prognosis – especially if low grade. These lesions can be controlled with large bloc resections. Further resection rather than radiotherapy is encouraged for patients with positive margins or recurrent disease (FU and PERZIN 1976 B).

Leiomyosarcomas, rhabdomyosarcomas, and osteogenic sarcomas tend to infiltrate extensively and metastasize rapidly and are therefore associated with a poor prognosis. Rhabdomyosarcoma is most frequently diagnosed in the first decade of life. They are also unusual in their propensity for lymph node metastases. The sarcoma botryoides subtype may have a better prognosis than the more common embryonal type. Leiomyosarcomas metastasize systemically at an early stage. Despite this, most patients die with some component of local disease. A combination of surgery and radiotherapy is the treatment most often advocated (FU and PERZIN 1975; 1976 A).

11.7.5 Lethal Midline Granuloma

Lethal midline granuloma (LMG) is a clinical descriptive term for a variety of conditions causing ulceration, necrosis and destruction of the nose and sinuses. These conditions include syphilis, tuberculosis, leprosy, various fungal and bacterial infections, diabetes, pemphigus, inflammatory and neoplastic disease. FAUCI et al. (1976) divide the inflammatory class of LMG into two major divisions, Wegener's granulomatosis and idiopathic midline granuloma. The former is a systemic vasculitis while the latter is localized to the sinonasal region only. They treated a series of 10 patients with midline granuloma using radiation doses of 5000 cGy to large fields. Seven patients enjoyed long-term remissions in what had previously been a uniformly fatal disease.

Among the neoplastic causes of LMG, malignant midline reticulosis (MMR) deserves further mention. This is a polymorphic lymphoproliferative disease. Histologically, a large proportion of normal appearing lymphocytes, plasma cells, and histiocytes are seen, throughout which are interspersed atypical, pleomorphic lymphocytes (FU and PERZIN 1976).

The malignant lymphocytes have been studied by ISHII et al. (1982) who demonstrated an identical cell surface phenotype to that of peripheral T-cells.

Whereas the more common lymphomata of the sinonasal region are easily controlled locally with radiation, Fu and PERZIN (1979) experienced local failures in all of their patients thus treated. In their review of the literature, however, they point out that most reported results were superior to their own. In the absence of much information on this topic, doses of 5000-6000 cGy are recommended.

Acknowledgement. The author wishes to acknowledge the work of Ms. Sandie Wnek and Ms. Beverly Kendall in the typing and preparation of the manuscript.

References

AJCC (1983) Manual for staging of cancer, 2nd ed J.B. Lippincott

Akanuma A (1977) High-dose rate intracavitary radiation therapy for advanced head and neck tumors. Cancer 40: 1071-1076

Amendola BE, Eisert D, Hazra TA, King ER (1981) Carcinoma of the maxillary antrum: surgery or radiation therapy? Int J Rad Onc Biol Phys 7: 743-746

Badib AO, Kurohara SS, Webster JH, Shedd DP (1969) Treatment of cancer of the nasal cavity. Am J Roentgenol 106: 824-830

Bailey BJ, Barton S (1975) Olfactory neuroblastoma. Arch Otolaryngol 101: 1-5

Barton RT (1980) Management of carcinoma arising in the lateral nasal wall. Arch Otolaryngol 106: 685-687

Bataini JP, Ennuyer A (1971) Advanced carcinoma of the maxillary antrum treated by cobalt teletherapy and electron beam irradiation. Br J Radiol 44: 590-598

Beatty CW, Pearson BW, Kern EB (1982) Carcinoma of the nasal septum: experience with 85 cases. Otolaryngol Head Neck Surg 90: 90-94

Berthelsen A, Anderson AP, Jensen S, Hansen HS (1984) Melanomas of the mucosa in the oral cavity and the upper respiratory passages. Cancer 54: 907-912

Blackstein ME, Chapnik JS (1976) Chemotherapy and palliative therapy in malignant disease of the maxillary sinus. Otolaryngol Clin North Am 9: 291-300

Boone MLM, Harle TS, Higholt HW, Fletcher GH (1968) Malignant disease of the paranasal sinuses and nasal cavity. Am J Roentgenol 102: 3, 627-636

Bosch A, Vallecillo L, Frias Z (1976) Cancer of the nasal cavity. Cancer 37: 1458-1463

Bush SE, Bagshaw MA (1982) Carcinoma of the paranasal sinuses. Cancer 50: 154-158

Catterall M, Blake PR, Rampling RP (1984) Fast neutron treatment as an alternative to radical surgery for malignant tumors of the facial area. Br Med J 289: 1653-1655

Chan RC, Shukovsky LJ (1976) Effects of irradiation on the eye. Radiology 120: 673-675

Chassagne D, Wilson JF (1984, p.3 "1974") Brachytherapy of carcinoma of the nasal vestibule. Int J Rad Onc Biol Phys 10: 761

Chaudhry AP, Gorlin RJ, Mosser DG (1960) Carcinoma of the antrum: a clinical and histopathologic study. Oral Surg 13: 269-281

Cheng VST, Wang CC (1977) Carcinomas of the paranasal sinuses. Cancer 40: 3038-3041

Cheng VST, Oral K, Aramamy MA (1982) The use of acrylic resin oral prosthesis in radiation therapy of oral cavity and paranasal sinus cancer. Int J Rad Onc Biol Phys 8: 1245-1250

Chung CT, Rabuzzi DD, Sagerman RH, King GA, Gacek RR (1980) Radiotherapy for carcinoma of the nasal cavity. Arch Otolaryngol 106: 763-766

Coia LR, Fazekas JT, Kramer S (1980) Postirradiation sarcoma of the head and neck. Cancer 46: 1982-1985

Cruz AB, McInnis WD, Aust JB (1974) Triple drug intra-arterial infusion combined with x-ray therapy and surgery for head and neck cancer. Am J of Surg 128: 573-579

Del Regato JA, Vuksanovic M (1962 p.6 "1961") Radiotherapy of carcinomas of the skin overlying the cartilages of the nose and ear. Radiology 79: 203-208

Deutch M, Oral K, Aramany MA (1981) Silicone radioactive seed carrier for nasal neoplasms. J Prosthet Dent 46: 88-90

Duncavage JA, Campbell BH, Kun LE, Toohill RJ, Hanson GA, Hansen RM, Malin TC (1983) Diagnosis of malignant lymphomas of the nasal cavity, paranasal sinuses and nasopharynx. Laryngoscope 93: 1276-1280

Elkon D, Hightower SI, Lim ML, Cantrell RW, Constable WC (1979) Esthesioneuroblastoma. Cancer 44: 1087-1094

Ellingwood KE, Million RR (1979) Cancer of the nasal cavity and ethmoid/sphenoid sinuses. Cancer 43: 1517-1526

Fauci AS, Johnson RE, Wolff SM (1976) Radiation therapy of midline granuloma. Annals Internal Med 84: 2, 140-147

Frazell EL, Lewis JS (1963) Cancer of the nasal cavity and accessory sinuses. Cancer 16: 1293-1301

Frich JC Jr (1982) Treatment of advanced squamous carinoma of the maxillary sinus by irradiation. Int J Rad Onc Biol Phys 8: 1453-1459

Frierson HF Jr, Mills SE, Innes DJ Jr (1984) Non-Hodgkins lymphomas of the sinonasal region: histologic subtypes and their clinicopathologic features. AJCP 721-727

Fu YS, Perzin KH (1975) Nonepithelial tumors of the nasal cavity, paranasal sinuses, and nasopharynx: a clinicopathologic study IV. smooth muscle tumors (leiomyoma, leiomyosarcoma). Cancer 35: 1300-1308

Fu YS, Perzin KH (1976A) Nonepithelial tumors of the nasal cavity, paranasal sinuses and nasopharynx: a clinicopathologic study. V. skeletal muscle tumors (rhabodomyoma and rhabdomyosarcoma). Cancer 37: 364-376

Fu YS, Perzin KH (1976B) Nonepithelial tumors of the nasal cavity paranasal sinuses, and nasopharynx: a clinicopathologic study VI. fibrous tissue tumors (fibroma, fibromatosis, fibrosarcoma). Cancer 37: 2912-2928

Fu YS, Perzin KH (1979) Nonepithelial tumors of the nasal cavity, paranasal sinuses and nasopharynx. A clinicopathologic study. X. malignant lymphomas. Cancer 43: 611-621

Galbraith DM, Aget H, Leung PMK, Rider WD (1985) Eye sparing in high energy x-ray beams. Int J Rad Onc Biol Phys 11: 591-595

Ghalichebaf et al. (1984) p 36

Goepfert H, Jesse RH, Lindberg RD (1973) Arterial infusion and radiation therapy in the treatment of advanced cancer of the nasal cavity and paranasal sinuses. Am J Surg 126: 464-468

Goepfert H, Guillamondegui OM, Jesse RH, Lindberg RD (1974) Squamous cell carcinoma of nasal vestibule. Arch Otolaryngol 100: 8-10

Harrison DFN (1972) The natural history of some cancers affecting the head and neck. J Laryngol Otol 86: 1189-1202

Harrison DFN (1978) Critical look at the classification of maxillary sinus carcinomata. Ann Otolaryngol 87: 3-9

Haynes WD, Tapley NV (1973) Radiation treatment of carcinoma of the nasal vestibule. Am J Roentgenol 120: 3, 595–602

Hintz BL, Kagan AR, Wollin M, Milles J, Chan PM, Nussbaum H, Rao AR, Ryoo MC (1984) Reassessment of technical and biological factors in paranasal sinus carcinoma. J Surg Onc 27: 59–66

Hopkin N, Mc Nicoll W, Dalley VM, Shaw HJ (1984) Cancer of the paranasal sinuses and nasal cavities. J Laryngol Otol 98: 585–595

"Ishii" et al. (1982

Ishll Y, Yamanaka N, Ogawa K, Yoshida Y, Takami T, Matsuura A, Isago H, Kataura A, Kikuchi K (1982) Nasal T-cell lymphoma as a type of so-called "lethal midline granuloma". Cancer 50: 2336–2344

Jackson RT, Fitz-Hugh GS, Constable WC (1977) Malignant neoplasms of the nasal cavities and paranasal sinuses: (a retrospective study). Laryngoscope 87: 726–736

Jacobs C, Hoppe RT (1985) Non-Hodgkins lymphomas of head and neck extranodal sites. Int J Rad Onc Biol Phys 11: 357–364

Jeans WD, Gilani S, Bullimore J (1982) The effect of CT scanning on staging of tumors of the paranasal sinuses. Clin Radiol 33: 173–179

Jensen KJ, Elbrond O, Lund C (1976) Olfactory esthesioneuroblastoma. J Laryngol Otol 90: 1007–1013

Jesse RH (1965) Preoperative versus postoperative radiation in the treatment of squamous carcinoma of the paranasal sinuses. Am J Surg 110: 552–556

Jing BS, Goepfert H, Close LG (1978) Computerized tomography of paranasal sinus neoplasms. Laryngoscope 88: 1485–1503

Kadish S, Goodman M, Wang CC (1976) Olfactory neuroblastoma: a clinical analysis of 17 cases. Cancer 37: 1571–1576

Kent SE, Majumdar B (1984) Metastases of malignant disease of the nasal cavity and paranasal sinuses. J Laryngol Otol 98: 471–474

Ketcham AS, Wilkins RH, Van Buren JM, Smith RR (1963) A combined intracranial facial approach to the paranasal sinuses. Am J Surg 106: 698–703

Ketcham AS, Chretien PB, Van Buren JM, Hoye RC, Beazley RM, Herdt JR (1973) The ethmoid sinuses: a re-evaluation of surgical resection. Am J Surg 126: 469–476

Lederman M (1969) Cancer of the upper jaw and nasal chambers. Proc R Soc Med 62: 65–72

Lederman M (1970) Tumors of the upper jaw: natural history and treatment. J Laryngol 84: 369–370

Lee F, Ogura JH (1981) Maxillary sinus carcinoma. Laryngol 91: 133–139

LeLiever WC, Bailey BJ, Griffiths C (1984) Carcinoma of the nasal septum. Arch Otolaryngol 110: 748–751

Lewis JS, Castro EB (1972) Cancer of the nasal cavity and paranasal sinuses. J Laryngol 86: 255–262

Lund VJ (1982) Malignant melanoma of the nasal cavity and paranasal sinuses. J Laryngol Otol 96: 347–355

Lund VJ, Howard DJ, Lloyd GAS (1983) CT evaluation of paranasal sinus tumours for cranio-fascial resection. Br J Radiol 56: 439–446

Mak ACA, Van Andel JG, Van Woerkom-Eijkenboom WMH (1980) Radiation therapy of carcinoma of the nasal vestibule. Eur J Cancer 16: 81–85

McGuirt WF, Thompson JN (1984) Surgical approaches to malignant tumors of the nasal septum. Laryngoscope 94: 1045–1049

McNicoll W, Hopkin N, Dalley VM, Shaw HJ (1984) Cancer of the paranasal sinuses and nasal cavities part II results of treatment. J Laryngol Otol 98: 707–718

Mendenhall NP, Parsons JT, Cassisi NJ, Million RR (1984) Carcinoma of the nasal vestibule. Int J Rad Onc Biol Phys 10: 627–637

Morita K, Kawabe Y (1979) Late effects on the eye of conformation radiotherapy for carcinoma of the paranasal sinuses and nasal. Radiology 130: 227–232

Moseley HS, Thomas LR, Everts EC, Stevens KR, Ireland KM (1981) Advanced squamous cell carcinoma of the maxillary sinus. Am J Surg 141: 522–525

Nakissa N, Rubin P, Strohl R, Keyes H (1983) Ocular and orbital complications following radiation therapy paranasal sinus malignancies and review of literature. Cancer 51: 980–986

Oberman HA, Rice DH (1976) Olfactory neuroblastomas: a clinicopathologic study. Cancer 38: 2494–2502

Ohngren LG (1933) Malignant tumors of the maxillo-ethmoidal region. Acta Otolaryngol (Suppl) 19

Parsons JT, Fitzgerald CR, Hood CI, Ellingwood KE, Bova FJ, Million RM (1983) The effects of irradiation of the eye and optic nerve. Am J Rad Onc Biol Phys 9: 609–622

Pope TH (1978) Surgical approach to tumors of the nasal cavity. Laryngol 88: 1743–1748

Redmond CK, Sass RE, Roush GC (1982) Nasal cavity and paranasal sinuses. In: Schottenfeld D, Fraumeni JF (eds) Cancer epidemiology and prevention. W. B. Saunders Company, Philadelphia, p 519–535

Robbins KT, Fuller LM, Vlasak M, Osborne B, Jing BS, Velasquez WS, Sullivan JA (1985) Primary lymphomas of the nasal cavity and paranasal sinuses. Cancer 56: 814–819

Robin PE, Powell DJ (1980) Regional node involvement and distant metastases in carcinoma of the nasal cavity and paranasal sinuses. J Laryngol Otol 94: 301–309

Robin PE, Powell DJ (1981) Diagnostic errors in cancers of the nasal cavity and paranasal sinuses. Arch Otolaryngol 107: 138–140

Rowe LD, Lane R, Snow JB Jr (1980) Adenocarcinoma of the ethmoid following radiotherapy for bilateral retinoblastoma. Laryngoscope 90: 61–69

Rubin P (1972) Cancer of the head and neck. JAMA 219: 3, 336–353

Sakai S, Fuchihata H, Hamasaki (1976) Treatment policy for maxillary sinus carcinoma. Acta Otolaryngol 82: 172–181

Sakai S, Hohki A, Fuchihata H, Tanaka Y (1983) Multidisciplinary treatment of maxillary sinus carcinoma. Cancer 52: 1360–1364

Samaan NA, Vieto R, Schultz PN, Maor M, Meoz RT, Sampiere VA, Cangir A, Ried HL, Jesse RH (1982) Hypothalamic, pituitary and thyroid dysfunction after radiotherapy to the head and neck. Int J Rad Onc Biol Phys 8: 1857–1867

Sato Y, Morita M, Takahashi H, Watanabe N, Kirikae I (1970) Combined surgery, radiotherapy and regional chemotherapy in carcinoma of the paranasal sinuses. Cancer 25: 571–579

Schaefer SD, Hill GD (1980) Epidermoid carcinoma of the nasal vestibule current treatment evaluation. Laryngol 90: 1631–1635

Shafir M, Raventos E (1983) Combined multimodality (surgery, radiotherapy, intra-arterial chemotherapy) treatment of advanced carcinoma of paranasal sinuses. Rec Results Cancer 86: 165–168

Shibuya H, Horiuchi J, Suzuki S, Shioda S, Enomoto S (1984) Maxillary sinus carcinoma: results of radiation therapy. Int J Rad Onc Biol Phys 10: 1021–1026

Shukovsky LJ, Fletcher GH (1972) Retinal and optic nerve complications in a high-dose irradiation technique of ethmoid sinus and nasal cavity. Radiology 104: 629-634

Sofferman RA, Cummings CW (1975) Malignant lymphoma of the paranasal sinuses. Arch Otolaryngol 101: 287-292

Steeves RA, Bataini JP (1981) Neoplasms induced by megavoltage radiation in the head and neck region. Cancer 47: 1770-1774

Tabb H, Barranco SL (1971) Cancer of the maxillary sinus. Laryngoscope 81: 818-827

Terz JJ, Young HF, Lawrence W Jr (1980) Combined craniofacial resection for locally advanced carcinoma of the head and neck. Am J Surg 140: 618-624

Wang CC (1976) Treatment of carcinoma of the nasal vestibule by irradiation. Cancer 38: 100-106

Wara WM, Irvine AR, Neger RE, Howes EL, Phillips TL (1979) Radiation retinopathy. Int J Rad Oncol Biol Phys 5: 81-83

Weimert TA, Batsakis JG, Rice DH (1978) Carcinomas of the nasal septum. J Laryngol Otol 92: 209-213

Weymuller EA Jr, Reardon EJ, Nash D (1980) A comparison of treatment modalities in carcinoma of the maxillary antrum. Arch Otolaryngol 106: 625-629

Young JR (1979) Malignant tumors of the nasal septum. J Laryngol Otol 93: 817-832

12 Chemodectomas

LAIRD E. OLSON and JAMES D. COX

12.1 Chemodectomas (Non-Chromaffin Paraganglioma)

12.1.1 Overview

Small collections of neuroepithelial cells are distributed widely throughout the body. When they are identifible grossly, they are called paraganglia. Those which do not secrete catecholamines, and thus are non-chromaffin, are related to the parasympathetic nervous system. Tumors which develop from these paraganglia are most frequently found in the temporal bone or the cervical region. The term "chemodectoma" has been applied to these tumors because of their lcoation in the vicinity of the carotid body, which is known chemoreceptor sensitive to pH, and concentrations of oxygen and car-

bon dioxide. Since only the tumors which arise in the vicinity of the aortic body or carotid body can be considered chemodectomas, the more general term, non-chromaffin paraganglioma, is preferred. However, much of the literature concerning these tumors uses "chemodectoma" in a broad sense, and the following discussion will use this term as synonymous with non-chromaffin paraganglioma.

Chemodectomas have been found in a wide variety of sites including (in decreasing order of frequency) the carotid body, glomus jugulare and tympanicum, intravagale, Zuckerkandl's body, aortic body, lung, larynx, retroperitoneum, orbit, tongue, urinary bladder, gallbladder, nasal cavity, heart, thyroid, and central nervous system (pineal region, parasellar region, and cauda equina) (ROSAI 1981).

Although histologically benign and very slowly growing, they may be locally destructive. They also metastasize occasionally. For these reasons, they should be considered together with the malignant tumors, of which they comprise approximately 0.3% (JACKSON and KOSHIBA 1974). Their clinical presentation, appropriate diagnostic evaluation and treatment, as well as prognosis, depend upon the site of origin.

12.1.2 Pathology

Histologically, chemodectomas closely resemble the glomus bodies from which they arise. There is marked capillary vascularity with nests of prominent epithelial cells (chief cells) within a sparse fibrous stroma. Mitoses are rare. In contrast to the adrenal medulla, the tumors do not stain with chromaffin, hence the name non-chromaffin paraganglioma. This was at first thought to indicate an absence of catecholamine secretion. More recent ultrastructural studies (CAPPS 1957; COLE 1979), as well as case reports of chemodectomas diagnosed in association with the clinical and biochemical signs of pheochromocytoma have shown, however, that they do have the potential for catecholamine secretion (DUKE et al. 1964; LEVIT et al. 1976). This

LAIRD E. OLSON, M.D., Assistant Professor, Department of Radiation Oncology, Medical College of Wisconsin, 8700 W. Wisconsin Avenue, Milwaukee, WI, 53226, USA

JAMES D. COX, M.D., Professor and Chairman, Department of Radiation Oncology, Columbia Presbyterian Medical Center, 622 W. 168th Street, New York, NY 10032, USA

aspect of their pathophysiology is poorly under-stood and is still under investigation.

12.2 Chemodectomas Arising in Temporal Bone Structures

In 1840, VALENTIN described a structure on the tym-panic nerve resembling a ganglion (VALENTIN 1840). In 1878, it was found by KRAUSE to be a vascular formation rather than a ganglion, closely resem-bling the carotid body histologically (KRAUSE 1878). For reasons which are probably due at least in part to their very small size (0.1 to 0.5 mm), the very ex-istence of these structures was questioned for many years. The careful temporal bone dissections of Guild in the early 1940's (GUILD 1941, 1953) how-ever, clearly established both their existence and an-atomical distribution. He noted that slightly more

Fig. 12-1. Distribution of paraganglia in relation to nerves, vessels, and temporal bone

than half of these paraganglia were found in the ad-ventitia of the dome of the jugular bulb, about one-fourth in the mucosa overlying the cochlear prom-ontory, one-fifth in the bony canal of the nerve of Jacobson, and a few along the course of the nerve of Arnold. Tumors arising from the paraganglia within the temporal bone were first reported by Rosenwasser in 1945 (ROSENWASSER 1951). Since that time, multiple reports have been published de-scribing their pathology, clinical presentation, surgi-cal and radiotherapeutic management, and out-come of treatment.

12.2.1 Anatomy

The distribution of glomus bodies within the tem-poral bone as well as their number varies between individuals. The most common location, i.e. in the adventitia of the superior bulb of the internal jugu-lar vein, along the course of the nerve of Jacobson (tympanic branch of IX), mucosa of the cochlear promontory, and nerve of Arnold (auricular branch

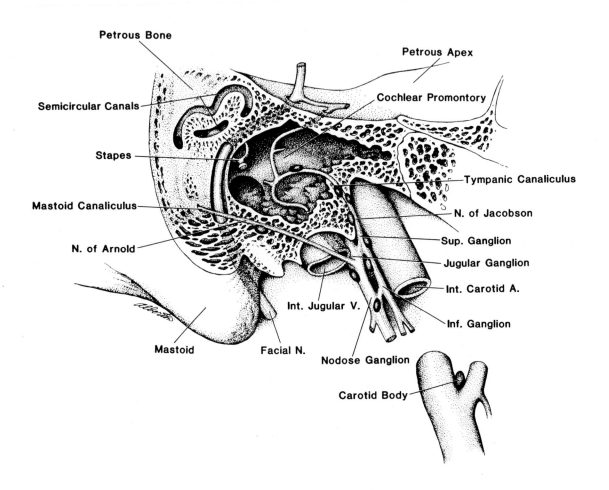

of X) are illustrated in Figure 12-1. Tumors arising in the middle ear are disgnated glomus tympanicum. Those arising from the jugular bulb are called glomus jugulare tumors. The intimate relationship of glomus jugulare tumors to the cranial nerves exiting the jugulare foramena (IX–XI) accounts for the frequent presence of cranial nerve palsies at presentation. Proximity to the anterior condylar foramen accounts for the occasional involvement of the XIIth nerve. Glomus tympanicum tumors may involve the tympanic membrane, ossicles, external auditory canal, labyrinth and mastoid, as well as the nerves of Jacobson and Arnold.

12.2.2 Patterns of Spread

Chemodectomas of the temporal bone are very invasive locally as shown in Fig. 12-2. They may extend superiorly to involve the petrous portion of the temporal bone, labyrinth, middle and posterior cranial fossa. They are thus capable of producing a great deal of erosion and destruction of bone. They may extend medially to involve the internal auditory canal and the VIIth and VIIIth cranial nerves. Laterally they may extend through the tympanic membrane to appear as masses in the external auditory canal. Glomus jugulare tumors may produce

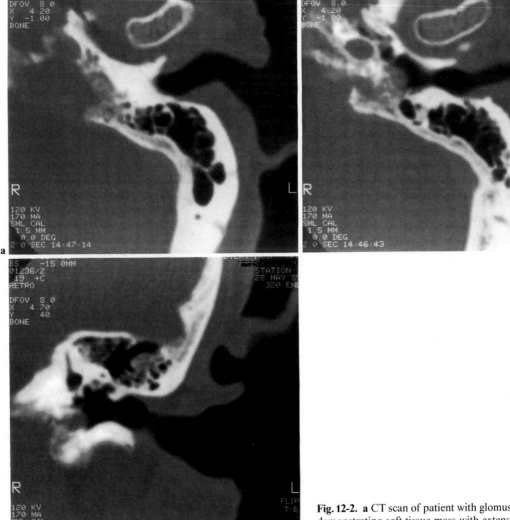

Fig. 12-2. a CT scan of patient with glomus jugulare tumor demonstrating soft tissue mass with extensive associated bone destruction *(axial plane)*. **b,c** CT of same patient. Note extension of tumor into middle ear *(axial plane)*

various cranial nerve syndromes by involvement of the jugular and anterior condylar foramina as well as intracranial extension. Distant metastases are very rare but have been reported (ROSENWASSER 1958). These may involve lung or bone. Lymphatic metastases are rare although neck masses can be caused by direct extension of the primary tumor. A staging classification has been proposed by McCabe and Fletcher (MCCABE and FLETCHER 1979) dividing chemodectomas of the temporal bone into three groups based on clinical and radiographic findings.

12.2.3 Clinical Presentation

Temporal bone paragangliomas show a female to male preponderance of approximately 5 to 1 (AL-FORD and GUILFORD 1953) in contrast to carotid body tumors which show roughly equal female to male incidence. Most patients are middle aged, with the average being about 55 years. The age range tends to be quite broad in most series, however. They are unusual in patients younger than 20 and can occur in patients in their 80's. Symptoms are typically longstanding and of insidious onset. The average duration of symptoms prior to diagnosis is about 3 years (SPECTOR et al. 1975). Signs and symptoms at presentation depend upon the location of the tumor. Tumors arising in the middle ear (glomus tympanicum) are accompanied by progressive hearing loss, usually conductive, in about 90% of all cases (ALFORD and GUILFORD 1953). Pulsatile tinnitus is also frequently present. Vertigo may occur. As the tumor enlarges, it may become visible as a bluish red mass bulging behind the tympanic membrane. An ear speculum fitted with an air bulb will sometimes allow the examiner to see blanching of the tumor and increased then diminished pulsation as the pressure is increased. The pulsations return when the pressure is released (Brown's sign). Eventually these tumors will grow through the tympanic membrane and a mass will become apparent in the external ear. Pain and otorrhea may accompany this. The danger of an erroneous diagnosis of chronic suppurative otitis exists. Peripheral facial nerve paralysis is not uncommon.

Tumors arising from the jugular bulb (glomus jugulare tumors) are more likely to cause extensive bone destruction and to be associated with multiple cranial nerve palses or even intracranial extension at presentation. The latter carries a grave prognosis. As previously mentioned, either the jugular foramen syndrome or other patterns of cranial nerve in-

volvement such as the Coloet-Sicard Syndrome (IX through XII) may occur. Paralysis of cranial nerves V through XII may occur with extension of tumor to the posterior cranial fossa. Ataxia and pulsatile occipital headache are also sometimes seen. Cranial nerves III through VI can be involved with tumor extension to the middle cranial fossa. Retro-orbital pain may also occur. Paroxysmal hypertension may occur rarely and may be associated with elevated levels of vanillyl mandelic acid (VMA) and methoxy hydroxy-phenyl-ethylene glycol (MHPG) in the urine.

12.2.4 Diagnosis and Evaluation

The aural and neurologic symptoms of chemodectomas of the temporal bone can also occur in a host of other inflammatory, infectious or neoplastic diseases. The differential diagnosis must include chronic serous otitis, mastoiditis, aural polyps, cholesteatoma, carcinoma of the middle ear or nasopharynx, metastatic carcinoma and acoustic neuroma. Because of the extreme vascularity of these tumors, biopsy may be frought with hazard. It may also result in the erroneous diagnosis of inflammatory granulation tissue if the biopsy is too superficial, as sometimes occurs with tumors extending into the external auditory canal, which mimic aural polyps. The epithelioid cells may shrink and become inconspicuous in poorly preserved specimens leading to a false diagnosis of vascular tumor or inflammatory granulation tissue (CAPPS 1957).

Fortunately, angiography is usually diagnostic and may obviate biopsy in many cases – see for example Fig. 12-3. It will also delineate tumor extent as well as blood supply (usually from the ascending pharyngeal branch of the external carotid artery). This information is essential if surgical resection is contemplated and is also necessary for treatment planning if radiation therapy is to be employed either primarily or in conjunction with surgery. Plain roentgenograms will frequently show clouding of the mastoid air cells. Enlargement of the jugular foramen may also be apparent. Tomograms of the temporal bone are required to assess the extent of bone destruction. Retrograde jugular venography may be useful since the tumor does have a propensity to invade the jugular vein directly. Similar information may be provided by the venous phase of the arteriogram. Computed tomography may be useful for delineation of the extent of the tumor involvement, especially intracranially. CT scanning with contrast enhancement contributes information

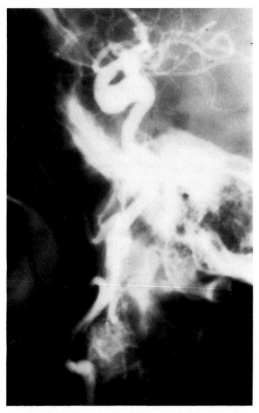

Fig. 12-3. Arteriogram of patient with glomus vagale tumor demonstrating marked vascularity typical of chemodectomas

about the soft tissue component of the tumor which may be useful for decisions regarding resectability and radiation therapy treatment planning. Angiography is desirable if a surgical procedure is planned, but CT may be sufficient if radiation therapy is to be definitive treatment. The role of digital angiography will probably increase.

12.2.5 Treatment of Chemodectomas of Temporal Bone

12.2.5.1 Selection of Treatment Modality

The very long natural history of these tumors and the lack of uniform criteria for measuring the success of treatment have led to considerable controversy over their optimum management. Patients may live with slowly progressive tumor for many years and die of other causes. Only a small proportion of patients actually die from their tumors, although mortality rates as high as 9% have been reported. Crude survival is therefore not a useful endpoint. Serial angiography and other radiograph-

ic studies may show apparent persistence of tumor for long periods of time. This has sometimes been used as an argument against the efficacy of radiation therapy (SPECTOR et al. 1975; 1976). The persistence of radiographic findings, however, does not indicate tumor activity, since they are not predictive of clinical recurrence (MARUYAMA 1972). The presence of morphologically intact tumor cells on serial biopsy likewise provides no evidence of tumor viability (SUIT and GALLAGHER 1964). Since the vast majority of these patients will eventually die of causes other than chemodectoma, whether they are treated by surgery, radiation therapy or a combination of the two, relief of symptoms with absence of clinically apparent progression during the patient's lifetime would appear to constitute a more practical definition of successful treatment. By this measure there is no question that radiation therapy is highly effective in the treatment of these tumors (COLE 1979; CUMMINGS et al. 1984; DICKENS et al. 1982; HATFIELD et al. 1972; HUDGINS 1972; KIM et al. 1980; MARUYAMA 1972; NEWMAN et al. 1973; REDDY et al. 1983; SIMKO et al. 1984; SPECTOR et al. 1976; TIDWELL and MONTAGUE 1975; WANG 1980).

It is clear that radiation therapy is the treatment of choice for advanced unresectable tumors. Its effectiveness in such cases has been clearly shown (HUDGINS 1972). This, combined with the high rates of disease control which have been observed following radiation therapy alone for less advanced tumors (COLE 1979; CUMMINGS et al. 1984; DICKENS et al. 1982; HATFIELD et al. 1972; KIM et al. 1980; MARUYAMA 1972; NEWMAN et al. 1973; REDDY et al. 1983; SIMKO et al. 1978; TIDWELL and MONTAGUE 1975; WANG 1980) has led some to advocate irradiation alone as the treatment of choice for all but the earliest ones (COLE 1977; DICKENS et al. 1982; MILLION and CASSISI 1984).

General agreement exists that early tumors confined to the middle ear should be resected (BATSAKIS 1979). Surgical techniques are still being developed and described for resecting even the most advanced tumors, including those with intracranial extension (BRAMMER et al. 1984). Potential complications of surgery include fatality due to hemorrhage, hemi-paresis, cerebrospinal fluid leak, injury to cranial nerves, and hearing loss. In view of the indolent nature of these tumors, caution should be exercised against giving excessively aggressive treatment, either surgical or radiotherapeutic. If resection is attempted and is incomplete, it should be followed by immediate postoperative irradiation. This will almost completely eliminate the risk of recurrence. If for some reason this is not done, radiation therapy will still frequently be the treatment of choice following post surgical recurrence.

12.2.5.2 Techniques of Irradiation

Superoinferior 45 degree wedge portals are generally best for encompassing the tumor with adequate margins while limiting the dose to the brain stem. Anterior and posterior wedged portals may sometimes be used, but exit dose to the contralateral eye may preclude this. A direct lateral beam may be added to the wedge pair in order to extend the high dose volume medially if this is desired. Cobalt 60, 4 or 6 MV x-rays should be used. A total dose of 4000 to 4500 cGy should be given at the rate of 180-200 cGy per day. Care should be taken to include the entire tumor volume as demonstrated on angiography and contrast-enhanced CT scanning with adequate margins. For more advanced tumors with extension toward the midline, such as those with intracranial involvement, parallel opposed lateral fields may be required. These may be weighted toward the site of the tumor in the ratio 2:1 or 3:2. Isodose distributions should be obtained and care taken to assure that the dose to the tumor is adequate and that the dose to the brain stem is acceptable.

12.2.5.3 Treatment Results

As previously stated, the measure of successful radiation therapy is relief of symptoms and absence of disease progression. Lengthy followup is necessary although post-irradiation recurrences usually take place within 3 years, in contrast to post surgical recurrrences which are not uncommon after 10 and 15 years. Numerous reports now indicate that control rates approaching 100% may be obtained with radiation therapy, whether it is used as the sole modality, for postoperative recurrence, or in the immediate postoperative period for known residual disease (BATSAKIS 1979). This is in contrast to results with surgery alone in which recurrence rates of 20 to 70% are reported for glomus jugulare tumors (HATFIELD et al. 1972; REDDY et al. 1983; SPECTOR et al. 1976). Recurrence rates for early tumors of the middle ear are much lower, of course. The dose required for permanent control has been well established. The recurrence rate in patients who received 4000 cGy in 4 weeks or higher was only 1.4% in an analysis by Kim of 142 patients so treated (KIM et al. 1980). CUMMINGS et al. report only 3 treatment

failures among 45 patients who received a total dose of 3500 cGy in 15 fractions over 3 weeks (CUMMINGS et al. 1984). The suggest that this is an adequate dose.

A total dose of 5000 cGy in 5 weeks has been advocated for larger, inoperable tumors (KIM et al. 1980; MILLION and CASSISI 1984), although there does not appear to be a great deal of evidence to support the need for a higher dose. Complete relief of pain following irradiation occurs almost invariably (CUMMINGS et al. 1984; HUDGINS 1972). Tinnitus usually abates completely. Some regression of the visible mass is generally apparent by the completion of treatment (CUMMINGS et al. 1984; HUDGINS 1972; KIM et al. 1980; MILLION and CASSISI 1984). Hearing loss may be persistent but rarely is it progressive (CUMMINGS et al. 1984). Cranial nerve palsies may stabilize or improve slightly, but complete recovery is unusual, as is any deterioration following treatment (CUMMINGS et al. 1984; KIM et al. 1980). Complications with properly fractionated irradiation at the doses previously mentioned are extremely rare. Bony sequestrum has sometimes been reported after postoperative irradiation. There are a few reports of brain stem necrosis which occurred many years ago when high doses were given or when large fractions were utilized. There have also been occasional reports of temporal bone necrosis. This is an easily avoidable complication with properly fractionated megavoltage irradiation. The risk of temporal bone necrosis is essentially zero when doses of less than 6500 cGy are given in 6.5 weeks (WANG and DOPPKE 1976). Thus, radiation therapy provides excellent tumor control with only a very small risk of complications when used in the treatment of chemodectomas of the temporal bone.

12.3 Carotid Body Tumors

The carotid body was first described by van Haller in 1743 (VAN HALLER 1945). Tumors of the carotid body are rare. They comprise approximately 0.01% of all malignant tumors (LACK et al. 1977). Nonetheless, the carotid body is the most frequent site of development of chemodectomas: approximately 900 cases have been reported to date (KRUPSKI et al. 1982). In contrast to chemodectomas which arise in the temporal bone, the incidence is nearly equal in men and woman. The average at onset has been reported to be between 41 and 49 years, but the range in age at presentation is very wide (17 to

80 years) (FARR 1980; JAVID et al. 1976; KRUPSKI et al. 1982; LACK et al. 1977). Familial cases are well described although most cases are sporadic. An increased frequency of bilateral tumors has been reported in familial cases, as has a higher frequency of multiple chemodectomas arising in several sites in the same individual. Grufferman et al. (GRUFFERMAN et al. 1980) colllected a total of 88 familial and 835 sporadic cases from the literature: the frequencies of bilateral tumors were 31.8 and 4.4 percent, respectively. An autosomal dominant mode of transmission with incomplete penetrance has been suggested.

The etiology of sporadic carotid body tumors is not known. Hypertrophy of the carotid body has been described in response to chronic hypoxemia, either pathologic or physiologic. Carotid body tumors are more common among populations which dwell at high altitudes (GRUFFERMAN et al. 1980).

Despite their rarity, carotid body tumors have generated an extensive literature, in part, due to the techical challenge which these highly vascular tumors presents to the surgeon, and in part, due to the controversy which exists over the relative merits of surgical resection and radiation therapy in the management of these tumors.

12.3.1 Anatomy

The carotid body is an ovoid structure measuring approximately $5 \times 5 \times 3$ mm lying within the adventitia of the common carotid artery on its posteromedial side. It extends superiorly just beyond the bifurcation of the artery. Its blood supply is predominately from the external carotid artery. Venous return is via the laryngopharyngeal and lingual veins. It derives sensory innervation from the glossopharyngeal nerve.

12.3.2 Patterns of Spread

Carotid body tumors usually grow very slowly. Their rate of growth has been estimated to be approximately 2 cm every 5 years (FARR 1980). The tumor characteristically surrounds and encroaches upon, but does not occlude, the carotid artery. It grows both superiorly and inferiorly along the artery, deriving its blood supply from the vasa vasorum. The tumor may also grow medially and produce a deviation of the pharyngeal wall; this has been observed in approximately half of the cases (FARR 1980). Eventually, the tumor may extend su-

periorly to involve the base of the skull. Metastasis to regional lymph nodes or distant sites is infrequent but the frequency may be underestimated due to insufficient periods of observation.

12.3.3 Clinical Presentation

The average duration of symptoms prior to diagnosis ranges from 4 to 8 years in various series, and there are multiple reports of symptoms being present for over 50 years (FARR 1980; KRUPSKI et al. 1982; LACK et al. 1977; VAN ASPEREN DE BOER et al. 1981). The great majority of these patients present with painless swelling at the bifurcation of the common carotid artery (KRUPSKI et al. 1982). The mass is frequently noted to be mobile in the anteroposterior but not in the superoinferior direction. A bruit is frequently present. Cranial nerve palsies may be present. These generally involve the IX, X and XII nerves. Hoarseness and vocal cord paralysis are relatively late findings, as are pain, tenderness, dysphagia and the carotid sinus syndrome. Other symptoms which are sometimes elicited include tinnitus, visual blurring, deafness and headache. The sympathetic nerves may become involved and Horner's syndrome may be present, although this is unusual (LACK et al. 1977). A staging classification based on degree of advancement has been devised by Shamblin (SHAMBLIN et al. 1971). Group I tumors are small and easily separated from the carotid vessel wall. Group II tumors partially surround the carotid artery, and Group III tumors are large and completely surround and adhere to the carotid bifurcation. This classification has been found useful in determining surgical management.

12.3.4 Diagnosis

A diagnosis of carotid body tumor should be suspected whenever a mass is found at the bifurcation of the carotid artery, especially if there is a long history and if the previously described presenting signs and symptoms are present. These tumors range in size from approximately 1 to 10 cm in diameter with an average of 4 cm. In one large series the diagnosis of carotid body tumor was made on admission in only 19% of all patients and was only considered in the differential diagnosis in 40% (LACK et al. 1977). In view of the potentially catastrophic consequences of failing to make the proper diagnosis prior to surgery a high index of suspicion is warranted. The differential diagnosis includes branchiogenic, lymphoma, metastatic carcinoma, salivary gland tumor, aneurysm, and tuberculous lymphadenitis. A thorough search for a primary carcinoma of the upper aerodigestive tract should therefore be made. Needle biopsy, while reasonably safe, is frequently not diagnostic. Because of the extreme vascularity of these tumors, an attempt at limited biopsy may be hazardous. Angiography has been reported by numerous authors to be the single most important diagnostic procedure. The accuracy rate is very close to 100% (FARR 1980; GRUFFERMAN et al. 1980; JAVID et al. 1976; LACK et al. 1977; SALDANA et al. 1973). In the absence of hypertension, testing for urinary catecholamine metabolites is probably not necessary, since functioning chemodectomas are uncommon.

12.3.5 Treatment Technique and Results

It is generally accepted that surgery is the treatment of choice for carotid body tumors when resection is possible. In view of the fact that they are locally quite invasive, early resection is indicated in spite of their generally slow rate of growth. As the tumors become more advanced, more radical operative procedures are required and the risk of complications increases. In a review of 8 series the incidence of operative complications was found to range from 2 to 40% (VAN ASPEREN DE BOER et al. 1981). Complications may be classified as neurologic or vascular. The former include damage to or sacrifice of cranial nerves VII through XII and damage to the sympathetic nerves. The latter include damage to the carotid arteries, which may require repair, as well as cerebrovascular accidents resulting in transient or permanent hemiparesis and even death. The risk of complications increases when the tumor extensively involves cranial nerves or the carotid arteries. The risk of vascular complications is extremely high when ligation of the common carotid artery is required, and may approach 50% under these circumstances (FARR 1980; DENT et al. 1976). The external carotid artery maybe sacrificed if necessary in order to obtain better exposure at the time of operation. Various techniques for reconstruction of the carotid arteries are available. Intraoperative shunting is sometimes indicated and may limit blood loss and simplify excision. It is essential to have a vascular surgeon available, especially when operating on the more advanced tumors, and to be certain that sufficient blood is on hand. In the majority of cases total excision is possible. When total

resection can be accomplished recurrence is uncommon (JAVID et al. 1976).

In spite of their greater frequency, much less information exists regarding the efficacy of radiation therapy for carotid body chemodectomas than for those which arise in the temporal bone. Since carotid body tumors have usually been resected, most of the radiotherapeutic experience has been with advanced, unresectable tumors (CONLEY 1965). Regressions of the tumors have been observed (MCGUIRT and HARKER 1975) but they have occurred slowly. Tumors which have remained stable for many years after irradiation have led to the conclusion that radiation therapy is ineffective (CHAMBERS and MAHONEY 1968; DENT et al. 1976; LACK et al. 1977; VAN ASPEREN DE BOER et al. 1981). Lybeert et al. (LYBEERT et al. 1984) reported the results of treatment of nine paragangliomas of the carotid body at the Rotterdam Radiotherapeutic Institute. Five patients were treated with total doses of 6000 cGy in 6 weeks, one received 5000 cGy in 5 weeks, and three received 4000 cGy in four weeks. All tumors were controlled, but regressions required months and asymptomatic palpable residua persisted; no complications were reported. This report and evidence from several other studies (FARR 1980; GRUFFERMAN et al. 1980; JAVID et al. 1976; KRUPSKI et al. 1982; LACK et al. 1977) indicate that paragangliomas of the carotid body behave in a manner similar to those in the temporal bone in regard to response to radiation therapy. Therefore, this treatment can be recommended for any patient who is medically inoperable or who has a tumor the resection of which would likely entail a high risk of morbidity.

References

Alford BR, Guilford FR (1953) A comprehensive study of tumors of glomus jugulare. Brain 76: 576

Batsakis JG (1979) Paragangliomas of the head and neck. In: Tumors of the head and neck, 2nd edn. Williams and Wilkins Company, Baltimore, pp 369–380

Brammer RE, Graham MD, Kemink JL (1984) Glomus tumors of the temporal bone: Contemporary evaluation and therapy. Otolaryngologic Clinics of North America 17: 499–512

Capps FCW (1957) Tumours of the glomus jugulare or tympanic body. J Facul Radiol 8: 312–324

Chambers RG, Mahoney WD (1968) Carotid body tumors. Am J Surg 115: 554–558

Cole JM (1977) Glomus jugulare tumor. Laryngoscope 87: 1244–1258

Cole JM (1979) Panel discussion: Glomus jugulare tumors of the temporal bone. Radiation of glomus tumors of the temporal bone. Laryngoscope 89: 1623

Conley JJ (1965) The carotid body tumor: A review of 29 cases. Arch Otolaryngol 81: 187–193

Cummings BJ, Beale FA, Garrett PG, Harwood AR, Keane TJ, Payne DG, Rider WD (1984) The treatment of glomus tumors in the temporal bone by megavoltage radiation. Cancer 53: 2635–2640

Dent TL, Thompson NW, Fry WJ (1976) Carotid body tumors. Surg 80: 365–372

Dickens WJ, Million RR, Cassisi NJ, Singleton GT (1982) Chemodectomas arising in temporal bone structures. Laryngoscope 92: 188–191

Duke WW, Boshell BR, Soteres P et al. (1964) A norepinephrine-secreting glomus jugulare tumor presenting as a pheochromocytoma. Ann Int Med 60: 1040–1047

Farr HW (1980) Carotid body tumors: A 40-year study. CA-A Cancer Journal for Clinicians 30: 260–265

Grufferman S, Gillman MW, Pasternek LR, Peterson CL, Young WG (1980) Familial carotid body tumors: Case report and epidemiologic review. Cancer 46: 2116–2122

Guild SR (1941) Anat Rec 79: 28

Guild SR (1953) Ann Otol, St. Louis 62: 1045

Hatfield PM, James AE, Schulz MD (1972) Chemodectomas of the glomus jugulare. Cancer 30: 1164–1668

Hudgins PT (1972) Radiotherapy for extensive glomus jugulare tumors. Radiol 103: 427–429

Jackson AW, Koshiba R (1974) Treatment of glomus jugulare tumors by radiotherapy. Proc R Soc Med 67: 9–12

Javid H, Chawla SK, Dye WS et al. (1976) Carotid body tumor. Arch Surg 111: 344–347

Kim JA, Elkon D, Lim ML, Constable WC (1980) Optimum dose of radiotherapy for chemodectomas of the middle ear. Int J Rad Oncol Biol Phys 6: 815–819

Krause W (1878) Zbl Med Wiss 16: 737

Krupski WC, Effeney DJ, Ehrenfeld WK, Stoney RJ (1982) Cervical chemodectoma. Technical considerations and mangement options. Am J Surg 144: 215–220

Lack EE, Cubilla AL, Woodruff JM, Farr HW (1977) Paragangliomas of the head and neck region. Cancer 39: 397–409

Levit SA, Sheps SG, Espinosa RE et al. (1976) Cathecholamine-secreting paraganglioma of glomus-jugulare region resembling phenchromocytoma. New Engl J Med 281: 805–811

Lybeert MLM, van Andel JG, Eijkenboom WMH, de Jong PC, Kengt P (1984) Radiotherapy of paragangliomas. Clin Otolaryngol 9: 105–109

Martin CE, Rosenfeld L, McSwain B (1973) Carotid body tumors. A 16-year followup of seven malignant cases. Southern Med J 66: 1236–1243

Maruyama Y (1972) Radiotherapy of tympanojugular chemodectomas. Radiol 105: 659–663

McCabe B, Fletcher M (1979) Selection of therapy of glomus jugulare tumors. Arch Otolaryngol 89: 182–185

McGuirt WF, Harker LA (1975) Carotid body tumors. Arch Otolaryngol 101: 58–62

Million RR, Cassisi NJ (1984) Chemodectomas (Glomus Body Tumors). In: Management of Head and Neck Cancer, A Multi-disciplinary Approach. J B Lippincott Company, Philadelphia, pp 567–578

Newman H, Rowe JF Jr, Phillips TL (1973) Radiation therapy of the glomus jugulare tumor. AJR 18: 663–669

Reddy EK, Mansfield CM, Hartman GV (1983) Chemodectoma of glomus jugulare. Cancer 52: 337–340

Rosai J (1981) Ackerman's surgical pathology 6th edn. The C V Mosby Company, St. Louis, pp 697–727

Rosenwasser H (1951) Arch Otolaryng 54: 453

Rosenwasser H (1958) Metastasis from glomus jugulare tumors. AMA Archives Otolaryngol 67: 197–203

Saldana MJ, Salem LE, Travezan R (1973) High altitude hypoxia and chemodectomas. Human Pathol 4: 251–263

Shamblin WR, ReMine WH, Sheps SG, Harrison EG Jr (1971) Carotid body tumor (chemodectoma). Clinicopathologic analysis of ninety cases. Am J Surg 122: 732–739

Simko TG, Griffin TW, Gerdes AJ, Parker RG, Tesh DW, Taylor W, Blasko JC (1978) The role of radiation therapy in the treatment of glomus jugulare tumors. Cancer 42: 104–106

Spector GJ, Campagno J, Perez CA, Maisel RH, Ogura JH (1975) Glomus jugulare tumors: Effects of radiotherapy. Cancer 35: 1316–1321

Spector GJ, Fierstein J, Ogura JH (1976) A comparison of therapeutic modalities of glomus tumors in the temporal bone. Laryngoscope 86: 690–696

Suit HD, Gallagher HS (1964) Intact tumor cells in irradiated tissue. Arch Pathol 78: 648

Tidwell TJ, Montague ED (1975) Chemodectomas involving the temporal bone. Radiol 116: 147–149

Valentin G (1840) Arch Anta Physiol LPZ: 287

van Asperen de Boer FRS, Terpstra JL, Vink M (1981) Diagnosis, treatment and operative complications of carotid body tumors. Br J Surg 68: 433–438

van Haller, cited by Dickinson AM, Traver CA (1945) Carotid body tumors. Review of the literature with report of two cases. Am J Surg 69: 9–11

Wang CC, Doppke K (1976) Osteoradionecrosis of the temporal bone – Consideration of nominal standard dose. Rad Oncol Biol Phys 1: 881–883

Wang CC (1980) What is the optimum dose of radiation therapy for glomus jugulare? Int J Radiat Oncol Biol Phys 6: 945–946

13 Tumors of the Major and Minor Salivary Glands*

Marsha D. McNeese and Gilbert H. Fletcher

CONTENTS

13.1 Introduction

Primary salivary gland tumors account for approximately 7% of all head and neck malignancies and less than 3% of all human tumors. The overall incidence in the general population is about 1.5/100,000. There do not appear to be any predisposing factors which can be identified, except for radiation induced neoplasms, such as those reported in the Hiroshima – Nagasaki survivors by Belsky et al. (1972), Takeichi et al. (1983), and Shore-Freedman et al. (1983). As a general rule, benign tumors tend to occur in younger patients and malignant tumors in the older age group. There is generally no sexual predilection except in the cases of Warthin's tumor, which is about 5 times more fre-

* This investigation was supported in part by Core Grants CA6294 and CA16672 awarded by the U.S. Department of Health and Human Services

Marsha D. McNesse, M.D., and Gilbert H. Fletcher, M.D., Department of Clinical Radiotherapy, The University of Texas, M.D. Anderson Cancer Center at Houston, Texas Medical Center, Houston, TX 77030, USA

quent in men as reported by Dorn & Cutler (1959).

Berg et al. (1968), Prior and Watherhouse (1977) and Abbey et al. (1984), and reported a possible association of the occurrence of salivary gland tumors with carcinoma of the breast. Berg et al. (1968) studied 396 patients with carcinoma of the major salivary gland and found that subsequent incidence of breast cancer was 8 times the expected figure, although Moertel and Elveback (1969) did not find any evidence to support that claim.

In addition to the major salivary glands, there are nests of salivary gland tissue located throughout the upper respiratory and digestive tract, and as a result tumors of minor salivary gland origin can be located at any site therein. The most common sites as reported by Spiro et al. (1973) and Guillamondegui et al. (1980) are the palate, base of tongue, and buccal mucosa. The majority of salivary gland tumors arise in the parotid glands, approximately half of which are benign mixed tumors. According to Eneroth and Hamberger (1974), a tumor arising in the submaxillary glands or in the glands of the mucous membranes is much more likely to be malignant than is one arising in the parotid glands. Because tumors of the major salivary glands are generally easily palpable, they frequently are diagnosed in earlier stages than tumors of the minor salivary glands. Treatment techniques, both from the surgical and radiotherapeutic standpoint, must be adapted to the clinical presentation.

13.2 Anatomy

The major salivary glands consist of the parotid, submaxillary, and sublingual glands. The largest glands are the parotid glands, which lie immediately anterior to the external auditory canal. Posteriorly the glands extend back to the mastoid process and superiorly over the temporal mandibular joint to the lower portion of the zygoma. The superficial lobes extend forward over the masseter muscle to its anterior border, and inferiorly into the subdigastric area. Each gland is basically a wedge-shaped structure, with the base positioned laterally and the apex in front of the anterior tonsillar pillar (Fig. 13-1).

Approximately 80% of the parotid gland is located in the superficial lobe, with only 20% of parotid tissue in the deep lobe. Accessory glandular tissue may be found along Wharton's duct in approximately 20% of the population as described by BATSAKIS (1974). Two medial extensions of the parotid gland are seen, one between the internal pterygoid muscle and the ascending ramus of the mandible, and a major portion extending into the lateral pharyngeal space in front of the styloid process. In close proximity to the deep lobe are the internal carotid artery, internal jugular vein, the glossopharyngeal, vagus, spinal accessory and hypoglossal nerves, as well as the cervical sympathetic chain. The facial nerve passes through the parotid gland, dividing it into superficial and deep lobes, and

branches of the nerve are frequently involved with tumor (Fig. 13-2). The auriculo-temporal nerve, a branch of the mandibular division of the fifth nerve, also enters the parotid compartment after circling behind the condylar process of the mandible. In addition to providing another route of spread to the base of the skull, this nerve, when invaded peripherally, can cause referred pain to the ear or superficial temporal region.

Because of the tough, dense superficial fascia overlying the parotid gland, benign or low-grade tumors may remain contained within the parotid bed until they become quite large. By contrast, the fascia which separates the deep lobe from the parapharyngeal space is relatively thin, and tumors involving the deep lobe may present with a mass bulging into the oropharynx, although such presentation is infrequent (ENEROTH and HAMBERGER 1974).

Multiple small lymph nodes are present within the parotid gland. The superficial parotid nodes re-

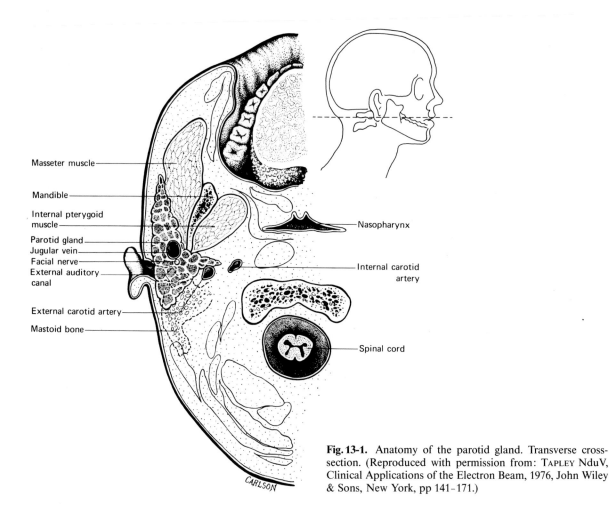

Masseter muscle

Mandible

Internal pterygoid muscle

Parotid gland
Jugular vein
Facial nerve
External auditory canal

External carotid artery

Mastoid bone

Nasopharynx

Internal carotid artery

Spinal cord

CARLSON

Fig. 13-1. Anatomy of the parotid gland. Transverse cross-section. (Reproduced with permission from: TAPLEY NduV, Clinical Applications of the Electron Beam, 1976, John Wiley & Sons, New York, pp 141–171.)

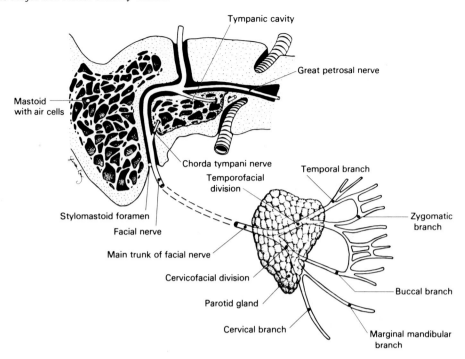

Fig. 13-2. Anatomy of the facial nerve in relation to the parotid gland. (Reproduced with permission from: McNaney D et al.: Int J Radiat Oncol Biol Phys 9: 1289–1295, 1983, Pergamon Press Inc)

ceive lymphatics draining the skin and subcutaneous tissues of the temporal area as well as the eyelids, brows, cheeks, and ears. The deep parotid lymph nodes course along the external carotid artery and drain portions of the external auditory canals, Eustachian tubes, and the parotid glands. These nodes then drain into the nodes at the angle of the mandible, upper posterior cervical chain, or the subdigastric nodes. Primary parotid malignancies frequently metastasize to regional nodes, depending on the type of the tumor (RAFLA-DEMETRIOUS 1973 and RAFLA 1977).

The submaxillary glands are the second largest salivary glands, each approximately the size of a walnut, and are situated in the submaxillary triangle of the neck beneath and anterior to the angle of the mandible. Each gland overlies the mylohyoid muscle and is in direct contact with the stylomandibular ligament posteriorly, with the lingual nerve just lateral and superior to the submaxillary duct. The hypoglossal nerve courses along the deep surface of the gland (Fig. 13-3). Wharton's duct arises from the deep surface of the gland and passes anteriorly for about 5 cm to an opening in the floor of the mouth, near the midline. Lymphatic channels are frequently invaded, particularly by high grade undifferentiated tumors, with the first level of nodal metastases generally being the nodes overlying the submaxillary gland itself, then to the subdigastric and high midjugular nodes. In the UT MDACC se-

ries (BYERS et al. 1973), nerve invasion was demonstrated in 50% of previously untreated malignant submaxillary gland tumors, and 44% had nodal metastases. One third of patients had direct extension to the mandible. Invasion of perineurial lymphatics may permit invasion of the mandible and/or spread along major nerves, to the base of the skull.

The smallest of the major salivary glands are the sublingual glands, located deep to the mucous membrane of the floor of the mouth (Fig. 13-4). Drainage of the glands is variable, with 10 to 12 small ducts emptying into the anterior floor of the mouth. Frequently at least one of the ducts may enter with Wharton's duct. Primary salivary gland tumors in this area are rather rare. (ENEROTH 1969; SPIRO et al. 1973; FU et al. 1976).

13.3 Pathology

13.3.1 Benign Tumors

Perhaps nowhere else is the histologic classification more important to proper treatment planning than in the group of salivary gland tumors. The majority

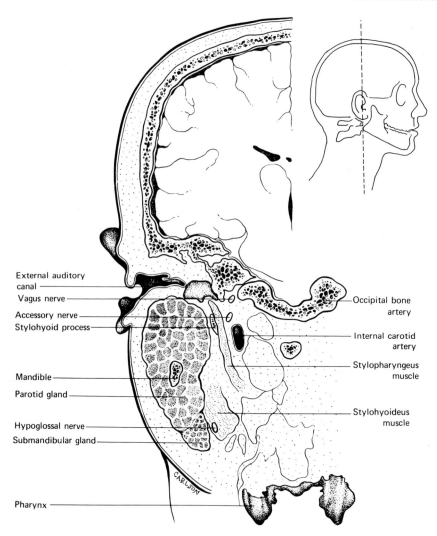

External auditory
canal
Vagus nerve
Accessory nerve
Stylohyoid process

Mandible
Parotid gland

Hypoglossal nerve
Submandibular gland

Pharynx

Occipital bone
artery

Internal carotid
artery

Stylopharyngeus
muscle

Stylohyoideus
muscle

Fig. 13-3. Anatomy of the parotid and salivary glands, sagittal cross-section. (Reproduced with permission from: TAPLEY NduV, Clinical Applications of the Electron Beam, 1976, John Wiley & Sons, New York, pp 141–171)

of tumors in the parotid glands are benign mixed tumors, more recently also called pleomorphic adenoma. Approximately 5% of benign mixed tumors undergo malignant transformation (BATSAKIS 1974; MARAN et al. 1984).

It is important to note that portions of a benign mixed tumor may be malignant, and it is therefore mandatory that multiple sections through the parotid tumor be done in order to obtain a correct diagnosis. A benign mixed tumor which suddenly exhibits rapid growth should be suspected of having undergone malignant transformation.

In BLANCK's series (1974) of 1378 benign parotid tumors, 93% were of the benign mixed type. Recurrence rates vary from 5% to as high as 30–40%, depending on the surgical approach used. Primary multicentric origin of such tumors is rare, and recurrences are generally felt to be due to tumor cells having been left behind at surgery. The time to recurrence can be extremely variable, ranging from a few months to several decades (RAFLA-DEMETRIOUS 1973).

Another type of benign tumor is the adenolymphoma or Warthin's tumor, also called papillary cystadenoma lymphomatosyum. This tumor is found only in the parotid glands, usually in the tail, occurs predominately in males in a 5:1 ratio to females, is occasionally familial and occurs bilaterally in approximately 10% of cases. It is generally slow-growing, cystic, and often multifocal. Surgical excision is usually curative (CHAUDHRY and GORLIN 1958).

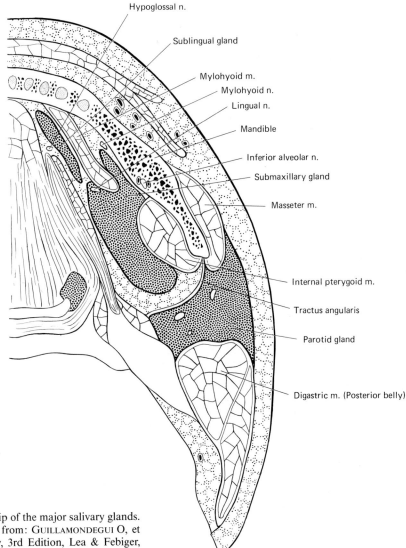

Hypoglossal n.

Sublingual gland

Mylohyoid m.

Mylohyoid n.

Lingual n.

Mandible

Inferior alveolar n.

Submaxillary gland

Masseter m.

Internal pterygoid m.

Tractus angularis

Parotid gland

Digastric m. (Posterior belly)

Fig. 13-4. Anatomic relationship of the major salivary glands. (Reproduced with permission from: GUILLAMONDEGUI O, et al., Textbook of Radiotherapy, 3rd Edition, Lea & Febiger, Philadelphia, PA, 1980, 426–443

13.3.2 Malignant Tumors

The basic histopathologic classification of salivary gland malignancies was first described by FOOTE and FRAZELL (1953). Certain malignant tumors are well-differentiated and carry a better prognosis than high-grade malignancies (FRAZELL 1954). Acinic (Acinous) cell carcinoma is a well-differentiated tumor accounting for 13% of all malignancies of the parotid glands and is rarely seen in other salivary tissues. This carcinoma ranks only behind Warthin's tumor in its frequency of bilateral parotid gland involvement, which is seen in approximately 3% of these patients. Multinodularity seen in primary lesions is felt to represent multifocal origin. Lymph node metastases occur in only 16% of pa-

tients. It has been demonstrated by several investigators that recurrences as well as metastases in this tumor may occur many years later (ENEROTH et al. 1966, BATSAKIS 1970; and SPIRO et al. 1978).

Adenoid cystic carcinoma, formerly called cylindroma, accounts for approximately 12% of parotid gland carcinomas, but approximately 58% of submandibular and minor salivary gland malignancies (CUMMINGS 1977; SCHELL et al. 1983). ENEROTH and HAMBERGER (1974) and SPIRO et al. (1979) demonstrated that the location of the primary was important to the survival rate, with patients presenting with lesions in the palate doing much better than patients with lesions in the parotid or submandibular glands. In the past, these tumors were frequently confused with malignant mixed tumors.

Late recurrences often occur (BLANCK 1974). Even though this tumor is considered low-grade histologically, one of the most outstanding features of this neoplasm is its marked tendency to invade nerves, observed in 46% of cases reviewed by LEAFSTEDT et al. (1971). Forty percent of patients may eventually develop regional or distant metastases or both, with the lungs being the most frequent site of metastatic involvement (LAMPE and ZATZKIN 1949; VIKRAM et al. 1984). Lymph nodes involvement is seen in approximately 15% of patients.

Of the malignant salivary gland tumors of the palate, parotid and submandibular glands, the mucoepidermoid carcinomas make up approximately 26, 21, and 10% respectively (HEALEY et al. 1979), and are the most common malignant salivary gland tumors associated with previous radiation exposure (BELSKEY et al.1972). Well-differentiated mucoepidermoid carcinomas are characterized by slow growth, a recurrence rate of only approximately 15%, and rare metastases. High grade mucoepidermoid malignancies, on the other hand, run a much more aggressive course with the rate of local recurrence reaching 60% (FRAZELL 1954). Approximately one-half the high grade mucoepidermoid carcinomas are associated with regional lymph node metastases, and one-third developed distant metastases (SPIRO 1975).

Adenocarcinomas account for about 12% of parotid malignancies. Some adenocarcinomas are classified as low grade malignancies depending on their histological appearance and clinical presentation. However the majority of adenocarcinomas of the major salivary glands are highly malignant neoplasms that metastasize to regional lymph nodes as well as distant structures, particularly bone and lungs. According to SPIRO (1975), 36% of patients with adenocarcinoma present with or develop lymph nodes involvement.

Malignant mixed tumors usually occur as carcinoma arising from a benign tumor, hence the term carcinoma ex-pleomorphic adenoma. Rarely, a true malignant mixed tumor composed of epithelial and mesenchymal cells may occur. At least one-fourth of these patients develop neck node metastases. Overall cure rates at 5 and 10 years were 63% and 39% respectively reflecting the aggressive nature of this tumor (SPIRO et al. 1977).

Undifferentiated carcinomas are rare, approximately 3% of all salivary gland tumors, and are usually highly malignant. Over one-third of the reported cases appear to have been superimposed on a previously diagnosed mixed tumor, often one of long standing. These lesions manifest a high frequency of metastases to cervical lymph nodes (50%) and an overall poor prognosis (RAFLA-DEMETRIOUS 1970 and SPIRO et al. 1975).

Primary squamous cell carcinomas of the parotid glands are rare, ranging from 0 to 3.4% of all parotid tumors (BATSAKIS and MCCLATCHEY 1976). However, due to the rich lymphatic network contained within the parotid glands, squamous cell carcinomas of the skin of the face, especially the forehead, temple or ear, frequently metastasize to the parotid nodes or gland (CONLEY and ARENA 1963). Before diagnosis of primary squamous cell carcinomas can be made, it is mandatory to exclude variants of mucoepidermoid carcinoma, as well as metastases from skin carcinomas. Patients with such a tumor should also have a complete head and neck examination in order to rule out the presence of a primary tumor in the oral cavity or oropharynx that has metastasized to the lymphatics of the parotid or submaxillary gland area. Fifty percent of patients with squamous carcinomas have positive neck nodes, and prognosis is poor.

13.4 Clinical Presentation

Quite frequently the presenting symptom is only a slowly enlarging mass in the area of the parotid or submaxillary glands or the submucosa of the upper oral or pharyngeal passages. Patients with a benign mixed tumor or a low-grade malignancy may have had the mass for many years. Pain is a rare symptom when the tumor is benign. Facial nerve weakness is rather rare as a presenting complaint reported at 12 to 14% but when present is an ominous sign more often associated with high grade malignant tumors. (ENEROTH and HAMBERGER 1974; CONLEY and HAMAKER 1975) The degree of fixation of the tumor to surrounding tissues is not a reliable indicator as to whether the tumor is benign or malignant.

Deep lobe presentations account for 12% of tumor presentations in the parotid gland (HANNA et al. 1968), and tumors involving the deep lobe of the parotid may produce symptoms of dysphagia, earache, or aural "stuffiness," trismus, and, rarely, progressive facial nerve palsy (CONLEY and SELFE 1981). Such tumors may bulge into the palate and lateral pharyngeal wall as a submucosal mass, and if the parapharyngeal space is invaded, cranial nerves IX, X, XI and XII may be involved as well. As in the superficial lobe, the majority of tumors of the deep lobe are benign mixed tumors, and only about 20% are malignant (HANNA et al. 1968; NIGRO and SPIRO 1977).

Neoplasms presenting in a submandibular gland usually develop as a painless swelling beneath the mandible, and nerve palsy is an infrequent phenomenon. Bimanual palpation should be used with one examining finger in the mouth to better determine tumor size and mobility.

13.5 Staging

The staging of salivary gland carcinoma, like that of almost any other tumor, depends on the size and location of the primary tumor, status of regional lymph nodes, and presence of distant metastases. The staging used is as recommended by the Salivary Gland Task Force of the American Joint Committee for Cancer Staging and End Results Reporting (LEVITT et al. 1981; BEAHRS and MYERS 1983).

T_X – Minimum requirements to assess the primary tumor cannot be met.

T_0 – No evidence of primary tumor.

T_1 – Tumor 2 cm or less in greatest diameter without significant local extension.*

T_2 – Tumor more than 2 cm but not more than 4 cm in greatest diameter without significant local extension.

T_3 – Tumor more than 4 cm but not more than 6 cm in greatest diameter without local extension.

T_{4A} – Tumor greater than 6 cm in greatest diameter without significant local extension.

T_{4B} – Tumor of any size with significant local extension.[1]

N_X – Minimum requirements to assess the regional nodes cannot be met.

N_0 – No evidence of regional lymph node involvement.

N_1 – Evidence of regional lymph node involvement.

---

[1] Significant local extension is defined as evidence of tumor involvement of skin, soft tissues, bone, or the lingual or facial nerves.

13.6 Treatment of Benign Salivary Gland Tumors

There is no question that the treatment of a benign mixed tumor is surgical excision. Radical irradiation as a primary treatment has been attempted in the past and shown to be less effective than surgery (MARAN et al. 1984), and the long-term risks of radiation should be carefully considered this patient population which tends to be younger than the population developing malignant disease.

However, the question of postoperative radiotherapy for residual or recurrent benign mixed tumor will occasionally arise, and may be attempted if the surgeon does not feel that the mass is completely resectable without major cosmetic deformity. WATSON (1965) showed good local control with doses ranging from 53 to 57 Gy over 5 weeks in 75 patients with limited postoperative residual benign mixed tumors, 5 of which recurred. DAWSON and ORR (1985) reported on 311 patients with pleomorphic adenoma (benign mixed tumors) followed for a minimum of 10 years, 172 of which were followed for 20 years after treatment with surgery and irradiation. Local recurrence rates were 1.5% at 10 years and 8% at 20 years. Early recurrences were all benign, but late recurrences were predominately malignant. Since radiotherapy may have increased the incidence of malignant transformation, the authors concluded that irradiation should be reserved for patients presenting surgical difficulties. However, 279 of these patients were treated by a radium needle implant, delivering 55–60 Gy at 0.5 cm over 6 days. How this would compare to external beam therapy is uncertain. Nevertheless, their conclusions seem to be prudent and valid.

External beam therapy is usually delivered by combining high energy electrons with photons delivering 55–60 Gy over 5½ to 6 weeks. Thirteen to 17 MeV electrons are generally adequate for superficial lobe tumors, although higher energies are generally needed for deep lobe presentations. Because of the higher surface doses with higher electron energies, the treatment is usually given with the electrons mixed with photons in a 3:1 or 4:1 ratio. Photon wedge techniques can also be used to avoid the contralateral parotid, but the volume of tissue is greater and care must be taken not to treat the eye or brainstem (Fig. 13-5). The field should be as circumscribed as possible, although the entire operative bed should be covered.

Above all, it is imperative that these patients receive follow-up for extended time periods, in view

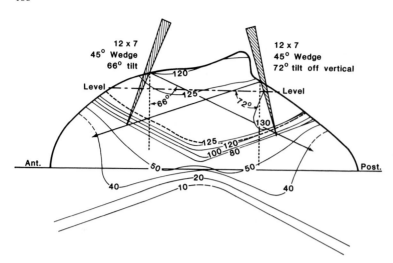

of the possibility of late recurrences and the malignant potential of these recurrences.

13.7 Treatment of Malignant Salivary Gland Tumors

13.7.1 Major Salivary Gland Tumors

13.7.1.1 Parotid Gland Tumors

Salivary gland tumors were for a long period of time considered unresponsive to radiotherapy, and therefore surgical treatment alone was the traditional treatment. There is no question that malignant major and minor salivary gland tumors are best treated by surgical removal, the extent of which varies according to tumor size, location, and histological type. For parotid malignancies, the minimal surgical procedure performed should be a superficial parotidectomy or a total parotidectomy, depending on tumor presentation. If the facial nerve does not appear to be involved, it is carefully spared. Most low grade tumors can be successfully removed in this way with minimal loss of function of the facial nerve. If there is an adequate surgical margin, no histological evidence of nerve invasion, and no previous excisions, such patients are at a low risk for local recurrence, and postoperative radiation therapy is generally not indicated (CHONG et al.1974).

The local extent of moderate and high-grade tumors frequently requires sacrifice of the facial nerve in parotid gland locations, and in submaxillary salivary gland tumors, removal of lingual and hypoglossal nerves or even the mandible may be required. This results in functional defects or cosmet-

ic deformities due to the radical surgical procedures. In addition, for the moderately malignant tumors, local recurrence rates in surgical series were 37.5% at 5 years and 54% for all histological types when margins were close (FU et al. 1970; KAGAN et al. 1976)

The UT MDACC reported in 1965 that malignant epithelial tumors of the major salivary glands exhibit the same radiosensitivity as squamous cell carcinomas (ALANIZ and FLETCHER 1965), and it became evident that postoperative radiotherapy could improve local control (KING and FLETCHER 1971). In the past, long segments of the facial nerve were removed if any part of the nerve was invaded by cancer, but with the use of postoperative radiotherapy, this approach has changed (GUILLAMON-DEGUT et al. 1975). The current policy at UT MDACC is to resect only gross tumor. If only one branch of the nerve is involved, that branch is resected, allowing the main trunk and other branches to remain intact. Radiotherapy is then administered to eradicate the subclinical disease in the high-risk patients.

The indications for radiotherapy are as follows: (TAPLEY and FLETCHER 1976; TAPLEY 1977).

1. Tumor removal with close surgical margins or with microscopically demonstrated positive margins, regardless of tumor grade, particularly if the deep lobe is involved.
2. All high-grade tumors or metastatic squamous cell carcinomas.
3. After removal of recurrent disease, regardless of histology and margins.
4. Invasion of skin, bone, nerve, or extraparotid tissue.
5. Regional nodal metastases after neck dissection.
6. Gross residual or non resectable tumor.

Fig. 13-6. This patient presented in 1970 at age 27 with a 2 cm preauricular mass that was excised and diagnosed as chronic inflammation, although the pathologist could not exclude the possibility of mucoepidermoid carcinoma. A new preauricular lesion measuring 1 cm developed in 1975 and was excised and read as low-grade mucoepidermoid carcinoma. Facial nerve function was normal, but there was considerable postoperative induration over the area of the parotid duct. Postoperative radiotherapy was given to the parotid bed using 18 MeV electrons and photons in a 3:2 ratio, with generous anterior margins. The spinal cord was excluded from the treatment volume. The parotid bed received 60 Gy tumor dose over a period of 6 weeks to a depth of 4.7 cm. The patient was well and free of disease in March 1986. (Reproduced with permission from McNaney D, et al., Int J Radiat Oncol Biol Phys, 9: 1289–1295, 1983)

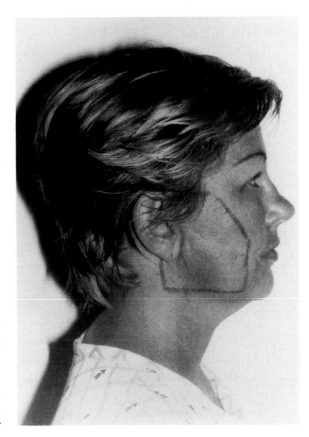

As previously described for benign mixed tumors, radiation therapy to the parotid bed may be given with either a photon wedge pair arrangement or a combination of electron and photon beams. The combination is generally preferable because less normal tissue is included in the treatment volume. In the past, there was some reluctance to use electrons when mastoid involvement was evident, or to use them in combinations with photons in ratios of more than 2:1 in favor of the electrons, because of possible dose pertubations caused by increased absorption of electrons by bone. However, with the advent of computerized tomography treatment planning and effective electron beam algorithms developed by Hogstrom et al. (1983) more confidence in the dosimetry has developed.

Radiotherapy fields are tailored according to the particular characteristics of the tumor, i.e., whether the tumor is locally aggressive with little tendency to metastasize to lymph nodes as in acinic cell carcinomas, or whether the tumor tends to infiltrate along nerves or spread to lymph nodes, as in the adenoid cystic or less differentiated tumors.

For the low grade tumors which are locally recurrent with no evidence of perineurial disease or lymphatic spread, radiotherapy of the parotid bed alone is adequate, without including the mastoid area or lower neck nodes (Fig. 13-6). For the less differentiated tumors, the portal covers the entire parotid bed from approximately 6 cm anterior to the ear to the mastoid area posteriorly, and from the zygomatic arch to the midjugular area (Fig. 13-7). Electron beam energies of 17–20 MeV are generally used, with photons added for skin-sparing, loaded 3:1 or 4:1 in generally used, with photons added for skin-sparing, loaded 3:1 or 4:1 in favor of the electrons. A low energy electron beam field is used to cover the lower portion of the neck as well as any scar extensions superior to the zygoma (McNaney et al. 1983).

In treatment planning, computerized tomography of the treatment area is useful in defining the tumor bed and depth for dosimetry. When doses of 60 Gy or more are to be delivered or for deep lobe lesions, CT-assisted computer dosimetry is extremely helpful. Care should be taken to limit the dose to the spinal cord to no more than 45 Gy.

Dose given to the primary bed generally range from 55 to 65 Gy, depending on the type of surgical procedure and the proportionate risk of disease left behind. For example, a low grade acinic cell tumor which has recurred after previous surgery and has been re-excised with clear margins and no evidence of nerve invasion can be treated adequately with 55 Gy. However, in a patient with a high grade mucoepidemoid carcinoma which has been dissected off the facial nerve, one can assume that there is microscopic residual disease, and doses in the range of 60 to 65 Gy are necessary.

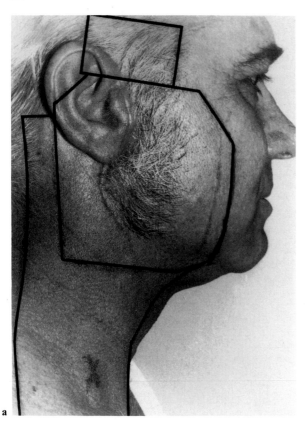

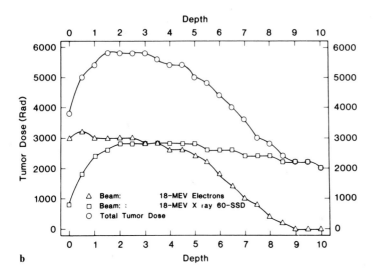

13.7.1.2 Submaxillary Salivary Gland Tumors

Clinical and pathological findings that adversely affect the control of submandibular gland cancer include invasion of the major nerves including the lingual, hypoglossal, and mylohyoid nerves, metastases to local and regional lymph nodes, periglandular soft tissue invasion, or invasion of the mandible (MILLION and CASSISI 1984). UT MDACC treatment policy for cancer of the submaxillary glands is as follows: the minimal biopsy procedure should be a total dissection of the submaxillary triangle with frozen section for histologic examination. If the nodes are negative and the lesion is of moderate grade potential, is confined within the capsule of the gland, and shows no evidence of nerve invasion, postoperative radiotherapy is generally not necessary. However, if the tumor has broken through the capsule and invaded nerves, connective tissue, periosteum or muscle, a wide resection is performed. A modified radical neck dissection is also done if enlarged lymph nodes are palpable. Postoperative radiotherapy of 55 to 60 Gy is administered to the operative bed and 50 to 55 Gy to the remainder of the ipsilateral neck. It the lesion extended to the submental region, the contralateral neck may also be irradiated. In addition, if major nerves were involved, the entire course of the nerve is followed to the base of the skull (Fig. 13-8). A higher energy electron beam such as 12-13 MeV is usually chosen for the primary bed and surrounding tissues and a lower energy of 7-10 MeV for the lower neck. A 10° cephalad tilt is frequently used to ensure adequate coverage of nodes under the mandible. High energy photons are used to treat the base of skull area.

13.7.2 Minor Salivary Gland Tumors

Due to the wide variety of presentations, treatment of these tumors varies depending on the area in which they are found. Generally, a conservative excision with a rather modest margin is performed in order to decrease the functional morbidity. In those lesions that are of low grade with no positive margins or nerve involvement, further treatment may not be necessary. For highly malignant lesions and in all lesions with nerve invasion, positive margins, or neck node involvement, postoperative radiotherapy to the primary site and to the neck is delivered. Doses are the same as those indicated for major salivary gland tumors.

13.7.3 Metastases to Parotid

For squamous cell carcinomas of the skin of the face, most frequently the forehead, temple or ear, that have metastasized to the parotid nodes or gland, the treatment is essentially the same as for a primary parotid tumor, with surgical removal, if possible, followed by irradiation to the parotid bed and entire ipsilateral neck due to the high probability of cervical node metastases (CASSISI et al. 1978; JACKSON and BALLANTYNE 1981; WANG 1982).

13.7.4 Gross Disease

While some reports of local control with radiotherapy for gross disease have been disappointing,

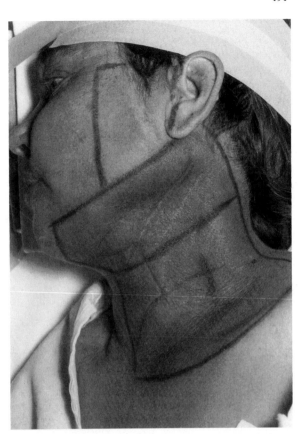

Fig. 13-8. This 51-year-old female had a mass excised from the right submaxillary gland in September 1968, revealing adenoid cystic carcinoma with extensive invasion of the lingual nerve. Fourteen lymph nodes were negative. She was referred to M. D. Anderson Cancer Center in November and received electron beam therapy to the entire right neck, using 12 MeV to deliver 60 Gy to the submaxillary gland area and 6 MeV to deliver 50 Gy to the lower neck. In addition, the path of the nerve up to the base of skull was treated to 60 Gy at 5 cm depth with a unilateral photon beam field. While undergoing radiotherapy, she experienced a small area of mandibular exposure along the lingual aspect just anterior to the photon field. In October 1969, she was noted to have persistent mandibular necrosis. Because this was a small area, attempts were made to treat her conservatively, but when she returned in February 1970, the necrosis had progressed, with associated trismus and pain. An intraoral resection of the portion of the mandible was performed, after which she did well until May 1971, when a small area in the lower lobe of the right lung, which was previously suspected of being a granuloma, was noted to have enlarged to approximately 2.5 cm in diameter, and a wedge resection revealed metastatic adenoid cystic carcinoma. She remained stable until September 1974, when a repeat chest x-ray showed 3 new lung nodules, an abnormal bone scan in the ribs and spine, and abnormal liver spleen scan. She expired of metastatic disease on April 10, 1977. (Reproduced with permission from: TAPLEY NduV, Clinical Applications of the Electron Beam, 1976, John Wiley & Sons, New York, pp. 141-171)

KING and FLETCHER (1971) reported local control of 81% in primary inoperable and postoperative recurrent groups, with several of the treatment failures due to marginal recurrences. Minimum dose to the midline was 60 Gy with the main bulk of the tumor receiving 70 Gy or more.

The possible role of fast neutrons in the treatment of salivary gland tumors was first published in 1975, when CATTERALL (1981) reported control rates as high as 90% for advanced tumors, with no complications, and later HENRY et al. (1979) reported 100% control in tumors measuring up to 6 cm. Studies of fast neutron therapy for such tumors is being carried out by several major institutions in the U.S., under the direction of the Radiation Therapy Oncology Group.

13.7.5 Dental Care

It is extremely important that the patient who is to receive radiation therapy to the salivary glands receive a dental evaluation prior to radiation. The

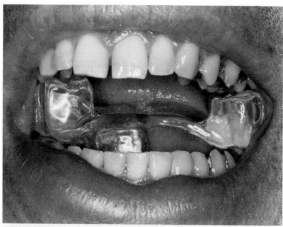

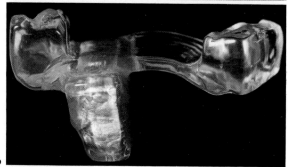

Fig. 13-9 a, b. Example of custom-made intraoral stent to protect tongue and opposite side of the mouth. (Reproduced with permission from: TAPLEY NduV, Clinical Applications of the Electron Beam, 1976, John Wiley & Sons, New York pp. 167)

doses necessary for tumor control will result in a severe decrease in salivary function. In addition to lubricating the oral cavity, saliva acts to buffer and dilute acids produced by fermentation, and washes the food particles and bacteria from the oral cavity. The altered thick saliva after radiation therapy is much less effective in these functions, and without proper precautions radiation caries will develop soon after radiation. Proper oral hygiene with fluoride treatments can prevent such sequelae. In addition, it has been shown (BEDWINEK et al. 1976) that the incidence of osteoradionecrosis can be decreased by performing any necessary dental extractions prior to radiation therapy and avoiding extractions after radiotherapy if at all possible. Any teeth to be extracted should be removed with minimal trauma and primary closure of the gingiva to minimize the healing period. Most patients are healed well enough to begin radiation therapy within 10 to 14 days. Intraoral stents containing metal, as described by FLEMING and RAMBACH (1983) are also useful to protect the tongue and other normal tissues, as demonstrated in Fig. 13-9. Active exercise for the temporomandibular joint is recommended to prevent trismus.

13.8 Treatment Results

13.8.1 Parotid Glands

The effectiveness of postoperative irradiation is indicated by a recent review of 116 patients treated at UT MDACC from 1954-1982. Of this group, 43 patients were followed from 2-5 years, 40 from 5-10 years, and 35 for more than 10 years. Those patients having more than two surgical procedures were excluded, as well as patients with squamous cell carcinoma, which could have been from skin origin. The mean age was 49 years, but ranged from 10 years to 83 years. Fifty-two males and 64 females were included in the study.

In this patient group, gross residual tumor was present in 18 patients and microscopic residual tumor in 42 patients. Of the 50 patients who had good margins, 30 had high-grade tumors, and the other 20 had tumors of undetermined grade. Six patients had low-grade tumors with questionable margins.

Total facial nerve resection was performed in 24 patients, partial resection in 32 patients, and no resection in 60 patients.

Tables 13-1 through 13-4 show the results in this patient group, analyzed for local failure and/or

Table 13-1. Primary parotid epithelial carcinomas. (From QUONG et al., Manuscript in preparation)

Histologic Grade	Total	P± DM	P+ N±DM	N± DM	DM only
Gross (any grade)	18	1	1	1	2
Microscopic (any grade)	42	3	0	1	5
High grade (good margin)	30	3	0	2	4
Unknown grade (good margin)	20	1	1	0	4
Low grade (questionable margin)	6	0	0	0	0
Total	116	8	2	4	15

Abbreviations: P, progressive disease; Dm, distant metastases; N, Nodal metastases

Table 13-2. Primary parotid epithelial carcinomas. (From QUONG et al., Manuscript in preparation)

Lymph nodes	Total	P± DM	P+N± DM	N± DM	DM only
Histologically positive	27	4	1	4	4
Histologically negative	43	2	0	0	7
Clinically negative (no nodal dissection)	46	2	1	0	4
Total	116	8	2	4	15

Table 13-3. Primary parotid epithelial carcinomas. (From QUONG et al., Manuscript in preparation)

Dose	Total	P±DM	P+N±DM
<5000	2	0	0
5000–6000	100	7	1
>6000	14	2	0
Total	116	9	1

Table 13-4. Primary parotid epithelial carcinomas. (From QUONG et al., Manuscript in preparation)

Extent of facial nerve resection	Total No.	P±DM	P±N±DM
Total	24	3	1
Partial	32	2	0
None	60	3	1
Total	116	8	2

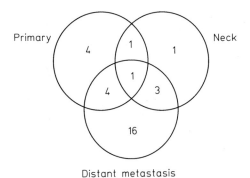

Fig. 13-10. Epithelial parotid malignancies – analysis August 1987 relationship of failures and location

distant metastases according to histology, nodal status, facial nerve sacrifice, and total dose of radiation. Of the ten patients who failed at the primary site, 2 also failed in the neck and 4 developed distant metastases. Of the four patients who failed in the neck but achieved control of the primary tumor, three developed distant metastases. The relationship of failures and their location is graphically illustrated in Figure 13-10. Regional failures were more frequent in patients with histologically positive nodes than in the histologically or clinically node negative patients.

Table 13-5 shows that in the patients who failed treatment, only 2 patients failed with distant metastases after 48 months, and the majority of local and distant failures occurred within 36 months of treatment. Determinate 5 year survivals in 107 patients according to histology are listed in Table 13-6, and correspond fairly well to the degree of tumor differentiation, with acinic cell tumors having the best prognosis, and undifferentiated tumor the worst.

13.8.2 Submaxillary, Sublingual and Minor Salivary Glands

In 1973 SPIRO et al. reported on 570 patients with minor salivary gland tumors seen at Memorial Hospital and reported that 88% of patients had malignant tumors, most frequently adenoid cystic. Ninety percent of patients were initially treated with surgery only with definitive radiotherapy given to only 20 patients, with no data available on these patients. This illustrates the rather scanty information available concerning the use of combined treatment. The determinate "cure" rate at 5, 10, and 15 years was 44.5%, 32.6%, and 21.4% respectively, reflecting the aggressive nature of this tumor.

Table 13-5. Parotid carcinomas. (From QUONG et al., Manuscript in preparation)

Months to failures	P	N	P+N	DM only
0–24	6	3	0	7
25–36	1	1	2	4
37–48	1	0	0	2
48–60	0	0	0	0
5–10 yrs	0	0	0	1 (76 mos)
>10 yrs	0	0	0	1 (181 mos)
Total	8	4	2	15

Table 13-6. Parotid cancer: 5-year determinate survival – 107 patients. (From QUONG et al., Manuscript in preparation)

Histology	No. of patients	5-yr. survival (%)
Acinic cell	11	100
Adenoid cystic	20	95
Mucoepidermoid (low grade)	10	90
Mucoepidermoid (high grade)	20	82
Adenocarcinoma	30	70
Malignant mixed	16	59

Table 13-7 shows the site of presentation and histology for 118 patients with malignant minor salivary gland tumors seen at the University of Texas M. D. Anderson Cancer Center. Because sublingual gland tumors are uncommon, they are analyzed with minor salivary gland tumors. The majority of the patients (57%) had adenoid cystic carcinoma, and because of the tendency for these tumors to invade nerves as well as adjacent tissues, patients with this histology are usually referred for postoperative irradiation depending on tumor size and location and adequacy of margins. A review of the lit-

erature suggests that patients with disease in the paranasal sinuses and nasal cavity tend to present with more advanced disease than in other locations (LEAFSTEDT et al. 1971; GOEPFERT et al. 1983) and combined treatment is particularly recommended for tumors in these locations. Although the number of patients with disease in paranasal sinuses is small, GOEPFERT et al. (1983) found a local control of 47% at 2 years with surgery alone (9/19) compared with 76% after surgery and irradiation (26/34). CONLEY (1972) in a review of 130 patients with malignant minor salivary gland tumors, found that for all histologies the 5-year disease-free surival was 55%, with adenoid cystic tumors showing only a 38% disease-free survival. Distant metastases developed in 27% of all histologies, compared to 46% in the adenoid cystic group. Local recurrence by histology was as follows: adenoid cystic 50%, adenocarcinoma 47%, malignant mixed tumor 33%, and mucoepidermoid carcinoma 30%. Thirty-seven percent of patients with malignant tumors received radiotherapy with unspecified doses for inadequate margins, preoperatively, or for recurrence at the primary site or neck.

BYERS et al. (1973) reviewed 36 patients treated at UT M. D. Anderson Cancer Center for malignant submaxillary gland tumors. Twenty-seven patients (75%) were found to have one or more of the following indicators of adverse prognosis: invasion of nerves, lymph node metastasis, invasion of periglandular soft tissue, high grade tumor or invasion of mandibular bone.

The most significant risk factor for all histologies noted was nerve invasion, which was seen in 19 patients, with only 7 of these patients having local

Table 13-7. Site of presentation and histology for 118 malignant minor salivary gland tumors (SCHELL et al. 1983)

Site	No. of patients	Adenoid cystic	Mucoepidermoid		Adeno-carcinoma	Malignant mixed	Acinic cell
			High-grade	Low-grade			
Lip	2	1	0	0	1	0	0
Buccal mucosa	16	9	1	3	3	0	0
Tongue	17	10	2	1	4	0	0
Floor of mouth	22	10	4	3	4	0	1
Gingivae	13	3	5	1	4	0	0
Palate	23	15	1	3	2	0	0
Paranasal sinuses and nasal cavity	20	16	1	1	2	0	0
Nasopharynx and pharynx	3	1	0	1	0	1	0
Trachea	1	1	0	0	0	0	0
Larynx	1	1	0	0	0	0	0
Total	118	67	14	13	20	1	1

Note: M. D. Anderson Cancer Center data; patients treated 1/70–2/78

Table 13-8

Histology	No. of pts.	Local control	No. NED
Adenoid cystic	21	10	5
Mucoepidermoid	8	4	2
Malignant mixed	5	1	1
Miscellaneous (1 SCC, 1 Adenoca)	2	2	2

control, and only 3 patients surviving. Minimum follow-up time was 7 years.

Table 13-8 shows an analysis of local control and survival by histology.

Because of the poor prognosis of these patients and high risk of local failure, it is recommended that all patients with adverse prognostic factors undergo en bloc dissection and postoperative radiotherapy in order to achieve maximal local control and also avoid extensive disfiguring surgery.

References

Abbey LM, Schwab BH, Landau GC, Perkins ER (1984) Incidence of second primary breast cancer among patients with a first primary salivary gland tumor. Cancer 54: 1439–1442

Alaniz F, Fletcher GH (1965) Place and technics of radiation therapy in the management of malignant tumors of the major salivary glands. Radiology 84: 412–419

Batsakis JG (1974) Tumors of the Head and Neck. In: Batsakis J (ed) Clinical and Pathological Considerations. Williams and Wilkins, Baltimore, p 388

Beahrs O, Myers MH (eds) (1983) American Joint Committee on Cancer Manual for Staging of Cancer. 2nd Ed. J B Lippincott, Philadelphia, p 250

Bedwinek JM, Shukovsky LJ, Fletcher GH, Daley TE (1976) Osteonecrosis in patients treated with definitive radiotherapy for squamous cell carcinomas of the oral cavity and naso- and oropharynx. Radiology 119: 665–667

Belsky JL, Tachikawa K, Cihak RW, Yamamoto T (1972) Salivary gland tumors in the atomic bomb survivors. Hiroshima – Nagasaki, 1957 to 1970. JAMA 219: 864–868

Berg JW, Hutter RVP, Foote FW (1968) The unique association between salivary gland cancer and breast cancer. JAMA 204: 771–774

Blanck C (1974) Carcinoma of the parotid gland; morphology and long-term prognosis. Acta Univ Upsaliensis 195: 1–114

Byers RM, Jesse RH, Guillamondegui OM, Luna MA (1973) Malignant Tumors of the Submaxillary Gland. Am J Surg 126: 458–463

Cassisi NJ, Dickerson DR, Million RR (1978) Squamous cell carcinoma of the skin metastatic to parotid nodes. Arch Otolaryngol 104: 336–339

Catterall M (1981) The treatment of malignant salivary gland tumors with fast neutrons. Int J Radiat Oncol Biol Phys 7: 1737–1738

Chaudhry AP, Gorlin RJ (1958) Papillary cystadenoma lymphomatosum (adenolymphoma): A review of the literature. Am J Surg 95: 923–931

Chong GC, Beahrs OH, Woolner LB (1974) Surgical management of, acinic cell carcinoma of the parotid gland. Surg Gynecol and Obstet 138: 65–68

Conley J, Selfe RW (1981) Occult neoplasms in facial paralysis. Laryngoscope 91: 205–210

Conley J, Hamaker RC (1975) Prognosis of malignant tumors of the parotid gland with facial paralysis. Arch Otolaryngol 101: 39–41

Conley J (1972) Analysis of 115 patients with tumors of the submandibular gland. Ann Otol Rhinol-Laryngol 81: 323–330

Conley J, Arena S (1963) Parotid gland as a focus of metastasis. Arch Surg 87: 757–764

Cummings CW (1977) Adenoidcystic carcinoma (cylindroma) of the parotid gland. Ann Otol Rhinol-Laryngol 86: 280–292

Dawson AK, Orr JA (1985) Long-term results of local excision and radiotherapy in pleomorphic adenoma of the parotid. Int J Radiat Oncol Biol Phys 11: 451–455

Dorn HF, Cutler SJ (1959) Public Health Monograph No 56. Washington, DC, Government printing office, Vol.13, p.201

Eneroth CM (1969) Incidence and prognosis of salivary gland tumors at different sites. A study of parotid, submandibular and palatal tumours in 2632 patients. Acta Otolaryngol 263: 174–178

Eneroth CM, Hamberger CA (1974) Principles of treatment of different types of parotid tumors. Laryngoscope 84: 1732–1740

Eneroth CM, Jakobsson PA, Blanck C (1966) Acinic cell carcinoma of the parotid gland. Cancer 1761–1772

Fleming TJ, Rambach SC (1983) A tongue-shielding radiation stent. J Prosthet Dent 49 (3): 389–392

Foote FW Jr, Frazell EL (1953) Tumors of the major salivary glands. Cancer 6: 1065–1133

Frazell EL (1954) Clinical aspects of tumors of the major salivary gland. Cancer 7: 637–659

Fu KK, Lichter A, Galante M (1976) Carcinoma of the floor of mouth: an analysis of treatment results and the sites and causes of failures. Int J Radiat Oncol Biol Phys 1: 829–837

Fu KK, Leibel SA, Levine ML, Friedlander LM, Boles R, Phillips TL (1977) Carcinoma of the major and minor salivary glands carcinoma of the major and minor salivary glands: analysis of treatment results and sites and causes of failures. Cancer 40: 2882–2890

Goepfert H, Luna M, Lindberg R, White A (1983) Malignant salivary gland tumors of the paranasal sinuses and nasal cavity. Arch Otolaryngol 109: 662–668

Guillamondegui OM, Byers RM, Tapley NduV (1980) Malignant tumors of the salivary gland. In: Textbook of Radiotherapy 3rd Edition, Lea & Febiger, GH Fletcher (ed), Philadelphia, 426–443

Guillamondegui OM, Byers RM, Luna MA, Chiminazzo H, Jesse RH, Fletcher GH (1975) Aggressive surgery in treatment for parotid cancer: the role of adjunctive postoperative radiotherapy. Am J Roentgenol Radium Ther Nucl Med 123: 49–54

Hanna DC, Gaisford JC, Richardson GS, Bindra RN (1968) Tumors of the deep lobe of the parotid gland. Am J Surg 116: 524–527

Healey WV, Perzin KH, Smith L (1970) Mucoepidermoid carcinoma of salivary gland origin: Classification, clinical-pathologic correlation, and results of treatment. Cancer 26: 368–388

Henry LW, Blasko JC, Griffin TW, Parker RG (1979) Evaluation of fast neutron teletherapy for advanced carcinomas of the major salivary glands. Cancer 44: 814–818

Hogstrom KR, Mills MD, Meyer JA, Palta JR, Mellenberg DE, Meoz RT, Fields RS (1984) Dosimetric evaluation of a pencil-beam algorithm for electrons employing a two-dimensional heterogeneity correction. Int J Radiat Oncol 10: 561–569

Jackson GL, Ballantyne AJ (1981) Role of parotidectomy for skin cancer of the head and neck. Am J Surg 142: 464–469

Johns M, Regazi J, Batsakis JG, McClatchey KD (1976) Primary squamous cell carcinoma of the parotid gland. Arch Otolaryngol 102: 355–357

Kagan AR, Nussbaum H, Handler S, Shapiro R, Gilbert HA, Jacobs M, Miles JW, Chan PYM, Calcaterra T (1976) Recurrences from malignant parotid salivary gland tumors. Cancer 37: 2600–2604

King JJ, Fletcher GH (1971) Malignant tumors of the major salivary glands. Radiology 100: 381–384

Lampe I, Zatzkin H (1949) Pulmonary metastases of pseudoadenomatous basal cell carcinoma (mucous and salivary and gland tumor). Radiology 53: 379–385

Leafstedt SW, Gaeta JF, Sako K, Marchetta FC, Shedd DP (1971) Adenoid cystic carcinoma of major and minor salivary glands. Am J Surg 122: 756–762

Levitt SH, McHugh RB, Gomez-Marin O, Hyams VJ, Soule EH, Strong EW, Seller AH, Woods JE, Guillamondegui OM (1981) Clinical staging system for cancer of the salivary gland: A retrospective study. Cancer 47: 2712–2724

Maran AGD, Mackenzie IJ, Stanley RE (1984) Recurrent pleomorphic adenomas of the parotid gland. Arch Otolaryngol 110: 167–171

McNaney D, McNeese MD, Guillamondegui OM, Fletcher GH, Oswald MJ (1983) Postoperative irradiation in malignant epithelial tumors of the parotid. Int J Radiat Oncol Biol Phys 9: 1289–1295

Million RR, Cassisi NJ (1984) Minor salivary gland tumors. In: Management of Head and Neck Cancer A Multidisciplinary Approach, RR Million and NJ Cassisi (ed) JB Lippincott Co, Philadelphia, p 547–557

Moertel CG, Elveback LR (1969) The association between salivary gland cancer and breast cancer. JAMA 210: 306–308

Nigro MF, Spiro RH (1977) Deep lobe parotid tumors. Am J Surg 134: 523–527

Prior P, Waterhouse JAH (1977) Second primary cancers in patients with tumors of the salivary glands. Br J Cancer 36: 362–368

Rafla S (1977) Malignant parotid tumors: Natural history and treatment. Cancer 40: 136–144

Rafla S (1970) Mucous and salivary gland tumors. Springfield Ill, Charles C Thomas Publisher

Rafla S, Rafla-Demetrious S (1973) Significance and treatment of lymph node metastases of malignant mucous and salivary gland tumors. Am J Roentgenol Radium Ther Nucl Med 117: 595–604

Schell S, Barkley HT Jr, Chiminazzo H Jr (1983) Treatment of malignant minor salivary gland tumors. Verbal Presentation MD Anderson Hospital data; patients treated 1/70–2/78

Shore-Freedman E, Abrahams C, Recant W, Schneider AB (1983) Neurilemomas and salivary gland tumors of the head and neck following childhood irradiation. Cancer 51: 2159–2163

Spiro RH, Huvos AC, Strong EW (1979) Adenoid cystic carcinoma: Factors influencing survival. Am J Surg 138: 579–583

Spiro RH, Huvos AG, Strong EW (1978) Acinic cell carcinoma of salivary origin – A clinicopathologic study of 67 cases. Cancer 41: 924–935

Spiro RH, Huvos AG, Strong EW (1977) Malignant mixed tumor of salivary gland origin a clinicopathologic study of 146 cases. Cancer 39: 388–396

Spiro RH, Huvos AG, Strong EW (1975) Cancer of the parotid gland. A clinicopathologic study of 288 primary cases. Am J Surg 130: 452–459

Spiro RH, Koss LG, Hajdu SI, Strong EW (1973) Tumors of minor salivary origin – a clinicopathologic study of 492 cases. Cancer 31: 117–129

Takeichi N, Hirose F, Yamamoto H, Ezaki H, Fujikura T (1983) Salivary gland tumors in atomic bomb survivors, Hiroshima Japan. Cancer 52: 377–385

Tapley NduV (1977) Irradiation treatment of malignant tumors of the salivary glands. Ear Nose and Throat J 56: 110–114

Tapley NduV, Fletcher GH (1976) Malignant tumors of salivary glands. In Clinical Applications of the Electron Beam, Tapley NduV (ed), John Wiley & Sons, New York, pp 141–171

Tortoledo ME, Luna MA, Batsakia JG (1984) Carcinoma ex pleomorphic adenoma and malignant mixed tumors. Arch Otolaryngol 110: 172–176

Vikram B, Strong EW, Shah JP, Spiro RH (1984) Radiation therapy in adenoid-cystic carcinoma. Int J Radiat Oncol Biol Phys 10: 221–223

Wang CC (1982) The management of parotid lymph node metastases by irradiation. Cancer 50: 223–225

Watson TA (1965) Irradiation in the management of tumors of the head and neck. Am J Surg 110: 542–548

14 Thyroid Cancer and its Management with Radiation Therapy

KATHERINE L. GRIEM and MELVIN L. GRIEM

CONTENTS

14.1 Incidence and Epidemiology

Carcinoma of the thyroid represents one of the more infrequent malignancies of the head and neck. Many of the nodular lesions of the thyroid are benign. Only a small percentage of the nodular thyroid disease represents malignancy and most of these tumors have a benign course with appropriate treatment. The majority of malignant tumors are well-differentiated and are readily managed with surgery and thyroid suppression. Tumors of the anaplastic type represent only a small fraction of thyroid tumors. Patients with these tumors have a very poor prognosis despite aggressive therapy. Combined surgery, radiation therapy and chemotherapy are suggested for management of these tumors. Management of thyroid tumors is based upon accurate histological assessment of the biopsy material.

In the United States there are approximately 10,000 cases of thyroid cancer per year and 1000 deaths from the disease (SILVERBERG and LUBERA 1986). There is a higher incidence in the United States in whites than blacks and thyroid cancer is three times more common in females than in males. Autopsy studies have found an incidence of occult disease of up to 8.6% (BONDESON and LJUNDSBERG 1981). Surveys in the United States have shown no variation in geographic incidence (MUSTACCHI and CUTLER 1956) though the incidence may be higher in areas of endemic goiter.

Carcinoma of the thyroid is rare in children and the incidence increases with age. Thyroid cancer generally presents in young and middle-aged adults with papillary tumors generally occur in younger patients (under age 40), follicular in a slightly older population, and anaplastic in patients over age 50 (DE GROOT et al. 1984). Medullary carcinoma of the thyroid occurs either sporadically or as part of two inherited endocrine syndromes, multiple endocrine neoplasia (MEN) type II A or II B. The MEN-associated cases of medullary thyroid carcinoma tend to present at a much earlier age (20-30) than do the sporadic cases which present in the 6th and 7th decade (DE GROOT et al. 1984).

14.2 Special Considerations

14.2.1 Carcinogenic Factors

Low dose radiation given for a variety of benign conditions during infancy and childhood has been shown to cause thyroid cancer (CLARK 1955, MO-

KATHERINE L. GRIEM, M.D., Department of Therapeutic Radiology, Rush Presbyterian - St. Lukes Medical Center, 1753 West Congress Parkway, Chicago, IL, 60612, USA.

MELVIN L. GRIEM, M.D., Department of Therapeutic Radiology, University of Chicago, Box 442, 5841 South Maryland Avenue, Chicago, IL, 60637 USA

DAN et al. 1977; REFETOFF et al. 1975). During the 1940's radiation was used for a wide variety of diseases: enlarged thymus in infants, tonsillitis, hemangiomas, and skin diseases such as tinea capitis in childhood and acne in the teenagers. Doses of between 300 cGy and 2000 cGy were used in dose fractions of less than 100 cGy to 300 cGy (CLARK 1955). The latent period between radiation and the appearance of tumor in the thyroid is 10 to 30 years. There appears to be no threshold dose and there is a dose-response curve through 1500 cGy (MAXON et al. 1977). Above 2000 cGy the thyroid gland tends to become sterilized by radiation with less chance for malignant transformation. Studies of the survivors of the atomic blasts at Nagasaki and Hiroshima have also demonstrated an increased incidence of thyroid carcinoma indicating that the adult thyroid is also sensitive to radiation though not as much as the child's thyroid. Though the practice of low dose radiation for benign conditions has largely been abandoned, patients with a diagnosis of thyroid tumor should be questioned for a history of irradiation and patients with a history of exposure should have careful assessment of the thyroid. The tumor type usually induced is of a well-differentiated histology with approximately 90% being of papillary histology. The behavior of these radiation-induced tumors is no different from spontaneous tumors. Radiation induced sarcomas of the thyroid have also been described after high dose radiation to the head and neck for other primary neoplasms. The latent period for development of these tumors is generally longer than for the epithelial neoplasms and, fortunately, sarcomas are quite rare.

14.2.2 MEN Syndromes

Medullary carcinomas constitute only 2 to 8% of all thyroid carcinomas and are derived from the "C" or parafollicular cells of the thyroid. All are calcitonin secreting (DE GROOT 1984). Approximately 10 to 20% arise as part of the MEN syndromes and are transmitted as autosomal dominant traits. MEN II A includes patients with medullary carcinomas of the thyroid, parathyroid hyperplasia or adenomas, and pheochromocytomas. MEN II B constitutes medullary carcinoma, mucosal neuromas, and pheochromocytomas. Members of families with these syndromes should be carefully screened. The thyroid tumor associated with this syndrome is of the medullary type, presumably arising from the calcitonin-secreting "C" cells of the thyroid. Only

20% of medullary carcinomas of the thyroid are familial, however.

14.3 Embryology and Anatomy

14.3.1 Embryology

The thyroid gland buds from the foramen cecum located at the level of the circumvallate papillae on the posterior aspect of the oral tongue. This forms the thyroglossal duct which during embryological development elongates at its distal end becomes bilobed and migrates to the neck to form the two lobes of the thyroid and the isthmus. By the seventh week, it reaches its final position in relation to the trachea and the larynx. Tumors may occasionally arise along this route of migration. The thyroid may also migrate to a substernal location, usually anterior to the trachea and may present as a widened mediastinum on chest x-ray. It is interesting that in the chicken the thyroid is found at the bifurcation of the trachea which may in part explain this unusual finding in mammals.

14.3.2 Anatomy

The thyroid gland is located anteriorly in the low neck draped on either side of the thyroid cartilage. It lies in close proximity to the larynx, esophagus, parathyroid glands, carotid sheath and recurrent laryngeal nerves. The thyroid gland consists of two pear-shaped lateral lobes connected by an isthmus. The lateral lobes usually extend from the level of the mid-thyroid cartilage superiorly to the level of the sixth tracheal ring inferiorly. The isthmus extends across the midline in front of the second, third and fourth tracheal rings. A pyramidal lobe is often present and projects upward from the isthmus.

Given its location in the neck, the thyroid lies close to several vital structures. The lobes of the thyroid lie posterior to the sternothyroid, sternohyoid and anterior border of the sternocleido-mastoid muscles. It lies laterally over the carotid sheath with the common carotid artery, internal jugular vein and vagus nerve (Fig. 14-1). Medially it is adjacent to the larynx, trachea and esophagus.

The recurrent laryngeal nerve lies in close proximity to the thyroid gland, in the groove between the esophagus and trachea, and great care must be taken that it is not injured during surgery on the

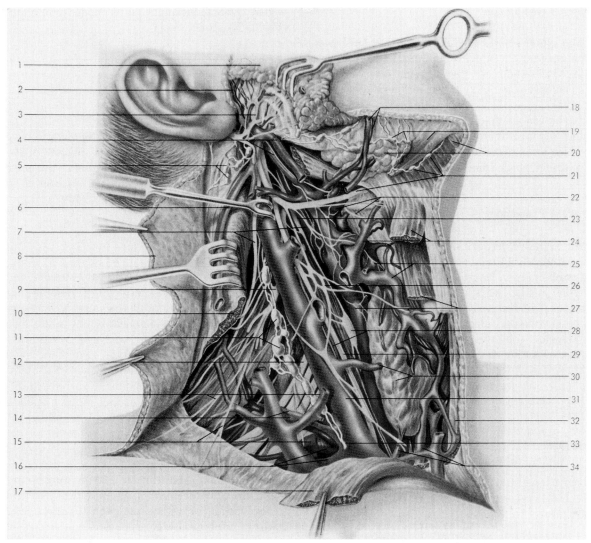

Fig. 14-1. Anatomy of the lower neck and thyroid (From Ciba symposia). *1* Parotid gland, *2* superficial temporal artery and vein, *3* temporal branch of facial nerve, *4* external carotid artery and posterior facial vein, *5* superficial cervical lymph nodes, *6* external jugular vein, *7* accessory nerve and internal carotid artery, *8* platysma muscle, *9* fourth cervical nerve, *10* superior position of sternocleidomastoid muscle, *11* deep cervical lymph nodes, *12* fifth cervical nerve, *13* posterior supraclavicular nerve and anterior jugular vein, *14* superficial cervical artery and vein, *15* middle supraclavicular nerve and subclavian artery, *16* transverse scapular artery and vein, *17* inferior position of sternocleidomastoid muscle, *18* external maxillary artery and anterior facial vein, *19* submaxillary lymph nodes and digastric muscle, *20* submaxillary gland and mylohyoid muscle, *21* submental lymph nodes and hypoglossal nerve, *22* superior laryngeal artery and nerve, *23* superior cervical ganglion, *24* superior laryngeal vein and omohyoid muscle, *25* superior thyroid artery and vein, *26* ansa hypoglossi, *27* common carotid artery and sternothyroid muscle, *28* middle cervical ganglion and phrenic nerve, *29* vagus nerve, *30* thyroid gland and middle thyroid vein, *31* internal jugular vein, *32* sternohyoid muscle, *33* jugular lymphatic trunk, *34* inferior thyroid veins

thyroid. The right recurrent laryngeal nerve courses around the aortic arch. Before the nerve enters the larynx, it lies just adjacent to the medial surface of the thyroid gland. Occasionally, the nerve may actually penetrate the thyroid gland. Injury of the recurrent laryngeal nerve produces a disabling injury; with paralysis of the vocal cords which may be fixed in the abducted or adducted position. The parathyroid glands lie lateral and posterior to the thyroid gland, but their location may vary. During total thyroidectomy, identification and preservation of at least one parathyroid gland is essential to maintain calcium homeostasis.

14.3.3 Blood Supply

The blood supply of the thyroid is extensive and comes from the superior and inferior thyroid arteries. Occasionally, the thyroidea ima artery is present as an accessory blood supply to the inferior thyroid artery.

The venous drainage of the thyroid comes from the superior thyroid and middle thyroid veins which drain to the internal jugular, and inferior thyroid vein which drains to the brachiocephalic vein.

14.3.4 Lymphatics

An extensive network of lymphatics drain the thyroid gland. From the lymphatics of the gland, lymph drains to several nodal sites including the internal jugular nodes, and the pretracheal and paratracheal nodes, and the Delphian node overlying the cricothyroid membrane. The latter serves as a "sentinel" for involvement by thyroid carcinoma. Spread may also occur to the supraclavicular as well as the anterior and superior mediastinal nodes (Fig. 14-2), (Rubin 1971).

14.4 Pathology

14.4.1 General

Various classification of tumors of the thyroid have been proposed. The Armed Forces Institute of Pathology (AFIP) classification represents the most widely used classification and is presented in Table 14-1. (Meissner and Warren 1969)

14.4.2 Papillary

Well-differentiated tumors, papillary tumors and follicular types as well as mixtures of these histologies, represent 75–80% of thyroid tumors. Papillary carcinomas are usually characterized by tumor cells surrounding a fibrovascular core and occasionally areas of follicular differentiation. Lymphatic invasion is common. Mitoses are infrequent but psammoma bodies are often abundant. Many of well-differentiated carcinomas are neither purely papillary or purely follicular but a mixture of both. The mixed tumor carries the clinical prognosis of the papillary variant. Characteristic of papillary thyroid carcinoma are optically clear nuclei, also referred to as "little Orphan Annie nuclei". The finding is a reliable artifact of formalin fixation and not seen in frozen section or with some other fixatives. The presence of optically clear nuclei in a neoplasm with follicular architecture warrants the diagnosis of a papillary carcinoma, follicular variant. The lesion will clinically behave like a papillary carcinoma.

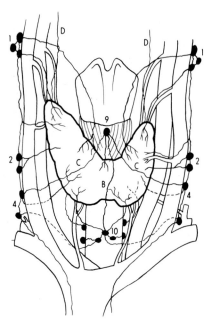

THYROID

Routes	1st Station
A. Median superior tr.	1. Jugulo-digastric
B. Median inferior tr.	2. Jugulo-omohyoid
C. Lateral tr.	9. Pretracheal
D. Posterior superior tr.	4. Transverse cervical
	10. Paratracheal

Fig. 14-2. Lymphatic anatomy of the thyroid (From Rubin P. Oncologic Anatomy)

Table 14-1. Classification of cancer of the thyroid

Carcinoma
  Papillary adenocarcinoma
  Follicular carcinoma
    Clear cell carcinoma
    Oxyphil carcinoma
  Medullary carcinoma
  Undifferentiated carcinoma
    Small cell carcinoma
    Giant cell carcinoma
  Epidermoid carcinoma
Other malignant tumors
  Lymphoma
  Sarcoma
  Malignant teratoma
  Secondary tumor

14.4.3 Follicular

Follicular carcinomas are often well-encapsulated and may be difficult to distinguish from follicular adenomas. The microscopic pattern may range from solid sheets of cells to well-differentiated follicles containing colloid. Capsular or vascular invasion must be present to allow a definitive histologic diagnosis. Follicular carcinoma most often metastasizes by hematogenous dissemination. Hurthle cell neoplasms may be a separate entity whereas others consider this entity simply as a variant of follicular thyroid carcinoma (WATSON et al. 1984) (TOLLEFSEN et al. 1975) (WOOLNER et al. 1961).

14.4.4 Medullary

Medullary carcinoma, as described earlier, arises from the "C" cells of the thyroid. In the sporadic form these tumors are usually unilateral while in the familial form associated with MEN-syndromes, they are usually bilateral. Microscopically the tumor cells are in solid groups and there may be considerable associated fibrosis. Deposits of amyloid may be seen and usually "make" the diagnosis of medullary carcinoma.

14.4.5 Anaplastic Carcinoma

Anaplastic or undifferentiated carcinoma occurs primarily in persons over 50 years of age. These carcinomas grow rapidly and local invasion may cause life-threatening problems with breathing or swallowing, and tracheotomy may be required. These tumors metastasize to lymph nodes and lung, but not characteristically to bone.

Histologically, these tumors contain neither papillary nor follicular elements. They are commonly subclassified into small and giant cell variants. The giant cell carcinoma is a highly malignant form and extracapsular invasion is common. Occasionally these tumors have been mistaken for a fibrosarcoma.

14.4.6 Rare Histologic Forms

Epidermoid or squamous cell carcinoma may arise in the thyroid as can malignant lymphomas. Primary sarcomas of the thyroid are rare lesions with cases of osteosarcoma, fibrosarcoma and other histologic types being reported. Many older reports of spindle cell tumors of the thyroid may reflect sarcomatoid anaplastic carcinomas (HEDINGER and SOBIN 1974). Malignant melanoma, lymphoma, bronchogenic carcinoma, renal cell and breast carcinoma may metastasize to the thyroid as well but these are usually found at autopsy and are rarely mistaken for primary thyroid cancer (IVY 1984).

The diagnosis of tumor in the thyroid may be based on a needle aspiration. At present, the diagnosis and subtyping of carcinoma of the thyroid is usually made via light microscopy. In the future, immunological techniques for identifying tumors with monoclonal antibodies may add to our ability to classify these tumors. In addition, newer imaging techniques may add to the ability to subclassify tumors. The use of positron emission tomography (PET), fluorescent scanning, magnetic resonance imaging (MRI), and ultrasound will add to our knowledge of the pathology of this disease.

14.5 Diagnosis

The management of thyroid nodules has been well-described recently in an excellent review by ROJESKI and GHARIB (1985). The approach to the problem of nodular thyroid disease has changed significantly in the past several years with the utilization of radionuclide imaging, high resolution ultrasound and the utilization of fine needle aspiration and cytology. The role of magnetic resonance imaging in thyroid disease has yet to be defined, however. Computerized tomography of the thyroid gland gives interesting images but does not have the fine resolution of ultrasound coupled with fine needle aspiration of palpable nodules in the neck. The later technique has dramatically improved the diagnostic accuracy and evaluation of early thyroid disease. High resolution ultrasound has the ability to image 1 mm nodules which is beyond the capabilities of other imaging procedures and even palpation (SCHEIBLE et al. 1979). Because this technique is a real time imaging procedure, it allows the physician to perform the needle aspiration simultaneously with the imaging of the nodule to be sampled (ROJESKI and GHARIB 1985).

The main limitation of needle aspiration is in the diagnosis of follicular tumors where differentiation between benign disease and malignancy cannot be established without obtaining an adequate surgical specimen for extensive evaluation by the surgical pathologist. The diagnosis of malignancy may require a search for invasion into the capsule or the presence of vascular or lymphatic invasion.

The use of thyroid hormone suppression may aid in the management of some thyroid nodules. Thyroid hormone may cause some reduction in the size of a nodule and may help in distinguishing a benign nodule from malignant. The lack of a response with thyroid hormone suppression is not specific for malignant disease, however (ROJESKI and GHARIB 1985). Other authors note the problems which may arise in using a trial of thyroid suppression (PARSONS and PFAFF 1984). They point out that if a nodule fails to regress with suppression, the decision on management has simply been postponed and if the nodule grows on suppressive therapy, then one has delayed definitive management.

14.6 Staging

Two staging systems for thyroid carcinoma are commonly used: The system listed in the AFIP fascicle on this subject (MEISSNER and WARREN 1969) and a second staging system proposed by the American Joint Committee (BEAHRS 1983) are presented in Table 14-2. Histologic type, the extent of local and regional disease, age and sex are prognostic

Table 14-2 a. Surgical and pathologic staging in thyroid carcinoma

Stage I	A Confined to one lobe B Bilateral, multicentric, or in isthmus
Stage II	Primary as in Stage I-A or Stage I-B with metastases in lymph nodes A Unilateral lymph nodes B Bilateral lymph nodes, lymph nodes in mediastinum, or midline lymph nodes
Stage III	Invasion of other tissues or structures in neck or adjacent mediastinum with or without lymph nodes
Stage IV	Distant metastases

Table 14-2 b. Modified UICC staging of thyroid cancer

Tumor (t), node (N) classification

T 1	Unilateral/single nodule
T 2	Unilateral/multiple nodules
T 3	Bilateral/isthmus nodule
T 4	Extension beyond gland
N 1	Homolateral movable
N 2	Contra-midline or bilateral movable
N 3	Fixed

factors in thyroid cancer (WOOLNER et al. 1961) (CADY et al. 1979) (TUBIANA et al. 1985 b). In Woolner's analysis, survival was mainly a feature of the histology and the presence or absence of lymphatic and vascular invasion, particularly in patients with medullary and follicular carcinomas respectively. Staging of thyroid carcinoma should, therefore, include not only the extent of local and regional disease, but the morphological findings as well in an attempt to guide the management more effectively.

14.7 Treatment

14.7.1 Papillary and Follicular Histology

14.7.1.1 Surgery

Surgery is the principal modality in the management of cancer of the thyroid and represents the first approach in establishing the regional distribution of disease in some situations. The extent of surgery will vary, however. Opinions vary on the extent of surgery necessary in these type of histology. Crile recommends limited surgery followed by thyroid suppression for well-differentiated tumors of papillary or follicular histology (CRILE 1968). Farrar reported on the results of 155 patients treated initially by surgery for papillary or follicular tumors and found no difference in survival or local recurrence rate between those treated with total thyroidectomy or partial thyroidectomy (FARRAR et al. 1982). The presence of lymph node metastases did not adversely affect prognosis in the Farrar series. Schroder and colleagues conducted a retrospective analysis of 109 patients with non-medullary thyroid carcinomas treated with partial or total thyroidectomy with the two groups being matched for prognostic indicators. They found no difference in cancer mortality or recurrence rates, though total thyroidectomy resulted in a significantly increased risk of postoperative complications, primarily transient or permanent hypocalcemia, when compared with partial thyroidectomy (SCHRODER et al. 1986). Cady analyzed the results of 792 patients treated for thyroid cancer at the Lahey Clinic over a 40 year period of which 90% of the tumors were well-differentiated (CADY et al. 1976). He recommends lobectomy only for patients with small carcinomas of well-differentiated histology. Certainly the presence of gross disease bilaterally requires a total thyroidectomy. In smaller, well-differentiated carcinomas, however, one could argue for lesser surgery since total thyroidectomy has not been shown to improve local control or survival and does have a higher incidence of postoperative complications including hypoparathyroidism. The incidence of permanent hypocalcemia may be as high as 30% in patients undergoing total thyroidectomy (MCCONAHEY et al. 1986). Furthermore, a recent series from the Mayo Clinic in which most patients underwent total or subtotal thyroidectomy found bilateral disease in only 14% of the patients (MCCONAHEY et al. 1986).

The approach to management of the neck in thyroid carcinoma has varied over the years (CADY et al. 1976). At present, elective neck dissection is not recommended as it has not been shown to improve survival and delayed therapeutic neck dissection has shown equal results. In patients presenting with gross nodal disease, however, modified neck dissection is recommended for removal of tumor. Thyroid carcinomas which present with more advanced local disease require individualization of surgical therapy as well. There may be theoretical reasons for "debulking" locally advanced disease before addition of radiation therapy or chemotherapy, but the goal of any such therapy must be removal of as much disease as possible while preserving normal function. Thus, if it appears that much gross disease will be left behind, one had best proceed to radiation therapy (either I-131 or external beam therapy) in hopes of making the local disease resectable at a later date.

In summary, although less than total thyroidectomy may be appropriate management for some well-differentiated tumors of the thyroid, most authors conclude that the operation for thyroid carcinoma must be individualized according to both the extent of disease and the histology as will be discussed later.

14.7.1.2 Thyroid Suppressive Therapy

All patients should be maintained on thyroid replacement therapy after surgery and/or thyroid ablation. This is both to restore euthyroidism and to maintain TSH suppression. Doses at or slightly above normal replacement levels may be used ranging from 0.15 to 0.25 mg of 1-T4 or the equivalent (DE GROOT et al. 1984).

14.7.1.3 I-131 Therapy

Radioactive I-131 therapy should be considered for either papillary or follicular thyroid carcinoma in patients with distant metastases. Potchin has shown

that approximately one half of the patients respond to therapeutic doses of I-131. A higher percentage of patients with pure papillary carcinomas will respond to this manipulation (POTCHIN 1971). Doses vary between 30 mCi given every other week (CLARK 1953) to 50-100 mCi given every several months. As the radioactive iodine is administered, the metastatic tumor and normal thyroid tissue take up the radioactive material and are treated – eliminating both tumor and normal thyroid tissue. After several doses of radioactive iodine, any tissue which has accumulated I-131 has been eradicated. As a consequence the patient becomes hypothyroid, the level of TSH becomes elevated and thyroid replacement is necessary (SCHIMPFF 1979; HARNESS 1974).

Radioactive iodine has been used for prophylactic treatment after complete surgical resection or when there is known gross or microscopic residual present. Cady (CADY et al. 1976) states that no improvement in survival was seen with the addition of I-131. This contradicts the reports by Varma (VARMA et al. 1970) who found an improvement in survival in patients over 40 year old treated with I-131 after total thyroidectomy when compared with a roughly matched historical group of patients. Maheshwari (MAHESHWARI et al. 1981) reports on the M. D. Anderson Hospital experience with routine use of I-131 after subtotal thyroidectomy for differentiated thyroid carcinomas as well, but no control group is avaiable for this study.

The recommendations for the amount of I-131 to be used for ablative radioactive therapy vary (VARMA et al. 1970; DE GROOT et al. 1984; BEIERWALTES 1978). Maxon and co-workers analyzed the relation between radiation dose and outcome of I-131 therapy for thyroid cancer (MAXON et al. 1977). They found a significantly higher rate of successful ablation in patients who received a total dose of 3000 cGy or more to the thyroid remmants. In the treatment of patients with metastatic foci of I-131 concentrating thyroid cancer, there was a significantly higher rate of response in patients receiving at least 80,000 cGy total dose to metastatic foci.

14.7.2 Medullary and Anaplastic Histology

14.7.2.1 General

Medullary and anaplastic carcinoma of the thyroid rarely take up radioactive iodine, and for this reason its use in their management is discouraged and other approaches will be discussed.

14.7.2.2 Medullary Carcinoma

Medullary carcinoma represents 5 to 10% of thyroid malignancies. This tumor frequently presents with lymph node metastases. Total thyroidectomy is the operation of choice because of the high incidence of multicentricity seen in this carcinoma. In addition, elective neck dissection should be performed even in the absence of nodal disease because nodal involvement is of prognostic importance in this histology. Medullary carcinomas will not concentrate radioactive I-131, and its use in the management is not likely to benefit the patient. External beam radiation therapy can be used in the management of locally advanced disease. A recent protocol for the management of medullary carcinoma of the thyroid from the Thyroid Cancer Treatment Cooperative Study Group is presented in Table 14-3 (DE GROOT 1985).

14.7.2.3 Anaplastic Carcinoma

Optimal management of anaplastic thyroid carcinoma has yet to be defined. These tumors are often locally advanced at presentation and surgery is performed accordingly. Often complete resection is not possible and the tumor can only be grossly resected. A tracheostomy is often required for the compromised airway from these locally invasive, rapidly growing tumors. Radiation therapy should be part of the management of any anaplastic carcinomas for these tumors can recur locally even after "com-plete" surgical removal. This tumor does not concentrate iodine and I-131 should not be used in its management.

Anaplastic carcinoma has a very poor prognosis as seen by the reported five year survival and five year disease-free survival of 0 to 10% (SMEDAL and MEISSNER 1961). In an attempt to improve this poor outlook, more aggressive radiation therapy and chemotherapy have been used in treatment of this histology. Aldinger reported on the use of radiation therapy and actinomycin-D after gross excision, but finds only 6/84 disease-free at five years (ALDINGER et al. 1978). Kim reports on the use of adriamycin and radiation therapy (160 cGy BID/three fractions per week to 5760 cGy) and finds that although 8/9 had complete disappearance of disease, only 1/9 was disease-free at 18 months (KIM and LEEPER). Simpson found some improvement in short term survival in patients treated with 100 cGy fractions three times a day to a total dose of 3600 cGy. Some of the patients in Simpson's series received adriamycin (SIMPSON 1980).

A recent protocol that was developed by the Thyroid Cancer Treatment Cooperative Study Group is presented in Table 14-4 (DE GROOT 1985), (Fig. 14-3).

Table 14-3. Medullary carcinoma protocol thyroid cancer tretment study group

Modified mantle radiotherapy (Fig. 14–3)

Technique:
The tumor volume includes the entire neck and upper half or two-thirds of the mediastinum, extending from the base of the skull to 4 cm below the carina.

Energy:
Cobalt-60 or 4–25 mV photons. Anterior compensators will be required for Cobalt-60 or 4–8 MV photons. The best iso-dose distribution is usually achieved by using an anterior field using Cobalt-60 or 4 MV photons, with a compensator, and a posterior field using 15–25 MV photons, uncompensated. A satisfactory distribution can be achieved with Cobalt-60 alone, but usually requires spinal cord shielding.

Dose:
TD 4000 cGy/20 treatments/4 weeks.

Note: A posterior spinal cord shield (2 cm) to be used to limit the spinal cord dose to 4000 cGy/4 weeks. Lung shields to be used throughout treatment.

Table 14-4. Anaplastic carcinoma protocol thyroid cancer treatment study group

Technique: Modified Mantle
The tumor volume includes the entire neck and upper half or two-thirds of the mediastinum, extending from the base of the skull to 4–8 cm below carina (Fig. 14-3).

Energy:
Co-60 or 4–25 mV photons. Anterior compensators will be required for CO-60 or 4–8 mV photons.

Dose:
(A) *Large Volume*
    Dose: TD 4000 cGy/20 treatments/4 weeks
    Note: Spinal cord shield (posterior field only) to be used to limit the spinal cord dose to 4000 cGy/4 weeks.
(B) *"Boost" Radiotherapy*
Following the modified mantle radiation, a "boost" dose will be given to the site of gross tumor present at the start of the radiation therapy. Appropriate techniques will vary with the size and location or the original disease – an anterior wedge pair, an anterior electron field, an A-P parallel pair with posterior spinal cord shielding, etc.
"Boost dose": 1500 cGy/8 treatments/1½ weeks.
In all cases, care must be taken to ensure that the spinal cord dose does not exceed a further 800 cGy/8 treatments/1½ weeks.

Shielding:
Lung shields throughout treatment. Spinal cord shield (2 cm width, post. field only) to prevent spinal cord dose from exceeding 4800 cGy/28 treatments/5½ weeks; the spinal cord dose to be calculated in all patients.

Fig. 14-3. Radiation fields used in medullary and anaplastic carcinoma protocols of the Thyroid Cancer Treatment Group

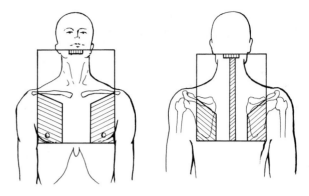

14.7.3 External Beam Radiation Therapy

14.7.3.1 Dose Considerations

The indications for the use of external beam radiation therapy in thyroid carcinomas are not well established. In well-differentiated tumors, however, many believe that radition therapy is indicated if residual disease remains after thyroidectomy, if there is tumor extension through the capsule of the gland, or if there is extranodal extension into surrounding soft tissues (SMEDAL 1967; SIMPSON and CARRUTHERS 1978; MAZZAFERRI 1977). The control of residual thyroid carcinoma with external radiation therapy requires doses used conventionally in squamous cell carcinoma of other head and neck sites. Chung and co-workers reported their results in the treatment of residual or recurrent primary thyroid carcinomas. Of the eight patients with well-differentiated thyroid carcinoma treated with local irradiation, only the four who received more than 1700 rets (6000 cGy in 6 weeks) were locally controlled (CHUNG et al. 1980). External beam radiotherapy has been combined with radioactive iodine as well (TUBIANA and LACOUR 1975). Tubiana failed to demonstrate any decrease in local recurrence with the addition of radioactive iodine to external radiation therapy following surgery for differentiated thyroid carcinoma. He did, however, find a significant difference in local recurrence between irradiated and non-irradiated patients after complete or incomplete surgical excision. Simpson's series from the Princess Margaret Hospital on patients with follicular carcinoma showed that in patients with gross disease, four of seven patients treated with both modalities had complete regression versus only five of fourteen patients treated with radiation alone (SIMPSON and CARRUTHERS 1978). These series would suggest that an adequate dose of ionizing radiation is required and that the addition of I-131 to

external beam treatment does not increase the complication rate of such treatment.

14.7.3.2 Treatment Planning

Planning external beam radiation therapy for carcinoma of the thyroid must take into account several important principles. In treating the thyroid gland and its draining lymph nodes, the dose limiting structures, particularly the cervical and upper thoracic spinal cord must be considered. Tolerance of the thoracic cord has been reported to be 5000 to 5500 cGy in 180 to 200 cGy fractions and cervical cord tolerance may be as high as 6000 cGy using the same fractionations (GILBERT 1980). In general, however, doses to the cord should be limited to 4500 to 5000 cGy (180 to 200 cGy daily fractions) because of concern over varying normal tissue tolerance for individual patients. In addition, data are available that some chemotherapeutic agents given after radiation therapy may increase the sensitivity of the central nervous sstem to injury from the interaction of radiation and chemotherapy (GRIEM 1987). If chemotherapeutic agents which penetrate the nervous system (i.e., methotrexate, adriamycin, platinum, Ara-C) are to be used as well, one may wish to limit the radiation dose even further.

Other normal tissues sensitive to radiation therapy include the salivary glands, and if these tissues are to be included in the radiation field, adequate measures must be taken to manage xerostomia. The pretreatment evaluation and management may include proper dental hygiene, particularly the use of fluoride for prevention of dental caries.

Necrosis of the thyroid cartilage and vocal cord injury are quite rare after radiation therapy of thyroid carcinoma (especially with the use of 180 to 200 cGy per fraction). Any altered fractionation

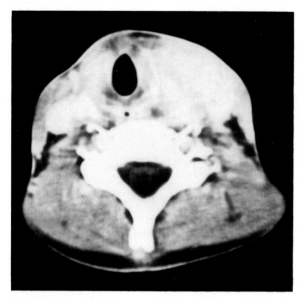

Fig. 14-4. CT scan of thyroid tumor

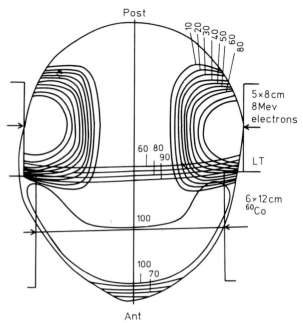

Fig. 14-6. Isodose distribution for anterior opposed laterally directed photon beams and posterior electron fields

scheme proposed for the treatment of anaplastic carcinoma must be careful to minimize late normal tissue injuries.

CT scanning coupled with the treatment planning computer allows the therapist to define a treatment plan which will include to thyroid and draining nodes but spare the spinal cord and lung (Fig. 14-4). The thickness of the neck tissues after surgery can be measured from the postsurgical CT scan and this is introduced into the planning computer. There should be adequate blocking of the spinal cord and if anterior fields are used to treat

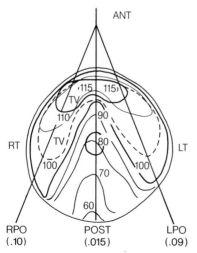

Fig. 14-5. Complex photon treatment planning with oblique beam angles, wedge filters and tissue compensation

the superior mediastinum, lung shielding should be provided. Oblique photon beams with appropriate wedge filters and tissue compensators can be used as shown in Fig. 14-5. Another approach can combine lateral photon beams for the anterior neck with posterior electron beams to give a high dose to the anterior structures (thyroid and lymph nodes) while sparing the spinal cord (Fig. 14-6) (GRIEM et al. 1979).

Other techniques may be useful in delivering a high dose of radition while preventing normal tissue damage. Electron beam therapy may be useful in treatment providing that adequate dosimetry for tissue inhomogenity is provided in the treatment plan. This must allow for the air containing cavities, particularly the hypopharynx which is immediately posterior to the thyroid, which may increase the penetration of the beam. Electron energies of from 10 to 15 MeV may be useful in the neck region when an anterior field is used to treat the thyroid and draining nodes (Fig. 14-7) (GRIEM et al. 1970). Because electron beam characteristics vary for different machines and for different field sizes, the electron beam energy to be used should be individually determined for each treatment situation.

After treatment with external beam radiation therapy, as with I-131, patients may require thyroid replacement and should have careful monitoring of their thyroid function.

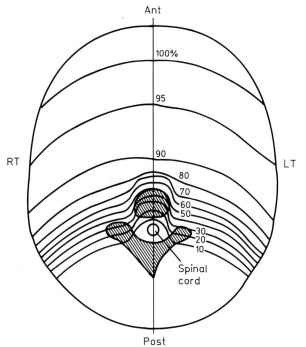

Fig. 14-7. Isodose distribution for anterior electron beam field to cover neck and superior mediastinum. The energy of the electron beam must be adjusted for the particular machine being used

14.8 Special Problems

14.8.1 Graves' Disease

Thyroid disease may produce exophthalmos which is so sufficiently severe that the eyelids no longer cover the cornea. This condition may ultimately result in loss of the globe due to corneal ulceration. Some patients may even be referred with the eyelids sewn shut to prevent ulceration. Although the exopthalmos associated with Graves' disease may regress with appropriate medical management, more emergent reversal of the eye symptoms is sometimes required. Under these circumstances, radiation therapy to the retro-orbital area may be very useful in relieving the exopthalmos (DONALDSON et al. 1973). In treatment planning for this situation, high resolution CT scanning of the orbits or magnetic resonance imaging (MRI) of this area will reveal the swelling of the extraoccular muscles (AUSTIN-SEYMOUR et al. 1985). Radiation should be directed to the muscle involvement with careful attempt to avoid irradiating the lens of the eye. Various treatment techniques have been published which consist of a method of beam direction, head

stabilization, and eye stabilization to provide the necessary requirements stated above (OLIVOTTO et al. 1985, AUSTIN-SEYMOUR et al. 1985). A total dose of 2000 cGy in 200 cGy daily fractions is well tolerated and should produce satisfactory improvement in the exopthalmos in most patients. Olivotto reported some response in 93% of patients and good to excellent response in 68% treated (OLIVOTTO 1985). If the situation persists, the course of treatment may be repeated.

14.8.2 Thyroid Sarcoma

Thyroid sarcomas are rare neoplasms. With the ability to use monoclonal antibodies to identify the tumor cells, many have been now reclassified as anaplastic thyroid carcinoma. These methods are specifically directed against different intermediate filament proteins, keratin, and common leukocyte antigens. Pathologists can now use these in addition to light microscopy to differentiate large cell anaplastic carcinoma from sarcoma even in fine needle aspirate specimens (DOMAGALA et al. 1986). Treatment of sarcoma of the thyroid should be individualized and should follow guidelines for treatment of sarcomas elsewhere. One study (MARCHEGIANI 1985) reports that two patients with sarcoma of the thyroid treated with total thyroidectomy died within one year of systemic disease, but does not state the staging of the patients nor whether they received any adjuvant therapy.

14.8.3 Thyroid Lymphoma

Lymphoma of the thyroid is rare and represents approximately 5% of thyroid neoplasms. Therapy has varied over the years and has included surgery, radiation therapy and chemotherapy. In recent years, several series have been published reviewing treatment and results in this rare disease. A series from the Royal Marsden Hospital analyzed 46 patients treated over a 32-year period. Sixty-one percent of patients underwent total macroscopic removal of tumor and most received radiotherapy as well. Because the patients undergoing complete removal of tumor surgically had a higher control rate and better long term survival, Tupchong and his associates advocate surgical eradication of disease if possible prior to radition therapy (TUPCHONG et al. 1986).

Blair and colleagues from the Mayo Clinic have published an analysis of 73 patients with malignant lymphoma of the thyroid. Of this series 38 patients completed treatment with radiotherapeutic management. Surgical management varied from needle biospy only to complete throidectomy. Most patients has residual disease following surgery. All patients received approximately 4000 cGy to the neck or neck and mediastinum. Four patients received chemotherapy as well. As in the English series, a marginal disease-free survival benefit was seen in patients without residual disease prior to radiotherapy. Their overall disease-free survival was 59% at five years. The most common site of failure was in the para-aortic lymph nodes. Stage IE and IIE primary lymphoma should be managed with radiotherapy in a continuous course technique to 4000 cGy and the field should include the neck, axillae and mediastinum (BLAIR et al. 1985).

The M. D. Anderson Hospital also has published its results in patients treated with radiotherapy, chemotherapy and radiotherapy or chemotherapy alone. For patients treated with radiotherapy only, results depended on stage and were excellent for Stage IE disease with survival and disease-free survival rates of 100% and 83% respectively (VIGLIOTTI 1986).

14.9 Results

The well-differentiated carcinomas have a long natural history and recurrences may not be manifested for many years. This means that series of results in treating thyroid carcinoma need sufficiently long follow-up to accurately assess treatment results. Both Cady's analysis from the Lahey Clinic and Carcangui's analysis from the University of Florence found a continuous increase in the probability of recurrence up to 15 to 30 years after diagnosis (CADY et al. 1976; CARCANGUI et al. 1985). Cady found that deaths due to cancer occurred up to 25 years after diagnosis. Nonetheless, the results of treatment of well-differentiated papillary and follicular carcinomas of the thyroid are favorable. A recent series from the Mayo Clinic reviewed 859 patients with papillary thyroid cancer. Most were treated with less than total thyroidectomy and thyroid suppression. With a median follow-up of 18.3 years, only 6.5% of their patients have died of papillary thyroid cancer and the overall mortality at 30 years was only 3% above that expected for a population of similar age (MCCONAHEY et al. 1986).

The report from the M. D. Anderson Hospital in which patients were treated with radioactive iodine thyroid ablation following thyroidectomy showed

only 12% of the patients dying from thyroid cancer. In this series, patients with Hurthle cell carcinoma did the poorest with a mortality rate of 38% (MAHESWARI 1980). Tubiana reports excellent results on a large series of patients from France where external beam radiation followed incomplete surgical resection in patients with both well-differentiated tumors and medullary carcinomas. He reports a five year survival of 68% for that group (TUBIANA et al. 1985).

The results of treatment of anaplastic carcinoma of the thyroid are poor as discussed. Medullary carcinoma of the thyroid has an intermediate prognosis with early detection in affected families being of greatest importance.

14.10 Summary

The presentation, management and prognosis of thyroid carcinoma depends on several factors, the most important of which is the histologic type. While well-differentiated tumors have a favorable prognosis with surgical management followed by radiation as indicated, the anaplastic form of thyroid cancer has a poor prognosis with current management using surgery, radiation and chemotherapy.

References

Aldinger KA, Samann NA, Ibane M, Hill CS (1978) Anaplastic carcinoma of the thyroid: a review of spindle and giant cell carcinoma of the thyroid. Cancer 41: 2267–2275

Austin-Seymour MM, Donaldson SS, Egberg PR, McCougall IR, Kriss JP (1985) Radiotherapy of lymphoid diseases of the orbit. Int J Radiat Onc Bio Phys 11: 371–379

Beahrs OH, Myers MH (1983) In: Manual for staging of cancer. JB Lippincott Co Philadelphia, PA

Beierwaltes WH (1978) The treatment of thyroid carcinoma with radioactive iodine. Sem Nucl Med 8: 79–84

Blair TH, Evans RG, Buskirk SJ, Banks PM, Earle JD (1985) Radiotherapeutic management of primary thyroid lymphoma. Int J Radiat Onc Biol Phys 11: 365–370

Bondeson L, Ljundsberg O (1981) Occult thyroid carcinoma at autopsy in Malmo Sweden. Cancer 47: 319–323

Cady B, Sedgwick CE, Meissner WA, Wool MS, Salzman FA, Werber J (1979) Risk factor analysis in differentiated thyroid cancer. Cancer 55: 810–820

Cady B, Sedgwick CE, Meissner WA, Bookwalter JR, Romagosa V, Werber J (1976) Changing clinical, pathologic, therapeutic, and survival patterns in differentiated thyroid carcinoma. Ann Surg 184: 541–552

Carcangui ML, Zampi G, Pupi A, Castagnoli A, Rosai J (1985) Papillary carcinoma of the thyroid. Cancer 55: 805–828

Chung CT, Sagerman RH, Ryoo MC, King GA, Yu WS, Dal-al PS, Emmanuel IG (1980) External irradiation for malignant thyroid tumors. Radiology 136: 753–756

Clark DE (1953) Treatment of thyroid cancer with radioactive iodine. In: Radioactive Isotopes in Medicine. pp 345–399, USAEC, Washington DC

Clark DE (1955) Association of irradiation with cancer of the thyroid in children and adolexcents, JAMA 159: 1007

Crile G Jr (1968) Treatment of carcinoma of the thyroid. In: Thyroid Neoplasia. Young S, Inman DR (eds) Academic Press, London, pp 39–50

De Groot LJ (1985) Personal communication

De Groot LJ, Frohman LA, Kaplan E, Refetoff S (1977) Radiation Induced Thyroid Carcinoma. Grune and Stratton, New York

De Groot LJ, Larson PR, Refetoff S, Stanbury JB (1984). Thyroid and Its Diseases. John Wiley and Sons, New York

Domagala W, Lubinski J, Weber K, Osborn M (1986) Intermediate filament typing of tumor cells in fine needle aspirates by means of monoclonal antibodies. ACTA Cytologica 30: 214–224

Donaldson S, Bagshaw MA, Kriss JP (1973) Supervoltage orbital radiotherapy for Graves' ophthalmology. J Clin Endocrinol Metab 37: 276–285

Farrar WB, Cooperman M, James AG (1982) Surgical management of papillary and follicular carcinoma of the thyroid. Ann Surg 192: 701–704

Gilbert HA, Kagan AR (1980) Radiation Damage to the Nervous System. Raven Press, New York

Goldberg RC, Chaikoff IL (1952) Induction of thyroid cancer in the rat by radioactive iodine. Arch Path 53: 22–28

Griem ML, Skaggs LS, Lanzl LH (1970) Radiation therapy of laryngeal and tracheal tumors with high energy electrons using pencil beam scanning. In: Symposium on High Energy Electrons – Madrid 1966. Graficas Canales, Madrid

Griem ML, Kuchnir FT, Lanzl LH, Skaggs LS, Sutton HG, Tokars R (1979) Experience with high-energy electron beam therapy at the University of Chicago. In: Proceedings of the Symposium on Electron Beam Therapy. Memorial Sloan-Kettering Cancer Center. Chu FCH and Laughlin JS (eds) Aubrion Press, New York, pp 99–104

Griem ML (1987) Treatment planning of tumors of the central nervous system. In: Treatment Planning in the Treatment of Cancer. Vaeth JM, Meyer J (eds) Karger, Basel, Switzerland

Harness JK, Thompson NW, Sisson JC, Beierwaltes WH (1974) Differentiated thyroid carcinomas: treatment of distant metastasis. Arch surg 108: 410–419

Hedinger C, Sobin LH (1974) Histological typing of thyroid tumours. International Histological Classification of Tumours, WHO, Geneva 11

Ivy HK (1984) Cancer metastatic to the thyroid. Mayo Clin Proc 59: 856–859

Kim JH, Leeper RD (1983) Treatment of anaplastic giant and spindle cell carcinoma of the thyroid gland with combination adriamycin and radiation therapy. Cancer 52: 954–957

Krishnamurthy GT, Blahd W (1977) Radioactive I-131 in the management of thyroid carcinoma: a prospective study. Cancer 40: 192–202

Leeper RD (1973) The effect of I-131 therapy on the survival of patients with metastatic papillary follicular thyroid carcinoma. J Clin Endocrinol Metab 36: 1143–1152

Lindsay S (1960) Carcinoma of the Thyroid Gland: A Clinical and Pathologic Study of 293 Patients. Charles C Thomas, Springfield, Illinois, USA

Maheshwari YK, Hill CR Jr, Haynie TP III, Hickey RC, Sa-mann NA (1981) I-131 therapy in differentiated thyroid carcinoma: MD Anderson Hospital experience. Cancer 47: 664–671

Maxon HS, Thomas SR, Saenger EL, Buncher CR, Kereiakes JG (1977) Ionizing radiation and the induction of clinically significant disease in the human thyroid gland. Am J Med 63: 967–978

Marchegiani C, Lucci S, DeAntoni E, Catania A, Grilli P, Pierro A, DiMatteo G (1985) Thyroid cancer: surgical experience with 332 cases. Internat Surg 70: 121–124

Mazzaterri EL, Young RL, Oertel JE, Kemmerer WT, Page CP (1977) Papillary thyroid carcinoma: the impact of therapy in 576 patients. Medicine 56: 171–176

McConahey WM, Hay ID, Woolner LB, van Heerden JA, Taylor WF (1986) Papillary thyroid cancer treated at the Mayo Clinic 1946–1970: initial manifestations, pathologic findings, therapy, and outcome. Mayo Clinic Proc 61: 978–995

Meissner WA, Warren S (1969) Tumors of the Thyroid Gland. Atlas of tumor pathology Second series. Fascicle 4 AFIP, Washington, DC

Modan B, Ron E, Werner A (1977) Thyroid cancer following scalp irradiation. Radiology 123: 741–744

Mustacchi P, Cutler SJ (1956) Some observations on the incidence of thyroid cancer in the United States. N Eng J Med 255: 889

Nel CJC, van Heerden JR, Goellner JR, Gharib H, McConahey WM, Taylor WF, Grant CS (1985) Anaplastic carcinoma of the thyroid: a clinicopathologic study of 82 cases. Mayo Clinic Proc 60: 51–58

Olivotto IA, Ludgate CM, Allen LH, Rootman J (1985) Supervoltage radiotherapy for Graves' ophthalmology: CCABC technique and results. Int J Rad Oncol Biol Phys 11: 2085–2090

Parsons JT, Pfaff WW (1984) Carcinoma of the thyroid. In: Management of Head and Neck Cancer: A Multidisciplinary Approach. Million RR, Cassisi NJ (eds) LP Lippincott, Philadelphia

Perzik SL (1976) The place of total thyroidectomy in the management of 909 patients with thyroid disease. Am J Surg 130: 399–404

Potchin EE (1971) Radioiodine therapy of thyroid carcinoma. Semin Nucl Med 1: 503–515

Refetoff S, Harrison J, Karanfilski BT, Kaplan EL, DeGroot LJ, Bekerman C (1975) Continuing occurrence of thyroid carcinoma after irradiation to the neck in infancy and childhood. N Eng J Med 292: 171–175

Rojeski MT, Gharib H (1985) Nodular thyroid disease: evaluation and management. N Eng J Med 313: 428–436

Ron E, Moden B (1984) Thyroid and other neoplasms following childhood scalp irradiation. In: Radiation Carcinogenesis. Boice JD Jr, Fraumeni JF Jr (eds) Raven press, New York

Rougier P, Pamentier C, Laplanche A, Lefevre M, Travagli JP, Caillou B, Schlumberger M, Lacour J, Tubiana M (1983) Medullary thyroid carcinoma: prognostic factors and treatment. Int J Rad Onc Biol Phys 9: 161–169

Rubin P (1971) Atlas of Oncologic Anatomy. University of Rochester Press, Rochester, New York

Scheible W, Leopold GR, Woo VL, Gosink BB (1979) High resolution real-time ultrasonography of thyroid nodules. Radiology 133: 413–417

Schimpff SC (1979) Well differentiated thyroid carcinoma: epidemiology, etiology and treatment. Am J Med Sci 278: 100–114

Schneider AB, Favus MJ, Stachura ME, Arnold J, Arnold MJ, Frohman LA (1978) Incidence prevalence and characteristics of radiation-induced thyroid tumors. Am J Med 64: 243-252

Schroder DM, Chambers A, Faance CH (1986) Operative strategy for thyroid cancer: is total thyroidectomy worth the price? Cancer 58: 2320-2328

Sheline GE, Galante M, Lindsay S (1966) Radiation therapy in the control of persistent thyroid cancer. Am J Roentgenol 97: 923-930

Shore RE, Woodard ED, Hempelmann LH (1984) Radiation-induced thyroid cancer. In: Radiation Carcinogenesis. Boice JD Jr, Fraumeni JF Jr (eds) Raven Press, New York

Simpson WJ (1975) Radiotherapy in thyroid cancer. Can Med Assoc J 113: 115-118

Simpson WJ (1980) Anaplastic thyroid carcinoma: a new approach. Can J Surg 23: 25-27

Simpson WJ, Carruthers JS (1978) The role of external radiation in the management of papillary and follicular thyroid cancer. Am J Surg 136: 457-460

Silverberg E, Lubera J (1986) Cancer Statistics, 1986. CA: A Journal for Clinicians 36: 9-25

Smedal MI, Meissner WA (1961) The results of x-ray treatment in undifferentiated carcinoma of the thyroid. Radiology 76: 927-935

Smedal MI, Salzman FA, Meissner W (1967) The value of 2 MV roentgen-ray therapy in differentiated thyroid carcinoma. Am J Rontgenol 99: 352-364

Tennvall J, Anderson T, Spegren K, Biorklund A, Ingemansson S, Landberg T, Akerman ML (1978) Undifferentiated giant and spindle cell carcinoma of the thyroid. Acta Radiologica Onc 18: 408-416

Tollefsen HR, Shah JP, Huvos AG (1975) Hurthle cell carcinoma of the thyroid. Am J Surg 130: 390-394

Trunnell JB (1953) Iodine therapy in thyroid carcinoma. In: Radioactive Isotopes in Medicine. USAEC, Washington DC, Chapter 26

Tubiana M, Haddad E, Schlumberger M, Hill C, Rougier P, Sarazin D (1985a) External radiotherapy in thyroid cancers. Cancer 55: 2062-2071

Tubiana M, Lacour J (1975) External radiotherapy and radio-iodine in the treatment of 359 patients with thyroid cancer. Br J Radiol 48: 894-907

Tubiana M, Schlumberger M, Rougier P, Laplanche A, Benhamou E, Gardet P, Caillou B, Travagli JP, Parmentier C (1985b) Long-term results and prognostic factors in patients with differentiated thyroid carcinoma. Cancer 55: 794-804

Tupchong L, Hughes F, Harmer CL (1986) Primary lymphoma of the thyroid; clinical features, prognostic factors and results of treatment. Int J Rad Oncol Biol Phys 12: 1813-1821

Varma VM, Beierwaltes WH, Nofal MM, Nishiyama RH, Copp JE (1970) Treatment of thyroid carcinoma: death rate after surgery followed by sodium iodide 131-I. JAMA 214: 969-974

Vigliotti A, Kong JS, Fuller L, Velasquez WS (1986) Thyroid lymphoma stages IE and IIE; Comparative results for radiotherapy only, combination chemotherapy only, and multimodality treatment. Int J Rad Oncol Biol Phys 12: 1807-1812

Watson RG, Brennan MD, Goellner JR, van Heerden JA, McConahey WM, Taylor WF (1984) Invasive Hurtle cell carcinoma of the thyroid. Mayo Clin Proc 59: 851-855

Woolner LB, Beahrs OH, Black BM, McConahey WM, Keating FR (1961) Classification and prognosis of thyroid carcinoma: a study of 885 cases observed in a thirty year period. Am J Surg 102: 354-387

15 Cervical Nodal Metastasis from an Unknown Primary Carcinoma

Judith Stitt Haas and James D. Cox

CONTENTS

15.1 Introduction

The diagnostic and therapeutic problems of cervical lymph node metastasis from an occult primary carcinoma are a dilemma for the oncologist. In general, patients who present with metastases and no obvious primary site of origin, have a median survival of three to four months (HOLMES and FOUTS 1970; RICHARDSON and PARKER 1975; SMITH et al. 1977). This poor prognosis is not altered by treatment unless a primary site can be identified, or the region that is the most probable primary site can be defined (NYSTROM et al. 1977). Autopsy studies of patients who have presented with metastasis from occult primary malignant tumors reveal the site of origin in only 15% of cases.

By contrast, patients who present with cervical lymph node metastasis from an unknown primary carcinoma, and receive local-regional therapy, have a relatively more favorable prognosis; 30–50% are alive five years after treatment (MILLION and CASSISI 1984; NORDSTROM et al. 1979). Clearly, some pa-

JUDITH STITT HAAS, M.D., Assistant Professor, Department of Radiation Oncology, Medical College of Wisconsin, 8700 W. Wisconsin Avenue, Milwaukee, WI 53226/USA

JAMES D. COX, M.D., Professor and Chairman, Department of Radiation Oncology, Columbia Presbyterian Medical Center, 622 W. 168th Street, New York, NY 10032/USA

tients can be cured since the cervical lymph node metastasis represents a regional rather than a distant manifestation of disease. The major problems in managing a patient with such a presentation are 1) to determine which diagnostic studies are appropriate to identify the primary site, and 2) if the primary remains unidentified after complete investigation, which treatment is most likely to eliminate both the primary and the regional disease.

This discussion will focus upon patients who present with cervical lymph node metastasis from squamous cell carcinomas in whom the search for a primary tumor is unsuccessful. With this definition, 2–3% of patients with carcinomas of the upper respiratory and digestive tract will be so classified (MILLION and CASSISI 1984).

15.2 Nodal Presentation

Johnson and Neuman reported the evaluation of 162 cervical masses; 46% were benign, 22% were malignant tumors of lymphoid structures, 22% were metastasis from primary tumors below the clavicle, 5% were thyroid carcinomas, and 5% were metastasis from squamous cell carcinomas (JOHNSON and NEWMAN 1981). The typical patient with a cervical metastasis from an unknown primary carcinoma of the upper aerodigestive tract is a 50 to 70 year old man with a solitary, painless, mass in the mid to upper cervical region. The lesion may have been present for as long as six months, but it is commonly described as having appeared suddenly. Bilateral cervical masses are found in 10% of patients, and multiple ipsilateral masses are seen in 15% (JESSE et al. 1973). Nordstrom evaluated 103 patients who presented with cervical lymph node metastasis; the primary tumor was identified in only one-third of cases after an extensive evaluation (NORDSTROM et al. 1979). In the group of 233 patients whose first sign of malignant disease was a cervical mass, Fitzpatrick found that 61% had no evidence of disease beyond the neck, 18% presented with cervical nodes plus other nodal involvement, and 21% had cervical node metastasis and distant metastasis (Fig. 15-1). In patients with cervical nodal disease, the right and left sides were involved with equal frequency. Patients with supraclavicular adenopathy more commonly had disease on the left as a result of involvement of the sentinel node related to the course of the thoracic duct (FITZPATRICK and KOTALIK 1974).

The histologic description of the cervical node mass may help direct the search for the primary process. Squamous cell histology in a high or mid cervical node is likely to represent metastasis from a head and neck site. However, lung or esophageal carcinomas may spread to supraclavicular or low anterior cervical chain lymph nodes. Adenocarcinomas of this area usually represent distant metastasis from breast, pancreas, bowel, ovary, prostate or lung. Yet, salivary gland, parotid and thyroid adenocarcinomas can produce local-regional lymph node disease. Of the 108 patients with cervical nodal disease in Fitzpatrick's series, anaplastic carcinoma and squamous carcinoma each made up nearly half of the population. For patients with supraclavicular nodes, anaplastic and adenocarcinoma were equally prevalent and accounted for most of the histologic types (FITZPATRICK and KOTALIK 1974) (Table 15-1).

The location of lymph node disease frequently gives an indication of a likely primary site (Fig. 15-2). The higher in the cervical chain, the more likely the chance of primary head and neck disease, and the better the survival. Patients with supraclavicular lymph nodes have a poorer prognosis, since this location usually represents metastatic disease from a distant primary. The specific anatomic location of the presenting mass within the cervical

Table 15-1. Histology of cervical and supraclavicular lymph nodes. Adapted from FITZPATRICK and KOTALIK 1974

	Cervical nodes	Supraclav nodes
Anaplastic carcinoma	54	12
Squamous carcinoma	50	8
Adenocarcinoma	1	15
Melanoma	2	0
Total	107	35

and supraclavicular lymph node chain can be a clue to the primary tumor site. The upper neck is the most common site of lymph node metastasis. The anterior cervical triangle is divided into high jugular, upper jugular, mid- and lower jugular lymph nodes. The high jugular lymph nodes are located between the angle of the mandible and the mastoid bone. Metastasis from the nasopharynx or oropharynx is most commonly seen in this region. The upper jugular (jugulodigastric) nodes drain lesions of the oral cavity, larynx, and hypopharynx. Mid-jugular lymph nodes may be involved if a primary lesion is present in the larynx, hypopharynx, or thyroid; esophageal and pulmonary carcinomas can give rise to metastasis in this region as well. The lower jugular lymph nodes may be the site of metastasis from the thyroid gland, cervical esophagus,

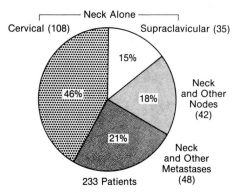

Fig. 15-1. Spectrum of disease in 233 patients whose first symptom of disease included a neck mass. (From: FITZPATRICK and KOTALIK, 1974)

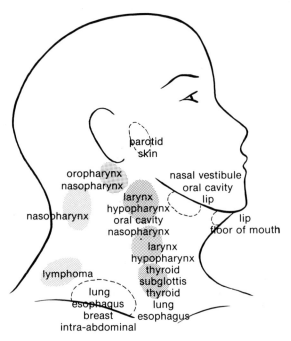

Fig. 15-2. Regions of nodal involvement in relationship to sites of potential primary disease

or lung. Primary tumors in the upper respiratory and digestive tracts can skip the upper echelon of lymph nodes and present with low anterior cervical metastasis. This is uncommon except for carcinoma of the anterior one-third of the tongue where lower cervical metastasis is well recognized (DEL REGATO et al. 1985). Pre-auricular lymphadenopathy suggests a primary carcinoma of the skin. Submental lymph node metastasis is seen with cancer of the lower lip, while involvement of the submandibular nodes directs attention to the oral cavity, nasal vestibule, or submandibular gland. Metastatic adenopathy in the superior posterior cervical nodes is characteristic of spread from a nasopharyngeal primary tumor. Adenopathy in the lower posterior cervical chain is usually related to a malignant lymphoma.

Bilateral adenopathy is most likely related to a midline tumor. Bilateral anterior upper jugular nodal metastases suggest a primary tumor in the nasopharynx, base of tongue, soft palate, supraglottic larynx, or posterior pharyngeal wall.

15.3 Initial Evaluation

15.3.1 Overview

The initial evaluation of patients who present with cervical adenopathy must include a detailed medical history and review of systems as well as a thorough physical examination including study of the oral cavity, oropharynx, larynx, hypopharynx and nasopharynx. The patient's age, sex, and racial background may provide important clues as to the site of the primary tumor. Children with cervical masses are more likely to have a developmental or infectious etiology, while cervical masses in adults are more frequently the result of a malignant tumor. Thyroid carcinomas are seen more frequently in females. The Southern Chinese have a much higher incidence of nasopharyngeal carcinoma. Previous removal of a mole or cutaneous carcinoma may be important.

Most patients with carcinomas of the upper respiratory and digestive tracts have a history of heavy tobacco and alcohol use and frequently have poor dentition. A history of earache suggests a tumor of the hypopharynx or oropharynx with the pain referred to branches of the vagus and glossopharyngeal nerves respectively. Carcinomas of the floor of the mouth may produce otalgia via the mandibular branch of the trigeminal nerve. Hoarseness suggests a primary tumor of the glottis, supraglottic larynx, or piriform sinus; it may also be the

result of laryngeal paralysis due to mediastinal involvement by a bronchial carcinoma. Involvement of the nasopharynx, paranasal sinuses, and nasal cavity may produce nasal stuffiness. Unilateral deafness may result from carcinoma of the nasopharynx or a paraganglioma of the temporal bone. Cranial nerve paralysis is very suggestive of nasopharyngeal carcinoma, extending through the foramen lacerum or involving the lateral retropharyngeal nodes near the jugular foramen. Facial pain or tooth ache are common symptoms resulting from paranasal sinus malignancies.

General physical examination should be detailed and it should always include a pelvic examination in women and a rectal examination in men. Observation of the scalp and skin of the face is important. A surgical scar may remind the patient of a forgotten important excision. An ill-defined scar with no history of an excision may be the site of a melanoma which has regressed spontaneously. The oral cavity should be examined with any dental appliances removed looking for ulceration, tumor formation, or leukoplakia. Palpation throughout the oral cavity and oropharynx is important to detect a submucosal mass with little mucosal abnormality. Indirect laryngoscopy and nasopharyngoscopy is mandatory. As indicated in Fig. 15-2, the location of the cervical lymphadenopathy may suggest the site of the primary tumor and should direct the examiner to evaluate these potential sites with particular care.

15.3.2 Laboratory Study

A complete blood count and biochemical panel are common procedures. Squamous carcinomas with metastatic adenopathy infrequently have any specific abnormalities in these studies. However, anemia, and elevations of lactic dehydrogenase (LDH), alkaline phosphatase, serum glutamic oxaloacetic transaminase (SGOT) may suggest an abdominal malignant tumor or malignant lymphoma. If the specific histopathology or cytologic studies suggest it, it may be appropriate to obtain determinations of carcinomembryonic antigen (CEA), prostatic acid phosphatase, alphafetoprotein, and the beta subunit of human chorionic gonadotropin.

15.3.3 Imaging Procedures

Imaging procedures are important in the search for the site of a primary tumor. Postero anterior and lateral chest films will assess primary pulmonary tumors and the possibility of pulmonary metastasis. Computed tomography of the thorax may be indicated depending upon the findings of the plain chest films. With a supraclavicular or lower cervical metastasis and a cytologic diagnosis of adenocarcinoma, computed tomography of the abdomen and pelvis may be revealing. If computed tomography is unrevealing, fluoroscopic and radiographic evaluation of the upper gastrointestinal tract, barium enema, and intravenous urography may be indicated.

A simple but frequently overlooked first imaging procedure for the upper respiratory and digestive tract is the lateral xeroradiogram or lateral soft tissue film. Pharyngo-esophagram is used to evaluate the pharynx and esophagus for evidence of primary lesions. Films of the paranasal sinuses may be indicated in patients who present with nasal stuffiness or facial pain. Computed tomography from the base of the skull to the clavicles may help delineate both a primary tumor and may further characterize the metastatic adenopathy in the cervical region. Radioisotope scans of the thyroid may be indicated, depending upon histopathologic and cytologic findings or if there is a thyroid abnormality on physical examination. Other radioisotope scans and radiographic procedures may be indicated to search for disseminated disease, but do not contribute to evaluation of the primary tumor or the cervical adenopathy.

15.3.4 Endoscopy

Unless the site of origin is determined to be below the clavicle by the previous procedures, panendoscopy is indicated. This should include nasopharyngoscopy and laryngoscopy as well as bronchoscopy and esophagoscopy. Biopsies of any suspicious lesions are warranted. Random biopsies are performed frequently. However, Fitzpatrick and Kotalik (FITZPATRICK and KOTALIK 1974) found that none of 86 patients who underwent random sampling had a positive biopsy.

15.3.5 Evaluation of the Cervical Mass

A thoughtful and logical sequence of steps is appropriate in the evaluation of a patient with a cervical mass. A cytologic evaluation can be made via fine needle aspiration or biopsy. This may be performed as an out-patient procedure without general anesthesia, major tissue planes are not interrupted with this biopsy, and subsequent surgical proce-

dures are not hampered. The diagnostic accuracy is high if experienced cytopathologists are available. Incisional or excisional biopsy is indicated if the fine needle aspirate suggests a malignant lymphoma. Detailed histopathologic classification as well as surface marker studies require several cubic centimeters of fresh tissue. The recent development of monoclonal antibody markers for tissues of epithelial origin provides a useful tool for further defining the origin of neck masses. Fresh tissue is also required by the pathologist.

It is unfortunately common that incisional biopsy is done without prior cytologic study as this may interfere with subsequent neck dissection. Special stains, electron microscopy, and other laboratory procedures may be indicated by the light microscopic findings.

15.4 Treatment Techniques

Radiation therapy with curative intent is predicated upon knowledge of the site of the primary tumor, the local and regional extensions, the potential for subclinical extension or metastasis, and the histopathologic diagnosis. The dilemma of treating patients with cervical lymph node metastases from an unknown primary site is the uncertainty as to the site of origin. The location of the lymphadenopathy is known and does suggest certain sites of origin as most probable. The histology, or course, is determined as part of the initial evaluation.

In several series in which the metastatic adenopathy has been treated by neck dissection or cervical irradiation only, the primary lesion has become manifest after treatment was completed. The most common anatomic locations for appearance of the primary tumor were the nasopharynx, oropharynx, (tonsillar fossa and base of tongue) and hypopharynx (BARRIE et al. 1970; FITZPATRICK and KOTALIK 1974; JESSE et al. 1973; LEIPZIG et al. 1981; SILVERMAN et al. 1983; YANG et al. 1983).

The site of the primary tumor was identified in 6 to 56% of patients reported, with approximately one-quarter to three-quarters of these patients having tumors which originated in the upper aerodigestive tract. Silverman described 18 of 83 patients (22%) in whom the site of the primary tumor developed following treatment for the nodal manifestation: Eleven of the 18 patients (61%) had primary tumors of the upper aerodigestive tracts and 7 of these were in the nasopharynx, oropharynx or hypopharynx (SILVERMAN et al. 1983). Jesse et al.

Table 15-2. Location of primary lesion appearing post-treatment 37/210 patients (18%). Adapted from JESSE et al. 1973

		Surgery	Radiation	Surgery + RT
1° Sites For Rx	Hypopharynx	6	1	1
	Tonsil/Faucial arch	4	0	1
	Base of tongue/Vallecula	4	0	0
	Nasopharynx	2	0	0
	A–E Fold/Epiglottis	1	0	1
		17/104 (16%)	1/52 (2%)	3/28 (10%)
	Oral cavity/salivary gland	2	2	0
	Maxillary antrum	0	0	1
	Cervical esophagus	1	0	0
	Thyroid	1	0	0
	Total head and neck	21/104 (20%)	3/52 (6%)	4/28 (16%)
	Total below clavicle	5	3	1

(JESSE et al. 1973) reported 104 patients treated by neck dissection of whom 20% developed evidence of the primary tumor after the operation: 16 of the 21 had primary tumors in the nasopharynx, oropharynx or hypopharynx. In the same series, (Table 15-2), 52 patients were treated with radiation therapy and 6% subsequently developed primary tumors in the upper aerodigestive tract. Only one patient treated radiotherapeutically had a tumor develop in the nasopharynx, oropharynx, or hypopharynx that had been irradiated. These data suggest that treatment of the sites which have the highest probability of an occult primary tumor may contribute to overall control of the disease. In addition, the risk of contralateral metastasis is reduced; treatment with unilateral radical neck dissection resulted in 16% of patients developing contralateral cervical metastases; no patient treated radiotherapeutically had contralateral metastasis. Finally, survival was 60% for patients who were treated and never developed evidence of the primary tumor, compared with 30% for patients who developed manifestation of disease in a primary site after treatment.

Treatment recommendation for patients who present with cervical adenopathy equal to or less than 3 cm in diameter (TX N1) is definitive radiation therapy. Parallel opposed lateral fields encompass the anterior and posterior and cervical nodal regions, the nasopharynx, oropharynx, and hypopharynx. Depending upon the site of nodal presentation, a choice may be made to limit the inferior border of this field to the superior border of the thyroid cartilage and then treat the lower cervical and supraclavicular regions with an anterior field. A minimal dose at the mid-sagittal plane from the

lateral fields or at a depth of 3 cm from the anterior field is 5000 cGy at 180-200 cGy per fraction, 5 fractions per week. A reduced volume which encompasses the nasopharynx, base of the tongue and pyriform sinus may be treated with an additional 1000-2000 cGy with the same fractionation. The dose to the spinal cord can be limited to 4000 to 4500 cGy the use of 7-10 MeV electrons as shown in Fig. 15-3.

Jesse and Perez recommend delivering 5000 cGy to the wide nodal regions as described above and boosting the nasopharynx with an additional 1000 cGy if the presenting nodal site is in the high anterior or posterior cervical chain (JESSE et al. 1973). The oral tongue, floor of mouth, gingiva, submaxillary and submental lymph nodes are all potential sites of primary or nodal disease, although the incidence of involvement is much less than in Waldeyer's ring, oropharynx, or hypopharynx. The addition of oral cavity sites to the volume of radiation will increase both the acute effects of treatment as well as chronic sequelae; therefore, routine inclusion of these regions is not recommended (JESSE et al. 1973; LEIPZIG et al. 1981; WANG 1983).

A neck dissection may complement the radiation therapy. Radiation therapy and a radical neck dissection were found to be equally effective if the cervical metastases were single and relatively small (N1) (JESSE et al. 1973; NORDSTROM et al. 1979). As the cervical nodes approach 2.5 to 3.0 cm in diameter, the addition of a neck dissection can contribute to control of the nodal disease. In patients with more advanced metastasis (N2-3), radiation therapy should be administered as described above, and

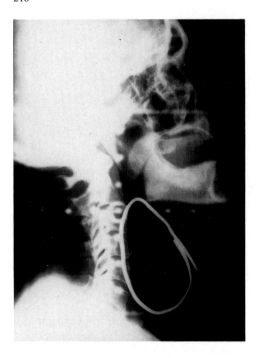

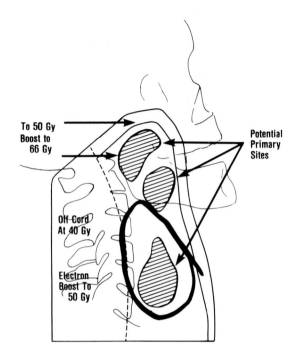

Fig. 15-3. Simulator film with wide field radiation fields and boost regions

a neck dissection should be added (LEIPZIG et al. 1981; WANG 1983).

Patients who present with supraclavicular adenopathy are unlikely to benefit from definitive radiation therapy to the upper aerodigestive tract. Supraclavicular metastases are usually manifestations of disseminated disease. Radiation therapy may be indicated for palliation, but long term survival is rare (MARCHETTA et al. 1963).

15.5 Results

"When secondary glandular metastases are present in malignant growths, the prognosis ordinarily is hopeless" according to a 1929 book Radium in General Practice (LARKIN 1929). Since that time, evaluation and management of the patient with occult primary malignancy involving the lymph nodes has improved so that the outlook is certainly less grim. The two-year survival for all patients presenting with metastatic cervical adenopathy has been reported between 53 and 66% (MILLION and CASSASI 1984; NORDSTROM et al. 1979). The five year survival rates are lower as shown in Table 15-3 (ACQUARELLI et al. 1961; COMESS et al. 1957; FRIED

et al. 1975; JESSE and NEFF 1966; MARCHETTA et al. 1963; PICO et al. 1971).

The prognosis by histopathologic diagnosis is similar to that for carcinomas of the nasopharynx. Wang (WANG 1983) found a three year survival rate of 30% when the nodal biopsy revealed squamous cell carcinoma, 54% for undifferentiated carcinoma, and 67% for lymphoepithelioma.

Table 15-3. Survival of unknown primary metastatic to cervical nodes

Author/year	No of patients	Survival time	Percent
COMESS 1957	103	unlimited	37
ACQUARELLI 1961	31	unlimited	23
MARCHETTA 1963	33	4 yr	30
JESSE/NEFF	127	3 yr	34
BARRIE 1970	123	3 yr 5 yr	30 25
PICO 1971	80	5 yr	21
JESSE/PEREZ 1973	210	3 yr	48
FITZPATRICK 1974	233	3 yr 5 yr	44 32
FRIED 1975	49	3 yr	49
NORDSTROM 1979	51	2 yr 5 yr	53 29
LEIPZIG 1981	48	3 yr	40
SILVERMAN 1983	83	5 yr	38
WANG 1983	50	3 yr	44
YANG 1983	113	5 yr	37
MILLION 1984	36	2 yr 5 yr	66 48

Table 15-4. Survival vs. nodal status (absolute 3 yr disease free survival – 184 patients). From JESSE et al. 1973

	Surgery		Radiation		Surgery + RT	
N_X	31/39	(79%)	8/9	(89%)	3/3	(−)
N_1	4/6	(67%)	1/3	(−)	1/3	(−)
N_2	10/22	(45%)	3/4	(75%)	5/9	(55%)
N_3	14/37	(38%)	13/36	(36%)	4/13	(31%)
	59/104[a]	(57%)	25/52[b]	(48%)	13/28[b]	(47%)

[a] Includes 8 patients salvaged with radiation and 6 patients salvaged with surgery.

[b] Includes 1 patient salvaged with surgery

There is some relationship between the volume of nodal disease and the prognosis (Table 15-4). When all evidence of tumor is eliminated by neck dissection, Jesse et al. (JESSE et al. 1973) reported a three year disease-free survival rate of 79%. The addition of radiation therapy resulted in a similar survival rate. By contrast, patients who would be classified as N3 had a 37% disease-free survival rate. Yang et al. (YANG et al. 1983) did not find a relationship between the size of the node and the survival rate. Patients with lymph nodes 7 cm or smaller had a five year survival rate of 56% compared to 50% for those with tumors larger than 7 cm. The prognosis was better for patients with unilateral as compared to bilateral adenopathy, independent of the volume of the lymph nodes. Jose et al. (JOSE et al. 1979) found the prognosis to be best in patients who presented with upper anterior cervical node metastasis (43% five-year survival); lower cervical node involvement was associated with a 6% five-year survival rate. Fitzpatrick et al. (FITZPATRICK and KOTALIK 1974) reported only 3 of 28 patients who presented with supraclavicular nodes were alive at 2 years and only one of fifteen lived five years.

Radiotherapeutic control of the cervical lymph node metastasis is related to the total dose administered. Failure within the cervical region is more likely if the dose is less than 5000 cGy. Yang (YANG et al. 1983) found only a slight improvement in control even with a dose of 6000 cGy. Patients with extra-capsular extension beyond the lymph node in the resected specimen have a decreased frequency of local control and an increased frequency of distant metastasis (SCHWARZ et al. 1981). Even with the administration of high total doses, approximately half the patients with extracapsular extension will have local recurrence in the cervical region.

Combining radiation with surgery appears to be superior in preventing local failure in N2-3 necks and in controlling the site of potential primary dis-

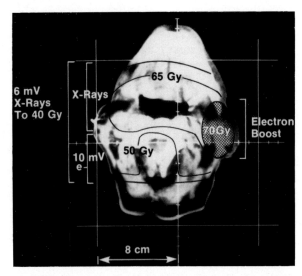

Fig. 15-4. Computed tomogram with isodose curves of wide field and nodal boost

ease. Either modality alone is effective for early nodal disease; however, if surgery is the only therapy, anatomic regions that might harbor occult primary disease will not be treated. The primary site of disease is more likely to appear when surgery is the only form of therapy (JESSE et al. 1973). In patients who subsequently developed a primary lesion, the three year survival was decreased from 53% to 31%. Development of local or regional recurrence does not necessarily prevent cures in these patients. Of the 97 three year survivors in Jesse's series of 184 patients, eight patients treated with surgery only were salvaged by radiation therapy and eight by additional surgery when they developed local or regional recurrence.

15.6 Summary

Squamous cell carcinoma presenting as cervical lymph node metastasis from an occult primary tumor is a complex problem that requires considerable judgement and individualization of treatment. Detailed investigations will reveal the primary tumor in most patients. For those in whom no primary site of disease can be identified, the most probable sites of origin are the nasopharynx, oropharynx, and hypopharynx. Comprehensive irradiation of these sites to modest doses with supplemental doses to the most likely site of the primary tumor based on the nodal presentation can result in long-term disease-free survival in 30 to 50% of patients. The addition of a neck dissection in patients with large N 1, N 2, and N 3 cervical metastases will improve regional control and enhance survival.

References

Acquarelli MJ, Matsunaga RS, Cruze K (1961) Metastatic carcinoma of the neck of unknown primary origin. Laryngoscope 71: 962-974

Barrie JR, Knapper WH, Strong EW (1970) Cervical nodal metastases of unknown origin. Am J Surg 120: 466-470

Comess MS, Beahrs OH, Dockerty MB (1957) Cervical metastasis from occult carcinoma. Surg Gyn Obstet 133: 0717

Fitzpatrick PJ, Kotalik JF (1974) Cervical metastases from an unknown primary tumor. Radiol 110: 659-663

Fried MP, Diehl WH, Brownson RJ, Sessions DG, Ogura JH (1975) Cervical metastasis from an unknown primary. Ann Otol 84: 152-157

Holmes FF, Fouts TL (1970) Metastatic cancer of unknown primary site. Cancer 26: 816-820

Jesse RH, Neff LD (1966) Metastatic carcinoma in cervical nodes with an unknown primary lesion. Am J Surg 112: 547-553

Jesse RH, Perez CA, Fletcher GH (1973) Cervical lymph node metastasis: Unknown primary cancer. Cancer 31: 854-859

Johnson JT, Newman RK (1981) The anatomic location of neck metastasis from occult squamous cell carcinoma. Otolaryngol Head Neck Surg 89: 54-58

Jose B, Bosch A, Caldwell WL, Frias Z (1979) Metastasis to neck from unknown primary tumor. ACTA Radiologica 18: 161-170

Larkin AJ (1929) Radium in General Practice. Paul B. Hoeber, Inc., New York, p 123

Leipzig B, Winter ML, Hokanson JA (1981) Cervical nodal metastases of unknown origin. Laryngoscope 91: 593-598

Marchetta FC, Murphy WT, Kovaric JJ (1963) Carcinoma of the neck. Am J Surg 106: 974-979

Million RR, Cassisi NJ (1984) The Unknown Primary. In: Management of Head and Neck Cancer. JB Lippincott Co, Philadelphia, pp 231-238

Nordstrom DG, Tewfik HH, Latourette HB (1979) Cervical lymph node metastases from an unknown primary. Int J Rad Oncol Biol Phys 5: 3-76

Nystrom JS, Weinder JM, Heffelfinger-Juttner J et al. (1977) Metastatic and histologic presentations in unknown primary cancer. Semin Oncol 4 (1): 53-58

Pico J, Frias Z, Bosch A (1971) Cervical lymph node metastases from carcinoma of undetermined origin. Am J Roentgenol Radium Ther Nucl Med 91: 95-102

del Regato JA, Spjut HJ, Cox JD (1985) In: Ackerman, del Regato (eds) Cancer: Diagnosis, Treatment, and Prognosis, 6th edn. CV Mosby Company, St. Louis, pp 257-272

Richardson RG, Parker RG (1975) Metastases from undetected primary cancers - Clinical experience at a radiation oncology center. West J Med 123: 337-339

Schwarz D, Hamberger AD, Jesse RH (1981) The management of squamous cell carcinoma in cervical lymph nodes in the clinical absence of a primary lesion by combined surgery and irradiation. Cancer 48: 1746-1748

Silverman CL, Marks JE, Lee J, Ogura JH (1983) Treatment of epidermoid and undifferentiated carcinomas from occult primaries presenting in cervical lymph nodes. Laryngoscope 93: 645-648

Smith PE, Krementz ET, Chapman E (1977) Metastatic cancer with a detectable primary site. J Surg 113: 663-637

Wang CC (1983) Management of squamous cell carcinoma in cervical node with "unknown primary". In: Radiation Therapy for Head and Neck Neoplasms. John Wright, Boston, pp 249-257

Yang ZY, Hu YH, Yan JH et al. (1983) Lymph node metastases in the neck from an unknown primary. ACTA Radiol (Onc) 22: 17-22

16 Overview of Clinical Trials and Basis for Future Therapies

Thomas W. Griffin and Joanne Mortimer

CONTENTS

16.1 Statement of Problem

The development of a research strategy investigating new approaches to the treatment of advanced head and neck cancers requires an extensive and complete data base. One must know the rate and pattern of distant metastasis and local treatment failure (how standard treatment fails) before one can develop new treatments. In order to develop such a data base, the Radiation Therapy Oncology Group (RTOG) established a prospective registry for head and neck cancer in 1977. Between February 1977 and April 1980, the following information was collected on all head and neck cancers treated at RTOG institutions: primary tumor site, T-stage, N-stage, M-stage, age, sex, Karnofsky performance score, tumor histology, tumor differentiation, extent of infiltration, treatment delivery, and outcome. All patients were staged according to the 1976 TNM staging system of the American Joint Committee for Cancer Staging and End Results Reporting. 2066 cases were entered into the registry. 992 of these had locally advanced inoperable disease treated by radiation therapy alone. The sites of treatment failure, including distant metastatic rates, were established for that group of patients.

Thomas W. Griffin, M.D., Joanne Mortimer M.D., Division of Medical Oncology, Department of Medicine, University of Washington Hospital/School of Medicine, Seattle, Washington 98195, USA

Tumor site, lymph node status and tumor differentiation all proved to be significant factors in the development of distant metastasis (Del Rowe et al. in press). Figure 16-1 illustrates the distant metastatic rate for advanced glottic and non-glottic carcinomas. The distant metastatic rate for non-glottic cancers is significantly worse ($p = 0.005$) than it is for glottic cancers. Likewise, patients with positive

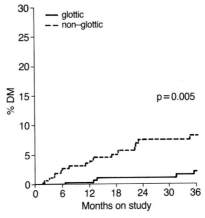

Fig. 16-1. The rate of distant metastasis for glottic and non-glottic head and neck cancer as a function of time

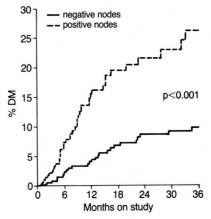

Fig. 16-2. The rate of distant metastasis for head and neck cancer with and without positive lymph nodes as a function of time

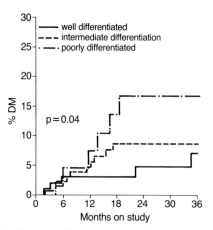

Fig. 16-3. The rate of distant metastasis for head and neck cancer as a function of tumor differentiation

lymph nodes had a significantly higher distant metastatic rate than patients with negative lymph nodes (p < 0.001, Fig. 16-2). Figure 16-3 illustrates the effect of tumor differentiation. Poorly-differentiated tumors have significantly higher distant metastatic rates than do intermediate and well differentiated tumors (p = 0.04). Overall, 92 of the 992 patients developed distant metastasis for a crude distant metastatic rate of 9.3%. The time-adjusted incidence rates were 10.5% at 3 years and 13.1% at 5 years. The yearly rates of developing distant metastasis decreased from 5.7% during the 1*st* year to 3.4% during the 2*nd* year and 0.7% during the 5*th* year.

The RTOG data base indicates that although distant metastases do develop in a significant number of cases, the overwhelming cause of treatment failure in advanced head and neck cancer is failure to control the loco/regional disease. The development of distant metastatic disease as a cause of treatment failure must be considered secondary in importance to the problem of loco/regional tumor control, and research strategies must address the loco/regional tumor problem if they are to be successful (PROBERT et al. 1984).

16.2 Altered Fractionation Radiation Therapy

16.2.1 Basic Rationale

Some of the earliest attempts to improve the results of treatment for advanced head and neck tumors involved altering the fractionation schemes for radi-

ation therapy (MARCIAL et al. in press). By manipulating the treatment factors of total radiation dose, dose per treatment fraction, number of treatment fractions, and total treatment time, it was hoped that tumor control could be improved, treatment complications could be reduced, or both. Clinical studies have investigated the use of accelerated fractionation, hyperfractionation, and split course radiation. Although the results of these studies have been variable, it has been found that if the dose per fraction is reduced (hyperfractionation), there is a relative sparing of late responding normal tissues compared to those which respond early. This difference can be detected either as a steeper slope on a log-log plot of total isoeffect dose vs number of fractions or as a difference in the relative magnitude of the linear (α) and quadratic (β) terms of a dose effect curve (WITHERS et al. 1983). This relationship can be described by the equation:

$$E = n(\alpha d + \beta d^2)$$

where E is a measured effect, n is the number of fractions and d is the dose per fraction. While the absolute values of α and β cannot usually be determined in terms of the radiosensitivity of a target cell, the α/β ratio can be determined from isoeffect doses in fractionation studies with different numbers and sizes of fractions. This ratio allows predictions of the relative change in effectiveness when dose per fraction is altered.

Low values of the α/β ratio (150-500 cGy) indicate rapidly bending survival curves at low doses per fraction, and predict that variations in fraction size within and below the usual clinical dose range should have a marked effect on isoeffect dose. High values of α/β (600-1400 cGy) indicating a predominance of the linear function predict that changes in fraction size would have a lesser effect on isoeffect dose. The dose per fraction at which the α component predominates and below which further fractionation will have no effect on the total isoeffect dose has been termed the flexure dose, and has been defined as an α/β ratio of 0.1. The values of 0.1 α/β obtained for both late (15-50 cGy) and acutely responding normal tissues (60-140 cGy) are all below the current clinical range of fraction size (180-300 cGy), and imply that hyperfractionation will spare late responding tissues more than acutely responding tissues (although both would be spared to some extent). Tumors are expected to behave like acutely responding tissues; this is one of the major reasons to expect a therapeutic gain from hyperfractionation relative to dose limiting late effects in normal tissues (WITHERS et al. 1983; WILLIAMS et al. 1985).

16.2.2 Clinical Trials

The first large altered fractionation study for advanced, inoperable squamous cell carcinomas of the head and neck was instituted by the RTOG in 1972. This study investigated split-course radiation therapy. Patients were first stratified by T-stage, N-stage, and sex, and then randomized to receive standard continuous course radiation therapy consisting of 6000–6600 cGy in 30 fractions over 6–7 weeks or split-course radiation therapy consisting of 3000 cGy in 10 fractions over 2 weeks, a 3-week rest period, and then an additional 3000 cGy in 10 fractions over 2 weeks. It was hoped that the split would reduce radiation-induced normal tissue damage and permit reoxygenation of the remaining tumor, increasing its radiosensitivity. An advantage of the protocol split-course schedule was that it would require ⅓ fewer daily fractions than the standard continuous schedule. 396 patients were analyzed. The split-course treatment failed to increase the complete response rate (58% vs 57%), prolong loco/regional tumor control, or increase survival. The 2- and 5-year survival rates were 47% and 27% for the continuous course, and 39% and 26% for the split course (Table 16-1). No significant differences were observed in either acute or late toxicities (MARCIAL et al. in press).

Hyperfractionation was first investigated by the RTOG in 1977. Pilot studies investigating twice-a-day fractionation schemes studied doses of 125 cGy and 150 cGy given twice daily with a 4-hour separation to a total dose of 6000 cGy. Tumor control was adequate with both fraction sizes; however, while

Table 16-1. RTOG Split course radiation therapy randomized study[a]

	Complete response (%)	Median survival (months)	2-Year survival (%)	5-Year survival (%)
Continuous radiation (N=201)	57	20.4	47	27
Split course radiation (N=195)	58	18.4	39	26

[a] 6000–6600 cGy, 30 fractions, 6–7 weeks vs 3000 cGy in 10 fractions, 2-week split, then another 3000 cGy in 10 fractions

Table 16-2. RTOG Hyperfractionation randomized study[a]

	Local control		Survival	
	Complete Response (%)	2-Year (%)	Median (months)	2-Year (%)
Standard fractionation (N=93)	60	29	11.5	28
Hyper-fractionation (N=94)	58	30	12.3	32

[a] 180–200 cGy, 33–41 fractions, 6600–7380 total dose vs 120 cGy b.i.d. to 6000 cGy total dose

acceptable acute and late normal tissue reactions were observed with 125 cGy fractions, excessive injury was seen with 150 cGy fractions. Based on these results, a Phase III randomized study was designed to compare a twice-daily 120 cGy dose to 6000 cGy hyperfractionation schedule to a conventional continuous course of radiation therapy consisting of 6600–7380 cGy in 33–41 fractions with 5 daily 180–200 cGy fractions per week. 187 patients were analyzed. The initial complete response rate was the same (statistically) for the 2 treatment arms. 60% of the standard fractionation and 58% of the hyperfractionation-treated patients received a complete response. The 2-year local control rates were 29% and 30% for the standard fractionation and hyperfractionation treatments (Table 16-2). The median survival and 2-year survival rates were 11.5 months and 28% for standard fractionation treatment and 12.3 months and 32% for hyperfractionation treatment respectively (p=n.s.). There was a higher frequency of acute treatment reactions with hyperfractionation (23% vs 13%), but the incidence of late reactions was similar in both treatment groups (MARCIAL et al. in press).

Other reports (PARSONS et al. 1984; MILLION et al. 1982) have indicated that the relative sparing of late normal tissue reactions by hyperfractionation permits total doses over 7000 cGy. Currently, the RTOG is conducting a dose-escalating study investigating twice-daily fractions of 120 cGy up to total doses of 8160 cGy. Once the maximum tolerated total dose with 2 daily fractions of 120 cGy is determined, a Phase III study will be designed to compare it with conventionally fractionated radiotherapy.

While hyperfractionation is designed to exploit differences in cellular repair mechanisms, accelerated fractionation is an attempt to limit the influence of tumor cell proliferation during treatment. Fractionation schemes have been developed to exploit some of the potential advantages of both accelerated fractionation and hyperfractionation. WANG et al. (1986) developed a treatment program which utilizes a split-course, accelerated hyperfractionation scheme. He delivered 160 cGy per fraction, 2 fractions per day, with a minimum of 4 hours between fractions, 5 days per week for 12 treatment days. After receiving 3840 cGy, the patients were given a 2-week break. Treatment was then resumed at 160 cGy b.i.d. to a total dose of 6400 cGy. In some cases, additional b.i.d. treatment was given, to 6720 cGy. The results obtained with this treatment were compared to historical controls from the Massachusetts General Hospital. Figures 16-4 and 16-5 graphically display the results in terms of local control in patients with Stages T_3 and T_4 primary tumors and patients with positive lymph nodes. The 3-year T_{3-4} local control rates were 66% for the altered fractionation scheme vs 33% for historical

controls (p = 0.004). The 3-year N_{1-3} local control rates were 76% for the altered fractionation scheme and 28% for the historical controls (p = 0.0004). The acute normal tissue effects of the altered fractionation scheme were moderately severe; however, the dose-limiting late normal tissue effects were no more severe than those seen following standard fractionation radiotherapy. This treatment protocol has been accepted as the new standard treatment for advanced head and neck cancer at the Massachusetts General Hospital. This scheme, however, has never been tested in a prospective, randomized study.

16.3 High LET Radiation

16.3.1 Basic Radiobiology

While altered fractionation studies attempt to maximize the effectiveness of conventional radiation therapy, high linear energy transfer (LET) radiation studies attempt to capitalize on the superior radiobiologic properties of high LET radiations (HALL 1978). The biologic effects of a radiation beam depend on the spatial distribution of ionizing events in tissue. The rate at which charged particles deposit energy per unit distance is known as the *linear energy transfer* (LET), expressed in keV/μm. Photons, electrons, protons and helium ions are sparsely ionizing, and are characterized by a low LET. Conversely, neutrons, pions and heavy ions are densely ionizing and are referred to as high LET radiations. Review of the possible causes of treatment failure in head and neck cancers with conventional low LET radiation therapy suggest that there are major areas in which high LET radiations offer a significant advantage.

Numerous studies in many biologic systems have shown that hypoxic cells are significantly more resistant to the effects of X-irradiation and gamma irradiation than are well-oxygenated cells (GRAY et al. 1953). Whereas cells in most normal tissues are well oxygenated, most solid tumors are thought to have hypoxic regions, which have outgrown their vascular supply. It has been postulated that these cells nevertheless remain viable and provide a focus for local tumor recurrence. The *oxygen enhancement ratio* (OER) is defined as the ratio of the dose of radiation required to produce a specified biologic effect under anoxic conditions to the dose required to produce the same effect under well-oxygenated conditions. With photons, the OER for most mammalian cells is 2.5 to 3.0. With neutrons,

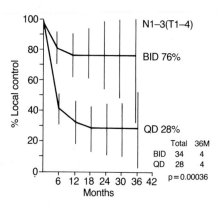

Fig. 16-4. Actuarial local control of T_{3-4} patients after b.i.d. and q.d. radiation therapy

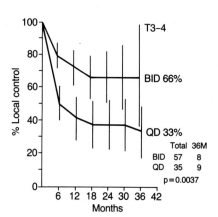

Fig. 16-5. Actuarial local control of N_{1-3} group (T_{1-4}) after b.i.d. and q.d. radiation therapy

heavy charged particles or pions, the OER is significantly smaller (1.4 to 1.7) and therefore, the protection conferred on tumor cells by hypoxia is diminished (CATTERALL and BEWLEY 1973; HALL 1978; GOLDSTEIN et al. 1981).

An area of therapeutic gain from high LET radiation also exists when tumor cells are relatively radioresistant because of increased capacity to accumulate sublethal radiation injury (GRAGG et al. 1977). This situation is reflected in a wide shoulder for the tumor cell survival curve. With neutrons and other high LET radiation, most cell killing results from single lethal events, leading to survival curves that are almost exponential in the range of clinical relevance. Head and neck tumors characterized by a large capacity to accumulate and repair sublethal radiation injury should be advantageously treated by high LET radiation.

Because of the variation in radiosensitivity between cells in different stages of the cell cycle, redistribution between dose fractions results in an effective sensitization of proliferating cells that is not shared by nonproliferating normal cells. The latter are probably responsible for late radiation sequelae, which are the usual dose-limiting factors in radiation therapy. The cell cycle-dependent variation of radiosensitivity is similar for neutrons and gamma rays, but the magnitude of the difference is smaller for neutrons. Whether this property constitutes a therapeutic advantage for high LET radiation cannot be predicted. Tumors whose cells redistribute poorly or whose spectrum is demonstrated by cells in resistant phases should be more effectively treated with high LET radiation (GRAGG et al. 1978).

The recovery from potentially lethal damage occurs over a period of hours in cells irradiated *in vitro* when the postirradiation conditions are suboptimal for growth. Repair of potentially lethal damage occurs following X-irradiation and gamma-irradiation but is observed less frequently after neutron irradiation. If, as has been suggested by HALL and KRALJEVIC (1976), potentially lethal damage repair after X-irradiation and gamma-irradiation occurs in nutritionally deprived head and neck tumor cells but not in normal tissue cells, then the use of high LET beams would be therapeutically advantageous in these tumors.

16.3.2 Salivary Gland Tumors

The biological properties of salivary gland tumors fit the criteria listed in the preceding paragraphs of a tumor system predicted to be advantageously treated by high LET radiations. Neutron irradiation was first used to treat advanced salivary gland tumors by STONE (1940), using a physics laboratory-based cyclotron in Berkeley, California. More recently, the results of fast neutron clinical trials have been reported from other treatment centers in Great Britain, Europe, the United States and Japan. Although instituted on a more-or-less empirical basis, these results have been consistently encouraging, and it has been suggested that salivary gland tumors are much more responsive to neutrons than to photons. The radiobiology results strongly support this conclusion.

The first radiobiological evidence that neutrons should be particularly effective in the treatment of salivary gland tumors came from BATTERMAN et al. (1981). The *relative biologic effectivenes* (RBE) of an ionizing radiation is the ratio of the dose of that radiation compared to the dose of a reference radiation required to produce a specific endpoint in a specific tissue. Batterman and coworkers measured the RBE of neutrons produced by a $d \Rightarrow T$ reaction relative to ^{60}Co radiation using human tumors metastatic to the lung. They determined the RBE for growth delay in terms of the time required for tumor mass to return to its preirradiation volume as evaluated on serial radiographs. Patients having 2 or more metastases had lesions simultaneously treated with the 2 types of radiation. The RBE for adenoidcystic carcinoma was 5.7 for a single radiation dose and 8.0 for fractionated radiation such as would correspond to clinical treatment schemes. The RBE's for most other tumors were in the range of 2.5 to 4.0.

Based on encouraging results from earlier nonrandom clinical trials, and the strong supporting evidence from Batterman's radiobiology studies, the Radiation Therapy Oncology Group (RTOG) in the United States and the Medical Research Council (MRC) of Great Britain sponsored a prospective, randomized study comparing fast neutron irradiation with low LET photon and/or electron treatment of inoperable malignant salivary gland tumors.

A total of 32 patients were entered on this study. Twenty-five were entered from the United States and 7 were entered from Scotland. Seventeen patients were randomized to receive neutrons and 15 were randomized to receive standard photon and/or electron radiation therapy. 61% of the neutron-treated patients and 75% of the photon-treated patients presented with inoperable or unresectable primary tumors, while 39% of the neutron-treated and 25% of the photon-treated patients presented with unresectable recurrent disease. The minimum followup period at the time of this analysis is 2 years.

The complete tumor clearance rates at the primary site were 85% for neutrons and 33% for photons following protocol treatment (p = 0.01). The complete tumor clearance rates in the cervical lymph nodes were 86% for neutrons and 25% for photons. The overall loco/regional complete tumor response rates were 85% and 33% for neutrons and photons respectively (Fig. 16-6). The loco/regional control rates at 2 years as illustrated in Fig. 16-7 for the 2 groups are 67% for neutrons and 17% for photons (p < 0.005). The 2-year survival rates as illustrated in Fig. 16-8 are 62% and 25% for neutrons and photons respectively (p = 0.10). There was no

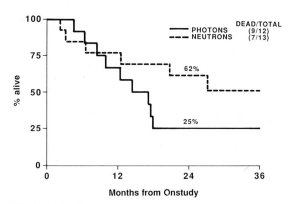

Fig. 16-8. Survival rates for neutron-treated and photon-treated patients. The difference is significant at the p = 0.10 level

significant difference between the normal tissue complication rates of the 2 groups.

Prior to this study, the results of neutron treatment of 289 patients with inoperable salivary gland tumors have been reported in the literature. This number excludes patients who were treated for presumed residual disease following surgery. Some of these patients were treated with "mixed beam" treatment (⅖ neutrons, ⅗ photons); others were treated with neutrons alone. Treatment was delivered in 12–38 fractions over 4–7 weeks. In spite of this variability, the results are remarkably consistent. Table 16-3 lists the reported neutrons experience in this tumor system. The composite local control rate is 67% (194/289). Local tumor control rates following low LET photon and/or electron irradiation of inoperable salivary gland carcinomas are less satisfactory. Table 16-4 lists the photon treatment results in this clinical situation. The composite local control rate following photons in these series is 24% (61/254).

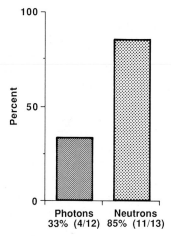

Fig. 16-6. Complete response rates for neutron-treated and photon-treated patients. The difference is statistically significant at the p = 0.01 level

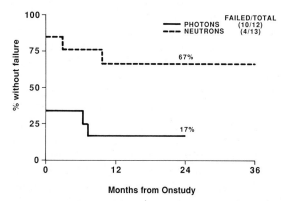

Fig. 16-7. Loco/regional tumor control rates for neutron-treated and photon-treated patients. The difference is statistically significant at the p < 0.005 level

Table 16-3. Neutron loco/regional tumor control rates for malignant salivary gland tumors

	No of patients	Loco/regional tumor control
Saroja (1987)	113	63% (71/113)
Catterall (1981)	65	77% (50/65)
Batterman et al. (1981)	32	66% (21/32)
Griffin et al. (1988)	32	81% (26/32)
Duncan et al. (1987)	22	55% (12/22)
Maor et al. (1981)	9	67% (6/9)
Ornitz et al. (1979)	8	38% (3/8)
Eichhorn (1981)	5	60% (3/5)
Skolyszewski (1982)	3	67% (2/3)
Total	289	67% (194/289)

Table 16-4. Low let (photon/electron) loco/regional tumor control rates for malignant salivary gland tumors

	No of patients	Loco/regional tumor control
Fitzpatrick (1979)	50	12% (6/50)
Vikram (1984)	49	4% (2/49)
Borthne (1986)	35	23% (8/35)
Rafla (1977)	25	36% (9/25)
Fu et al. (1977)	19	32% (6/19)
Stewart et al. (1968)	19	47% (9/19)
Dobrowski (1986)	17	41% (7/17)
Shidnia et al. (1980)	16	38% (6/16)
Elkon (1979)	13	15% (2/13)
Rossman (1975)	11	54% (6/11)
Total	254	24% (61/254)

Table 16-5. Comparison of the RTOG-MRC study results with historical results

	No of patients	Loco/regional tumor control (%)
Low LET		
Low LET historical experience	254	24
RTOG/MRC photon controls	12	17
Neutron		
Historical neutron experience	289	67
RTOG/MRC neutron results	13	67

Table 16-5 compares the randomized study results with the historical results. Taken as a whole, the data from the radiobiological studies, the nonrandom clinical studies and the prospective randomized clinical trial overwhelmingly support the contention that fast neutron radiotherapy offers a significant advance in the treatment of inoperable and unresectable primary and recurrent malignant salivary gland tumors. There was no observable difference in tumor response to neutron therapy according to histology.

16.3.3 Squamous Cell Carcinomas

The results obtained with squamous cell head and neck cancers have been less consistent. The first randomized study in this tumor system was conducted by Catterall and coworkers (1973) in the 1960's at Hammersmith Hospital in London and reported a significant advantage for neutrons over conventional photon treatment. Using the low-energy MRC cyclotron, they observed a 76% (53 of 70)

local control rate for neutrons, compared to a 19% (12 of 63) local control rate for photons in a group of patients with advanced disease. The survival rates were poor in both treatment groups. Their early work led to many followup studies in Europe, Japan and the United States (Griffin et al. 1978, 1979; Duncan et al. 1982; Laramore et al. 1983).

A second randomized study of fast neutrons in head and neck cancer has recently been reported by Duncan et al. (1984) on a group of patients with earlier stage disease. They reported the results of a randomized, cooperative study conducted at the Antoni van Leeuwenhoek Ziekenhuis in Amsterdam, the Department of Clinical Oncology in Edinburgh, and the Universitatsklinikum in Essen. No significant advantage for neutrons over photons could be demonstrated in this study. The complete rate for neutrons was 70% (70 of 100), and the complete response rate for photons was 66% (63 of 95). The ultimate local control rates were 44% (44 of 100) for neutrons and 40% (38 of 95) for photons. There was no significant difference in the overall survival rates between the 2 groups. These results stand in contrast to the results obtained at Hammersmith Hospital.

A third major randomized study of neutrons in head and neck cancer was carried out in the United States by the RTOG. More than 300 patients were entered in this study, which compared both neutrons used alone and neutrons used in a "mixed beam" treatment schedule (⅔ neutrons and ⅓ photons) against photons for inoperable squamous cell carcinomas. There were no significant differences between the mixed beam and photon control treatments in terms of either primary tumor control or survival; however, significant advantages were seen for neutrons given alone (Griffin et al. 1984). The complete response rates were 52% for neutrons compared with 17% for photons (p = 0.035), with a major complication rate of 18% for neutrons and 33% for photons. Figure 16-9 illustrates the survival rates adjusted for prognostic factors for the 3 randomizations. This study demonstrated a 37% improvement in 5-year survival for neutron-treated patients over photon-treated patients, which is significant at the p = 0.04 level.

The patient populations in these 3 randomized studies were distinctly different as evidenced by differences in photon local control rates and the percentage of patients with neck node involvement (83% for the RTOG neutron-only study [Griffin et al. 1983]; 66% in the Hammersmith study; approximately 50% in the Edinburg study). Advantages for fast neutron radiation therapy in squamous cell car-

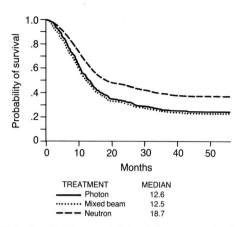

TREATMENT   MEDIAN
—— Photon   12.6
········· Mixed beam   12.5
– – – Neutron   18.7

Fig. 16-9. Survival curves balanced for prognostic factors from randomized RTOG studies of neutron and mixed beam irradiation in squamous cell carcinoma of the head and neck

Table 16-6. Randomized fast neutron studies of squamous cell carcinomas of the head and neck

Study	Neutron local control (%)	Photon local control (%)
CATTERALL et al. (1977)	76	19
DUNCAN (1984)	44	40
RTOG mixed beam	35	35
RTOG neutrons alone	30	10

cinomas of the head and neck were seen only in the clinical trials studying patients with more advanced disease. The results of these randomized studies are summarized in Table 16-6.

Further studies are ongoing with high LET pions, neon ion beams, and hospital-based, high-energy, isocentric neutron beams.

16.4 Chemotherapy

The role for chemotherapy is best accepted in the setting of metastatic disease. A number of single agents have activity in squamous cell cancers arising in this region as summarized in Table 16-7. Methotrexate and cisplatin are generally considered the most active single agents and of equal efficacy (HONG et al. 1983). Methotrexate has been given in high doses with leukovorin rescue assuming that higher drug concentrations will lead to higher response rates with calcium leukovorin used to rescue normal tissue toxicity. Trials comparing the standard weekly intravenous administration of methotrexate with high dose methotrexate with leukovorin rescue have failed to show an advantage in

Table 16-7. Single agent activity in advanced head and neck cancer

Agent	Response rate
Cytoxan (LIVINGSTON and CARTER 1970)	28/77 (36%)
Methotrexate (LIVINGSTON and CARTER 1970)	101/232 (43.5%)
5-Fluorouracil (LIVINGSTON and CARTER 1970)	1/12 (8%)
Hydroxyurea (LIVINGSTON and CARTER 1970)	7/18 (39%)
Vinblastine (LIVINGSTON and CARTER 1970)	10/35 (29%)
Procarbazine (LIVINGSTON and CARTER 1970)	3/31 (10%)
Bleomycin (Cancer Treatment Symposia 1985)	8/34 (24%)
Cisplatin (Cancer Treatment Symposia 1985)	83/305 (27%)
VP-16 (Cancer Treatment Symposia 1985)	2/16 (12.5%)

response rate or survival with the high dose method (DE CONTI and SCHOENFELD 1981; TAYLOR et al. 1984). Lesser toxicity and lower cost favor the standard weekly administration. A dose response has not been observed when cisplatin was given as 120 mg/M^2 compared with 60 mg/M^2 in a randomized trial in Italy (VERONISI et al. 1985). In general, single agents will produce a $>50\%$ tumor regression ins 20–40% of patients with squamous cell cancers of head and neck for a median of 4 months.

Combinations of active agents will generally result in higher response rates than those observed with single agents. Various permutations of these agents have been tested in the setting of disseminated disease. Response rates to chemotherapy are highest in patients without previous therapy, whether surgery and/or radiation therapy. These interventions may result in alteration of the normal blood supply to the region, thereby affecting drug delivery to the region (AMER et al. 1979). Table 16-8 summarizes the response rates observed with combination chemotherapy based on prior treatment. Additionally, not all tumor sites are equally responsive to chemotherapy. Tumors originating in the oral cavity and nasopharynx are most chemosensitive and laryngeal primaries the least sensitive (HILL et al. 1986). A number of prospective randomized trials have compared the efficacy of single agent to combination therapy. These trials are summarized in Table 16-9: The higher response rates initially reported in Phase II studies did not impact on survivial in these trials. However, in widely disseminated disease, combination therapy has been shown to result in significantly higher response rates than patients with locally advanced disease. Median survivals for combination chemotherapy are disappoint-

Table 16-8. Combination therapy in disseminated disease

Investigator chemotherapy		Advanced disease				Neoadjuvant therapy	
		Prior therapy		No prior therapy			
		RR	CR	RR	CR	RR	CR
ERVIN et al. (1981)	CDDP/Bleo	7/22 (30%)	1/22 (5%)	54/71 (76%)	16/71 (23%)		
HONG et al. (1979)	CDDP/Bleo X 2					30/39 (79%)	8/39 (20%)
AMREIN and WEITZMAN (1985)	FU/CDDP	15/30 (50%)	5/30 (17%)	26/31 (84%)	7/31 (23%)		
ROONEY et al. (1985)	FU/CDDP X 3					57/61 (93%)	33/61 (54%)
AMREIN et al. (1983)	CDDP/VCR Bleo	1/6 (17%)	0	25/37 (67%)	2/37 (5%)		
ROONEY et al. (1985)	CDDP/VCR Bleo X 2					61/77 (80%)	22/77 (29%)

Table 16-9. Randomized trials of single agent and combination chemotherapy in advanced head and neck cancer

Investigator	Chemotherapy	No of pts.	Response rate	Results
DRELICHMAN et al. (1983)	CDDP/VCR/Bleo versus MTX	27 24	41% (11% CR) 33% (8% CR)	Survival and response duration were comparable. Myelosuppression greater with MTX
VOGL et al. (1985)	MTX/Bleo/CDDP versus MTX	85 83	48% (16% CR) 35% (8% CR)	Significantly higher response rate with combination. p=0.04 Median survival and time to progression are equal.
WILLIAMS et al. (1986)	CDDP/VLB/Bleo versus MTX	92 98	24% (1% CR) 16% (0 CR)	Overall response rates equal. In widely disseminated disease combination is superior. Remission durations are equal.
DECONTI et al. (1981)	High dose MTX/CF versus MTX versus MTX/CF/CTX/Ara-C	80 81 76	24% (3% CR) 26% (7% CR) 18% (3% CR)	Duration of response significantly better for MTX. Survival favored MTX with p=0.06.
JACOBS et al. (1983)	CDDP versus CDDP/MTX/CF	40 39	18% (8% CR) 33% (15% CR)	No difference in response, response duration or survival.

MTX, Methotrexate; *MTX/CF,* High dose methotrexate with citrovorum factor rescue; *CDDP,* Cisplatin; *Bleo,* Bleomycin; *CTX,* Cyclophosphamide; *Ara-C,* Cytosine arabinoside; *VCR,* Vincristine; *VLB,* Vinblastine

ingly similar to single agents. The weekly administration of methotrexate appears equally effective to cisplatin-containing regimens without the toxicity, expense or need for hospitalization. Combination chemotherapy may offer an advantage in patients with widely disseminated disease.

The 5-year survival for Stages III and IV squamous cell cancers of the head and neck is less than 50%, with 90% having uncontrolled local disease at the time of death (HONG et al. 1985). Realizing that

response rates are highest in previously untreated patients, investigators have used chemotherapy in the initial management of these patients as part of a planned sequence. Chemotherapy has been used either in combination with radiation therapy where these agents serve as radiation potentiators, or as initial therapy prior to definitive surgery and/or radiation therapy, so-called neoadjuvant therapy.

For a disease which requires improved local control, potentiation of a local modality such as radiation therapy is appealing. Anal cancer, another squamous cell cancer, sets a precedent for this approach: fluorouracil and mitomycin-C in conjunction with radiation therapy is curative in 80–85% of patients, limiting the use of radical surgery in the initial therapy of this tumor (LEICHMAN et al. 1985; BOMAN et al. 1984). The mechanism of action postulated for this combined modality approach is that the chemotherapy serves as a radiopotentiator and may also affect metastatic disease. A number of agents are recognized as potentiators of radiation therapy. The imidazoles, misonidazole and metronidazole, are hypoxic cell sensitizers. Other mechanisms proposed for "radiopotentiation" by the

chemotherapeutic agents include: inhibition of the repair of sublethal and potentially lethal damage, alterations of the slope of hypoxic cell radiation dose-response curves or alterations in cell kinetics with synchronization of cells into the proliferative (radiosensitive) phases of the cell cycle (FU 1985; TUBIANA et al. 1985). Encouraging data from Phase I-II trials of chemotherapy and radiation therapy have resulted in a number of subsequent randomized trials which are summarized in Table 16-10. Although RICHARDS et al. (1969) reported that patients treated preoperatively with hydroxyurea and radiation had a higher incidence of node-negative neck dissections at surgery, the com-

Table 16-10. Randomized trials of chemotherapy with radiation therapy

Reference	No	Radiation therapy	Chemotherapy	Conclusions
STEFANI et al. (1971)	48	600–1000 cGy + boost +	Hydrea 80 mg/kg twice weekly	Increased mucositis with chemotherapy esp with boost. No difference in response distant metastasis or survival
		versus		
	42	600–1000 cGy + boost		
RICHARDS and CHAMBERS (1969)	20	600–1000 cGy + Preop +	Hydrea 80 mg/kg q 3 days	Higher incidence of N_o necks at surgery in the combination arm
	20	versus		
		600–1000 cGy Preop		
ANSFIELD et al. (1970)	68	6500 cGy	5 FU 10 mg/kg D_{1-3} then 5 mg/kg q MWF	Median survival and 5 year survival superior with chemotherapy p = 0.006. Advantage especially in T_3 lesions.
		versus		
	66	6500 cGy		
Lo et al. (1976)	68	6000–7000 cGy +	5 FU 10 mg/kg/d D_{1-3} 5 mg/kg/d D_4 then q MWF	Improved overall survival for all patients (p = 0.05) though not significant for tonsil and soft pallate. 2 yr NED superior in combination P < 0.05. No difference in metastases.
		versus		
	68	6000–7000 cGy		
		versus		
GOLLIN et al. (1972)	76	5000–10000 cGy +	5 FU 10 mg/kg/d D_{1-3} 5 mg/kg/d D_4 then q MWF	Overall survival superior for chemotherapy arm, p < 0.03 (Most significant for oropharyngeal)
		versus		
	79	5000–10000 cGy		
CACHIN et al. (1977)	99	5000–7000 cGy	Bleo 15 mg twice/ week X 5 wks	No difference in response of primary or lymph nodes, or survival. Mucositis increased in combination arm.
		versus		
	87	5000–7000 cGy		
KNOWLTON et al. (1975)	28	6000–6600 cGy	MTX 0.2 mg/kg/d X 5	No improvement in survival or local control
	20	6000–6600 cGy	MTX 240 mg/M^2 + CF $D_{1,5,9}$	
		versus		
		6000–6600 cGy		
FU et al. (1986)	52	5000–7000 cGy	Bleo 5 mg twice/wk + MTX 25 mg/M^2/wk X 16 post-radiation	Improved 2 year local control 64% vs. 24% P < 0.001 and relapse-free survival p = 0.04 in chemotherapy arm. No improvement in overall survival
		versus		
	52	5000–7000 cGy		

bination with postoperative radiation or with definitive radiation therapy is associated with a higher incidence of local reactions without an improvement in survival (RICHARDS et al. 1969). In 3 separate randomized trials, the concomitant use of fluorouracil and radiation showed benefit in certain subsets of patients. ANSFIELD et al. (1970) found a survival advantage for T_3 lesions while LO et al. (1976) and GOLLIN et al. (1972) reported overall improvement in survival for all patients treated. LO et al. (1976), however, did not find this survival advantage for patients whose tumors arose from the tonsil or palate. Concomitant radiation with bleomycin or methotrexate in head and neck tumors consistently resulted in an increased incidence of mucositis when compared to radiation therapy alone. In a Northern California Oncology Group (NCOG) study using bleomycin with radiotherapy followed by 16 weekly injections of methotrexate, improved local control and relapsefree survival were observed in the combined modality arm. This did not, however, result in a significant survival advantage (FU et al. 1987).

The term "neoadjuvant" refers to therapy given prior to definitive treatment. A number of Phase II studies have been performed in this mode with complete response rates following chemotherapy ranging from 26–63% (DECKER et al. 1983; KRASNOW et al. 1984; WEICHSELBAUM et al. 1985; SPAULDING et al .1980; SPAULDING et al. 1986). Of these patients who achieve a complete clinical remission with neoadjuvant chemotherapy and then undergo surgery, 30–60% will be histologically tumor free (KIES et al. 1985; SHAPSHAY et al. 1980). Other pathologic findings in these specimens may include evidence of increased tumor differentiation, tumor necrosis or only microscopic residual disease. Lymph nodes which are still palpable following chemotherapy may show only nodal hyperplasia (SHAPSHAY et al. 1980). Therefore, the clinical response may not accurately predict the pathologic response.

The most commonly used neoadjuvant combination is the Wayne State regimen of fluorouracil and cisplatin which produced a maximum number of complete responses when administered monthly for 3 cycles (ROONEY et al. 1985). Because response rates of 70–90% are gratifying, neoadjuvant therapy has become almost common practice in some communities. To date, however, only 4 randomized trials have looked at neoadjuvant therapy compared with surgery and radiation therapy, and only 1 has involved fluorouracil and cisplatin. These results are summarized in Table 16-11. The National Can-

cer Institute sponsored a 3-arm trial in patients with advanced squamous cell cancers. The control arm was surgery followed by radiation therapy. Two arms contained 1 cycle of preoperative cisplatin and bleomycin followed by surgery and radiation. One of these arms also contained 6 monthly cycles of cisplatin upon completion of radiation therapy. Objective tumor response was achieved in 37% and only 3% of patients achieved a complete response after 1 cycle of preoperative chemotherapy (H & N Contract Program 1987). In assessing local control and survival, no advantage could be identified in the chemotherapy arms. However, the incidence of distant metastases and time to development of distant disease were significantly less in the maintenance chemotherapy arm when compared with the control arm. Several problems occurred in the conduct of this study. Lack of compliance was a major problem in the chemotherapy arms with only 50% of patients completing induction therapy. Less than ⅓ of patients received > 50% of the intended maintenance in arm 3. High dose metaclopramide was not routinely used as an anti-emetic during the time period of the study's conduct which probably affected compliance related to side effects from cisplatin. The most serious flaw in the study's design is the use of only 1 cycle of cisplatin and bleomycin. In the Wayne State experience using 5-fluorouracil and cisplatin, the maximum number of complete remissions is achieved with 3 cycles of neoadjuvant therapy (ROONEY et al. 1985).

TAYLOR et al. (1985) reported the results of 3 cycles of high dose methotrexate with leukovorin rescue before surgery and radiation therapy compared to local therapy alone. Following completion of radiation therapy, patients received additional chemotherapy with either high dose methotrexate and leukovorin or cisplatin and adriamycin. No difference in local control or survival was observed.

The Medical College of Wisconsin compared standard surgery and postoperative radiation therapy or definitive radiation therapy alone with chemotherapy prior to radiation therapy and/or surgery. The chemotherapy consisted of 2 cycles of bleomycin, cyclophosphamide, methotrexate and fluorouracil. No difference in disease-free or overall survival was observed by the addition of this chemotherapy combination. At 2 years, there is a trend for improved survival in favor of the control arm for local control of tumor ($p < 0.06$) (KUN et al. 1986). Although high response rates have been reported with this particular combination, the highest response rates in this disease are with cisplatin-containing regimens. Wayne State has reported signifi-

Table 16-11. Randomized trials of neoadjuvant chemotherapy in head and neck cancer

Investigators	Patients	Therapy	No of pts.	Results
H & N Contract Program (1987)	Resectable Stage III and IV	Bleo/CDDP X 1 Surg. + Radiation versus	140	No difference in relapse-free or overall survival. Incidence and time to distant relapse prolonged in maintenance arm compared to standard therapy (P=0.02)
		Bleo/CDDP X 1 Surg. + Radiation CDDP q mo X 6 versus	151	
		Surg. + Radiation	152	
TAYLOR et al. (1985)	Advanced Local Disease	MTX/CF X 3, +/−Surg.+6500 cGy, MTX/CF or CDDP/Adria X 4 versus	41	No difference in local control, response or survival.
		+/−Surg.+6500 cGy	41	
KUN et al. (1986)	Advanced Local Disease	B-CMF X 2, 5000-7000 cGy +/− Surgery versus	38	Local region control at 2 yrs 53% vs. 35% favoring control (p<0.06). Complete response and survival similar.
		5000-7000 cGy +/− Surgery	40	
HAAS et al. (1986)	Advanced Resectable Disease	5 FU/DCCP X 3, 5000 cGy + Surgery versus	27	52% vs 24% D.O.G. or tumor progression (p<0.05) favoring standard theapy. By two years 70% chemotherapy and 44% of the control patients were dead of disease or had uncontrolled cancer (p<0.05). The study was closed early.
		5000 cGy + Surgery	33	

CDDP/Bleo, Cisplatin + Bleomycin
MTX/CF, High-dose Methotrexate with Citrovorum Factor Rescue
CDDP/Adria, Cisplatin + Adriamycin
B-CMF, Bleomycin + Cyclophosphamide + Methotrexate + Fluorouracil
FU/CDDP, Fluorouracil + Cisplatin

cantly higher response rates with infusion fluorouracil than bolus injection fluorouracil as administered in this program (KISH et al. 1985).

A trial from the University of Wisconsin randomized patients with advanced resectable squamous cell cancers to either radiation followed by surgery or 3 cycles of fluorouracil and cisplatin prior to radiation and surgery. The disease-free survival, overall survival and local control rate were statistically superior in the control arm. The study was terminated with 63 patients when this significant result was realized (HAAS et al. 1986).

If one analyzes the data for neoadjuvant therapy according to response rate, it becomes apparent that only a complete response predicts for improved survival. In reviewing 3 separate neoadjuvant programs at Wayne State, survival for patients achieving a partial response is only slightly longer than that for non-responding patients. An additional correlate with response to neoadjuvant chemotherapy is that lack of chemotherapy response seems to predict lack of response to radiation therapy (HILL et al. 1986). As in disseminated disease, response to preoperative chemotherapy

may be predicted by primary tumor site with tumors arising from the oropharynx and nasopharynx being most sensitive and laryngeal the least. However, SPAULDING et al. (1986) recently observed that primary hypopharyngeal tumors responded less well to the combination of cisplatin, vinblastine and fluorouracil than to bleomycin-containing chemotherapy. A high response rate was observed for tumors of the oral cavity and oropharynx. The heterogeneity of head and neck cancers may necessitate site-specific chemotherapy in the future.

The final role for chemotherapy is in the adjuvant setting. Here chemotherapy is utilized as "maintenance" following treatment of the primary tumor in patients at high risk for recurrence. To date, this therapy has been addressed in only 3 randomized trials (DECKER et al. 1983; WOOLFE et al. 1984; TAYLOR et al. 1985). Medical and social problems uniquely associated with head and neck cancer seem to predict noncompliance. Although compliance was a problem in the NCOG study, local control at 2 years favored the chemotherapy arm. However, overall survival was not affected due to an increase in cardiovascular deaths in that arm

(DECKER et al. 1983). Not enough information is available from any of these trials to draw conclusions about adjuvant chemotherapy in head and neck cancers.

A number of well-designed studies are ongoing which will attempt to avoid some of the problems that arose with previous combined modality trials. The Southwest Oncology Group (SWOG), Eastern Cooperative Oncology Group (ECOG) and the Radiation Therapy Oncology Group (RTOG) are involved in a combined modality study in patients with operable lesions. Following complete surgical excision, patients are randomized to receive either postoperative radiation therapy or 3 cycles of fluorouracil and cisplatin prior to radiation therapy. The Veterans Administration Hospitals are involved in a trial for laryngeal cancer. Patients receive 3 cycles of fluorouracil and cisplatin. Complete responders are randomized to receive either radiation therapy or laryngectomy followed by radiation therapy. The routine use of chemotherapy in the preoperative management of head and neck cancers should be discouraged until the results of controlled studies are available.

16.5 Future Directions

In addition to the areas previously discussed, head and neck cancer treatment investigations are ongoing into the value of hyperthermia, intraoperative radiation therapy, photodynamic therapy, hypoxic cell sensitizing agents, radioprotective agents, and biological response modifiers. All of these areas hold promise. Including altered fractionation studies, high LET studies and chemotherapy studies, there are currently 59 National Cancer Institute-sponsored clinical studies investigating new treatment strategies for this group of diseases. It is hoped that this effort will result in an improvement in the quality and length of life available to patients suffering from cancers of the head and neck region.

References

Amer MH, Al-Sarraf M, Vaitkevicius M (1979) Factors that affect response to chemotherapy and survival of patients with advanced head and neck cancer. Cancer 43: 2202–2206

Amrein PC, Figert H, Weitzman SA (1983) Cisplatin-vincristine-bleomycin therapy in squamous cell carcinoma of the head and neck. J Clin Oncol 1: 421–427

Amrein PC, Weitzman SA (1985) Treatment of squamous cell carcinoma of the head and neck with cisplatin and 5-fluorouracil. J Clin Oncol 3: 1632–1639

Ansfield FJ, Ramirez G, Davis HL, Korbitz BC, Vermund H, Gollin FF (1970) Treatment of advanced cancer of the head and neck. Cancer 25: 78–82

Batterman JJ, Breuer K (1981) Results of fast neutron teletherapy for locally advanced head and neck tumors. Int J Radiat Oncol Biol Phys 7: 1045–1056

Batterman JJ, Breuer K, Hart BAM et al. (1981) Observations on pulmonary metastases in patients after single doses and multiple fractions of fast neutrons and cobalt-60 gamma rays. Eur J Cancer 17: 539–545

Boman BM, Moertel CG, O'Connell MJ, Scott M, Weiland LH, Beart RW, Gunderson LL, Spencer RJ (1984) Carcinoma of the anal canal. A clinical and pathologic study of 188 cases. Cancer 54: 114–125

Borthne A, Kjellevold K, Kaalhus O, Vermund H (1986) Salivary gland malignant neoplasms: treatment and prognosis. Int J Radiat Oncol Biol Phys 12: 741–754

Brennan JT, Phillips TL (1971) Evaluation of past experience with fast neutron teletherapy and its implications for future applications. Eur J Cancer 7: 219–234

Cachin Y, Jortay A, Sancho H, Eschwege F, Madelain M (1977) Preliminary results of a randomized EORTC study comparing radiotherapy and concomitant bleomycin to radiotherapy alone in epidermoid carcinomas of the oropharynx. Europ J Cancer 13: 1389–1395

Cancer Treatment Symposia (1985) (Table 16-7)

Carter SK (1977) The chemotherapy of head and neck cancer: Semin Oncol 4: 413–424

Catterall M, Bewley DK (1973) Fast neutrons in the treatment of cancer, pp 14–27. London, Academic Press

Catterall M (1974) The treatment of advanced cancer by fast neutrons from the Medical Research Council's cyclotron at Hammersmith Hospital, London. Eur J Cancer 10: 343–449

Catterall M, Bewley DK, Sutherland I (1977) Second report on a randomized clinical trial of fast neutrons with X or gamma rays in the treatment of advanced cancers of the head and neck. Br Med J 1: 1942–1954

Catterall M (1981) The treatment of malignant salivary gland tumors with fast neutrons. Int J Radiat Oncol Biol Phys 7: 1737–1745

Decker DA, Dreilichman A, Jacobs J, Hoschner J, Dinzie J, Loh JJK, Weaver A, Al-Sarraf M (1983) Adjuvant chemotherapy with cis-diamminodichloroplatinum II and 120-hour infusion 5-fluorouracil in Stages III and IV squamous cell carcinoma of the head and neck. Cancer 51: 1353–1355

DeConti RC, Schoenfeld D (1981) A randomized prospective comparison of intermittent methotrexate, methotrexate with leukovorin and methotrexate combination in head and neck cancer. Cancer 48: 1061–1072

Del Rowe J, Pajak TF, Davis LW, Brady L, Mohiuddin M, Rubin P, Marcial V, Stetz J (in press) The role of distant metastasis as a site of failure in cancers of the head and neck region. Int J Radiat Oncol Biol Phys

Dobrowsky W, Schlappack O, Karcher KH, Pavelka R, Kment G (1986) Electron beam therapy in treatment of parotid neoplasm. Radiother Oncol 6: 293–299

Drelichman A, Cummings G, Al-Sarraf M (1983) A randomized trial of the combination of cis-platinum, oncovin and bleomycin vs methotrexate in patients with advanced squamous cell carcinoma of the head and neck. Cancer 52: 399–403

Duncan W, Arnott SJ, Orr JA et al. (1982) The Edinburgh experience of fast neutron therapy. Int J Radiat Oncol Biol Phys 8: 2155–2164

Duncan W, Arnott SJ, Batterman JJ et al. (1984) Fast neutrons in the treatment of advanced head and neck cancers: the results of a multi-centre randomly controlled trial. Radiother Oncol 2: 293–305

Duncan W, Orr JA, Arnott SJ, Jack WJC (1987) Neutron therapy for malignant tumors of the salivary glands: a report of the Edinburgh experience. Radiother Onc 8: 97–104

Eichhorn HJ (1981) Pilot study on the applicability of neutron radiotherapy. Radiobiol Radiother 3: 262–292

Elkon R, Colman J, Hendrickson FR (1928) Radiation therapy in the treatment of malignant salivary gland tumors. Cancer 41: 502–506

Ervin TJ, Miller D, Weichselbaum R, Fabian RL, Meshad M (1981) Chemotherapy for advanced carcinoma of the head and neck. Arch Otolaryng 107: 237–241

Fitzpatrick PJ, Theriault C (1986) Malignant salivary gland tumors. Int J Radiat Oncol Biol Phys 12: 1743–1747

Fu KK, Leibel SA, Levine MG et al. (1977) Carcinoma of the major and minor salivary glands: analysis of treatment results and sites and causes of failure. Cancer 40: 2882–2889

Fu KK (1985) Biologic basis for the interaction of chemotherapeutic agents and radiation therapy. Cancer 55: 2123–2130

Fu KK, Phillips TL, Silverberg IJ, Jacobs C, Chun C, Friedman MA, Kohler M, McWhirter K, Carter SK (1986) Combined radiotherapy and chemotherapy with bleomycin and methotrexate for advanced inoperable head and neck cancer: update of a Northern California Oncology Group (NCOG) randomized trial. Proc ASCO 5: 145–153

Fu KK, Phillips TL, Silverberg IJ, Jacobs C, Goffinet DR, Chun C, Friedman MA, Kohler M, McWhirter K, Carter SK (1987) Combined radiotherapy and chemotherapy with bleomycin and methotrexate for advanced inoperable head and neck cancer: update of a Northern California Oncology Group randomized trial. J Clin Oncol 5: 1410–1418

Goldstein LS, Phillips TL, Fu KK (1981) Biological effects of accelerated heavy ions. I. Single doses in normal tissues, tumors and cells in vitro. Radiat Res 86: 529–541

Gollin FF, Ansfield FJ, Brandenburg JH, Ramirez G, Vermund H (1972) Combined therapy in advanced head and neck cancer: a randomized study. Rad Ther & Nucl Med 114: 83–88

Gragg RL, Humphrey RM, Meyn RE (1977) The response of Chinese hamster ovary cells to fast neutron radiotherapy beams. II. Sublethal potentially lethal damage recovery capabilities. Radiat Res 71: 461–469

Gragg RL, Humphrey RM, Thomas HW et al. (1978) The response of Chinese hamster ovary cells to fast neutron radiotherapy beams. I. Variations in RBE with position in the cell cycle. Radiat Res 76: 283–294

Gray LH, Conger AE, Ebert M et al. (1953) Concentration of oxygen dissolved in tissues at time of irradiation as factor in radiotherapy. Br J Radiol 26: 638–646

Griffin BR, Laramore GE, Griffin TW, Eenmaa J (in press) Fast neutron radiotherapy for advanced malignant salivary gland tumors. Cancer

Griffin TW, Laramore GE, Parker RG, Gerdes AJ, Hebard DW, Blasko JC, Groudine MT (1978) An evaluation of fast neutron beam teletherapy of metastatic cervical adenopathy from squamous cell carcinomas of the head and neck region. Cancer 42: 2517–2520

Griffin TW, Blasko JC, Laramore GE (1979) Results of fast neutron beam pilot studies at the University of Washington. Eur J Cancer (Suppl): 23–29

Griffin TW, Davis R, Laramore GE, Hussey DH, Hendrickson FR, Rodriguez-Antunez A (1983) Fast neutron irradiation of metastatic cervical adenopathy: the results of a randomized RTOG study. Int J Radiat Oncol Biol Phys 9: 1267–1270

Griffin TW, Davis R, Hendrickson FR (1984) Fast neutron radiation therapy for unresectable squamous cell carcinomas of the head and neck: the results of a randomized RTOG study. Int J Radiat Oncol Biol Phys 10: 2217–2221

Haas C, Anderson T, Byhardt R, Cox J, Duncavage J, Grossman T, Haas J, Libnoch J, Malin T, Ritch P, Toohill R (1986) Randomized neo-adjuvant study of 5-fluorouracil and cis-platinum for patients with advanced resectable head and neck squamous cancer. Proc AACR 27: 185–198

Hall EJ, Kraljevic J (1976) Repair of potentially lethal radiation damage: comparison of neutron and X-ray RBE and implications for radiation therapy. Radiology 121: 731–749

Hall EJ (1978) Radiobiology for the Radiologist, Ed 2. Hagerstown, Maryland, Harper & Row

Head and Neck Contract Program (1987) Adjuvant chemotherapy for advanced head and neck squamous carcinoma: final report of the head and neck contracts program. Cancer 60: 301–311

Henry LW, Blasko JC, Griffin TW (1979) Evaluation of fast neutron teletherapy for advanced carcinomas of the major salivary glands. Cancer 44: 814–818

Hill BT, Price LA, MacRae K (1986) Importance of primary site in assessing chemotherapy response and 7-year survival data in advanced squamous cell carcinomas of the head and neck treated with initial combination chemotherapy without cisplatin. J Clin Oncol 4: 1340–1347

Hong WK, Shapshay SM, Bhutani R, Craft ML, Ucmakli A, Yamaguchi KT, Vaughn CW, Strong MS (1979) Induction chemotherapy in advanced squamous head and neck carcinoma with high dose cis-platinum and bleomycin infusion. Cancer 44: 19–25

Hong WK, Schaefer S, Issell B, Cummings C, Luedke D, Bromer R, Fofonoff S, D'Aoust J, Shapshay S, Welch J, Levin E, Vincent M, Vaughan C, Strong S (1983) A prospective randomized trial of methotrexate vs cisplatin in the treatment of recurrent squamous cell carcinoma of the head and neck. Cancer 52: 206–210

Hong WK, Bromer RH, Amato DA, Shapshay S, Vincent M, Vaughn C, Willett B, Katz A, Welch J, Fofonoff S, Strong S (1985) Patterns of relapse in locally advanced head and neck cancer patients who achieve complete remission after combined modality therapy. Cancer 56: 1242–1245

Howlett JF, Thomlinson RH, Alper T (1975) A marked dependence of the conformative effective causes of neutrons on tumor line and its implications for clinical trials. Br J Radiol 48: 40–46

Jacobs C, Meyers F, Hendrickson C, Kohler M, Carter S (1983) A randomized Phase III study of cisplatin with or without methotrexate for recurrent squamous cell carcinoma of the head and neck. Cancer 52: 1563–1569

Kaul R, Hendrickson F, Cohen L, Rosenberg I, Haken RT, Awschalom M, Mansell J (1981) Fast neutrons in the treatment of salivary gland tumors. Int J Radiat Oncol Biol Phys 7: 1667–1675

Kies MS, Hauck WW, Gordon LI, Krespi Y, Ossoff RH, Pecaro BC, Yuska C, Lamut CH, Brand WN, Chang SK, Shetty R, Sisson GA (1985) Analysis of complete responders after initial treatment with chemotherapy in head and neck cancer. Oto Head & Neck Surg 93: 199–205

Kish JA, Ensley JF, Jacobs J, Weaver A, Cummings G, Al-Sarraf M (1985) A randomized trial of cisplatin (CACP)+5-fluorouracil infusion and CACP+5-FU bolus for recurrent and advanced squamous cell carcinoma of the head and neck. Cancer 56: 2740–2744

Knowlton AH, Percarpio B, Bobrow S, Fischer JJ (1975) Methotrexate and radiation therapy in treatment of head and neck tumors. Radiology 116: 709–712

Krasnow SH, Cohen MH, Johnston-Early A, Citron ML, Fossieck BE, Mauk CM, Yenson A, Banda FP, Lunzer S, deFries HO (1984) Combined therapy for Stages II–IV head and neck cancer: preliminary results. J Clin Oncol 2: 804–810

Kun LE, Toohill RJ, Holoye PY, Duncavage JA, Byhardt RW, Ritch PS, Grossman TW, Hoffmann RF, Cox JD, Malin T (1986) A randomized study of adjuvant chemotherapy for cancer of the upper aerodigestive tract. J Radiat Oncol Biol Phys 12: 173–178

Laramore GE, Griffin TW, Tesh DW, Wong HH, Parker RG (1983) Phase I pilot study on fast neutron teletherapy for advanced carcinoma of the head and neck region: final report on local control rate and survival. Cancer 51: 192–199

Leichman L, Nigro N, Vaitkevicius VK, Considine B, Buroker T, Bradley G, Seydel H, Olchowski S, Cummings G, Leichman C, Baker L (1985) Cancer of the anal canal. Model for preoperative adjuvant combined modality therapy. Am J Med 78: 211–215

Livingston RB, Carter SK (1970) Single agents in cancer chemotherapy. New York, Plenum Press, pp 1–405

Lo TCM, Wiley AL, Ansfield FJ, Brandenburg JH, Davis HL, Gollin FF, Johnson RO, Ramirez G, Vermund H (1976) Combined radiation therapy and 5-fluorouracil for advanced squamous cell carcinoma of the oral cavity and oropharynx: a randomized study. 126: 229–235

Maor MH, Hussey DH, Fletcher GH et al. (1981) Fast neutron therapy for locally advanced head and neck tumors. Int J Radiat Oncol Biol Phys 7: 155–173 (private communication also)

Marcial VA, Pajak TF, Kramer S, Davis LW, Stetz J, Laramore GE, Brady LW (in press) Radiation therapy oncology group studies in head and neck cancer. Int J Radiat Oncol Biol Phys

Million HR, Cassisi NJ, Wittes RE (1982) Cancer in the head and neck. In: Cancer: principles and practice of oncology. De Vita VY, Hellman S, Rosenberg SA (eds). Philadelphia, JB Lippincott Co, pp 301–395

Morita S, Tsunemoto H, Kurisu A et al. (1978) Results of fast neutron therapy at NIRS. Proc Fourth High LET Radiotherapy Seminar, pp 127–141

Ornitz R, Herskovic A, Bradley E (1979) Clinical observations of early and late normal tissue injury and tumor control in patients receiving fast neutron irradiation. In: High LET radiations in clinical radiotherapy. Barendsen GW, Broerse J, Breur K (eds). New York, Pergamon Press, pp 44–50

Parsons JT, Cassisi NJ, Million RR (1984) Results of twice-a-day irradiation of squamous cell carcinomas of the head and neck. Int J Radiat Oncol Biol Phys 10: 2041–2049

Probert JC, Thompson RW, Bagshaw MA (1984) Patterns of spread and distant metastases in head and neck cancer. Cancer 33: 127–133

Rafla S (1977) Malignant parotid tumors: natural history and treatment. Cancer 40: 136–148

Reddy EK, Mansfield CM, Hartman GV et al. (1979) Malignant salivary gland tumors: role of radiation therapy. JAMA 71: 959–971

Richards GJ, Chambers RG (1969) Hydroxyurea: a radiosensitizer in the treatment of neoplasms of the head and neck. Amer J Roentgenol 105: 555–565

Rooney M, Kish J, Jacobs J, Kinzie J, Weaver A, Crissman J, Al-Sarraf M (1985) Improved complete response rate and survival in advanced head and neck cancer after three-course induction therapy with 120-hour 5-FU infusion and cisplatin. Cancer 55: 1123–1128

Rossman KJ (1975) The role of radiation therapy in the treatment of parotid carcinomas. Am J Radiol 123: 492–499

Saroja KR, Mansell J, Hendrickson FR, Cohen L, Lennox A (1987) An update on malignant salivary gland tumors treated with neutrons at Fermilab. Int J Radiat Oncol Biol Phys 13: 1319–1325

Shapshay SM, Hong WK, Incze JS, Sismanis A, Bhutani R, Vaughn CW, Strong WS (1980) Prognostic indicators in induction cis-platinum-bleomycin chemotherapy for advanced head and neck cancer. Am J Surg 140: 543–547

Shidnia H, Hornback NB, Hamaker R et al. (1980) Carcinoma of major salivary gland. Cancer 45: 693–699

Skolyszewski J, Byrski E, Chrzanowski A, Gasinska A, Reinfus M, Huczkowski J, Lazarska B, Michalowski A, Meder J (1982) A preliminary report on the clinical application of fast neutrons in Krakow. Int J Radiat Oncol Biol Phys 8: 1781–1786

Spaulding MB, Klotch D, Grillo J, Sanani S, Lore JM (1980) Adjuvant chemotherapy in the treatment of advanced tumors of the head and neck. Am J Surg 140: 538–542

Spaulding M, Ziegler P, Sundquist N, Klotch D, Lee K, Khan A, Lore J (1986) Induction therapy in head and neck cancer. A comparison of two regimens. Cancer 57: 1110–1114

Spaulding MB, Vasquez J, Khan A, Sundquist N, Lore JM (1983) A non-toxic adjuvant treatment for advanced head and neck cancer. Arch Otolaryngol 109: 789–791

Stefani S, Eells RW, Abbate J (1971) Hydroxyurea and radiotherapy in head and neck cancer. Radiology 101: 391–396

Stewart JG, Jackson AW, Chew MK (1968) The role of radiation therapy in the management of malignant tumors of salivary glands. Am J Roentgenol 102: 100–112

Stone RS (1940) Neutron therapy and specific ionization. Am J Roentgenol 59: 771–784

Taylor SG, McGuire WP, Hauck WW, Showel JL, Lad TE (1984) A randomized comparison of high-dose infusion methotrexate vs standard-dose weekly therapy in head and neck squamous cancer. J Clin Oncol 2: 1006–1011

Taylor SG, Appelbaum E, Showel JL, Norusis M, Holinger LD, Hutchinson JC, Murthy AK, Caldarelli DD (1985) A randomized trial of adjuvant chemotherapy in head and neck cancer. J Clin Oncol 3: 672–679

Tubiana M, Arriagada R, Cosset J (1985) Sequencing of drugs and radiation. The integrated alternating regimen. Cancer 55: 2131–2139

Veronisi A, Zagonel V, Tirelli U, Galligioni E, Tumolo S, Barzan L, Lorenzini M, Comoretto R, Grigoletto E (1985) High-dose vs low-dose cisplatin in advanced head and neck squamous carcinoma: a randomized study. J Clin Oncol 3: 1105–1108

Vikram B, Strung EW, Shah JP, Spiro RH (1984) Radiation therapy in adenoid-cystic carcinoma. Int J Radiat Oncol Biol Phys 10: 221–223

Vogl SE, Schoenfeld DA, Kaplan BH, Lerner HJ, Engstrom PF, Horton J (1985) A randomized prospective comparison of methotrexate with a combination of methotrexate, bleomycin and cisplatin in head and neck cancer. Cancer 56: 432–442

Wang CC, Suit HD, Phil D, Blitzer PH (1986) Twice-a-day radiation therapy for supraglottic carcinoma. Int J Radiat Oncol Biol Phys 12: 3–14

Weichselbaum RR, Clark JR, Miller D, Posner MR, Ervin TJ (1985) Combined modality treatment of head and neck cancer with cisplatin, bleomycin, methotrexate-leukovorin chemotherapy. Cancer 55: 2149–2155

Williams MV, Denekamp J, Fowler JF (1985) A review of α/β ratios for experimental tumors: implications for clinical studies of altered fractionation. Int J Radiat Oncol Biol Phys 11: 87–95

Williams SD, Velez-Garcia E, Essesse I, Ratkin G, Birch R, Einhorn LH (1986) Chemotherapy of head and neck cancer: comparison of cisplatin + vinblastine + bleomycin vs methotrexate. Cancer 57: 18–23

Withers HR, Thames HD, Peters LJ (1982) Biological bases for high RBE values for late effects of neutron irradiation. Int J Radiat Oncol Biol Phys 8: 2071–2082

Withers HR, Thames HD, Peters LJ (1983) A new isoeffect curve for change in dose per fraction. Radiother & Oncol 1: 187–198

Woolfe GT, Makuch RW, Baker SR (1984) Predictive factors for tumor response to preoperative chemotherapy in patients with head and neck squamous carcinoma. Cancer 54: 2869–2877

Subject Index

Medical Radiology
Diagnostic Imaging
and
Radiation Oncology

Edited by: L. W. Brady, Philadel-
phia; M. W. Donner, Baltimore;
H.-P. Heilmann, Hamburg;
F. Heuck, Stuttgart

C. W. Scarantino, Wake Forest University (Ed.)

Lung Cancer

Diagnostic Procedures and Therapeutic Management – With Special Reference to Radiotherapy

1985. 42 figures. XI, 173 pages. Hard cover.
ISBN 3-540-13176-0

Contents: Epidemiology of Lung Cancer. – Approach to the Patient with Lung Cancer. – Lung Cancer: Considerations Related to Gross Anatomy. – Pathologic Aspects of Lung Cancer. – Diagnostic Work-up. – Radiation Therapy in Cancer of the Lung. – Results of Clinical Trials and Basis for Future Therapeutics. – Redefining Clinical Research. – Subject Index.

This up-to-date reference book covers a broad range of topics regarding lung cancer.
There is an extensive review of recent epidemiological and early detection studies, as well as of current histological observations of the tumor heterogenity of lung cancer. It presents an up-to-date examination of the latest clinical developments in diagnosis and treatment as well as results of clinical trials employing irradiation, chemotherapy and surgery. Also included is a discussion on the need for alternative approaches to treatment, with half-body radiation offered as a model, and a consideration of the application of basic research to clinical management.

Springer-Verlag Berlin
Heidelberg New York London
Paris Tokyo Hong Kong

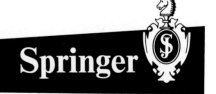

Springer

Medical Radiology
Diagnostic Imaging and
Radiation Oncology

Edited by: L. W. Brady, Philadel-
phia; M. W. Donner, Baltimore;
H.-P. Heilmann, Hamburg;
F. Heuck, Stuttgart

H. R. Withers, University of California;
L. J. Peters, University of Texas (Eds.)

Innovations in Radiation Oncology

1988. 111 figures. XVII, 329 pages. Hard cover.
ISBN 3-540-17818-X

The book contains up-to-date reports of areas of growth in radiation oncology written for the practising radiation oncologist. Early chapters review conservative treatments that preserve the function and maintain or improve tumor control rates in breast, rectum, anus, head and neck, soft tissues and bones, and the eye. This followed by a section dealing with extended field therapy encompassing total body irradiation, half body irradiation and systemic therapy with radionuclide-labeled antibodies. The potential roles of three new diagnostic imaging technologies (CT, MRI and PET) in radiotherapy are considered. Various modifications of treatment are reviewed, including hyperfractionation, accelerated treatment, accelerated hyperfractionation and neutron therapy. Also discussed is the clinical use of adjuvants to radiotherapy, such as radio-sensitizers, cytotoxic drugs, interstitial and external hyperthermia and bone fixation in metastatic disease. Current innovations for predicting tumor responses are described and a national survey of the quality of radiotherapy in the U.S.A. is reviewed. Finally, two chapters consider the quality of patient survival.

Springer-Verlag Berlin
Heidelberg New York London
Paris Tokyo Hong Kong

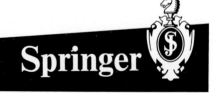

Springer